MAIN ISSUES IN MENTAL HEALTH AND RACE

Main Issues in Mental Health and Race

Edited by
DAVID NDEGWA
South London and Maudsley NHS Trust

DELE OLAJIDE
South London and Maudsley NHS Trust

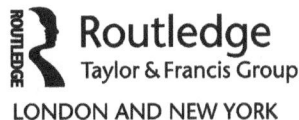

Routledge
Taylor & Francis Group

LONDON AND NEW YORK

First published 2003 by Ashgate Publishing

Reissued 2019 by Routledge
2 Park Square, Milton Park, Abingdon, Oxon, OX14 4RN
52 Vanderbilt Avenue, New York, NY 10017

Routledge is an imprint of the Taylor & Francis Group, an informa business

A Library of Congress record exists under LC control number:

ISBN 13: 978-1-138-71383-3 (hbk)
ISBN 13: 978-1-138-71381-9 (pbk)
ISBN 13: 978-1-315-19808-8 (ebk)

Contents

List of Contributors

Dr Susan Collinson MA PhD is a Lecturer in Medical Education at St Bartholemew's and Royal London School of Medicine and Dentistry.

Dr Trevor Turner is a Consultant Psychiatrist and Clinical Director of Research and Development at City and Hackney NHS Trust. He is also Chair of the London Region of the Royal College of Psychiatrists.

Professor Valentine Y. Mudimbe is William R. Kenan Jr Professor of French Comparative Literature and Classics at Stanford University.

Dr David Barker is a Lecturer in Forensic Psychiatry at the John Howard Centre, City and Hackney NHS Trust.

Dr Gargi Bhattacharyya is a Lecturer in Cultural Studies at the University of Birmingham.

Dr John Gabriel is Professor of Sociology in the Department of Cultural Studies at Guildhall University, London.

Dr Kate Miriam Loewenthal is Reader in Psychology at the Royal Holloway and Bedford College, University of London.

Dr Marco Cinnirella is a Lecturer in Psychology at the Royal Holloway and Bedford College, University of London.

Dr Prakash Shah is a Lecturer in Law at the School of Oriental and African Studies.

Dion Hanna is completing a PhD in Law at the School of Oriental and African Studies.

Dr William Obomanu is a Consultant Forensic Psychiatrist at the South London and Maudsley NHS Trust.

Dr Tami Kramer is a Senior Lecturer in Child and Adolescent Psychiatry at Imperial College School of Medicine.

Dr Matthew Hodes is a Senior Lecturer in Child and Adolescent Psychiatry at the Imperial College School of Medicine.

Dr Ros Ramsay is a Consultant Psychiatrist at South London and Maudsley NHS Trust.

Dr C. Gorst-Unsworth is a Consultant Psychiatrist.

Dr Zelpha Kittler is a Specialist Registrar working in addictions at South London and Maudsley NHS Trust.

Dr Vincent Kirschner is a Senior Registrar in Psychiatry at Newham Community Health Services NHS Trust.

This book project was made possible by a grant from the Department of Health to Dr David Ndegwa.

Contributor affiliations shown above were correct in 1999 and 2000.

Foreword

David Ndegwa and Dele Olajide

This book arose out of our concerns at the current British academic psychiatry's preoccupation with an alleged 'epidemic' of schizophrenia in black people of African descent. Black people in contact with psychiatric services are predominantly categorised as suffering from schizophrenia but do not seem to attract other diagnostic categories. This diagnostic pattern also seems to determine the differential treatment options available to them when compared with their white counterparts.

Their over-representation in psychiatric institutions and in the coercive end of psychiatric services has been further explained by this alleged epidemic of schizophrenia. We felt that the current psychiatric approach to the study of mental illness in black people is conceptually restrictive and a hindrance to the full understanding of the multi-factorial causality of psychosis. It is our view that academic psychiatry's preoccupation with the study of psychosis has stunted research in the search for an effective understanding of mental disorders in the black community and the development of a more robust intervention which will harness the strength of the community in collaboration with other agencies charged with the task of providing effective and appropriate care. We feel that psychosis as manifested in this population may well be an end stage of environmental factors in the biologically predisposed. We were curious to find out how other disciplines not traditionally allied to psychiatry conceptualised this observed phenomenon.

Unfortunately in the UK, unlike in the United States of America, African or black studies has not received much academic interest and it was difficult to identify many disciplines other than psychiatry who could bring additional insights into our inquiry.

We invited colleagues who have shown an interest in broadening the debate to review the available literature in order to determine what their disciplines could contribute to our understanding. We asked our contributors to carry out a broad based critical review of a particular area using the technology that has been developed for conducting systematic literature reviews. Most of that technology has much to say about quantitative studies although our intentions had been to review mix quantitative and qualitative studies. What the contributors found useful in that technology was the methodology for ensuring a comprehensive search of both published and unpublished literature. We wanted the reviewers to distil insights from a given subject by looking at the range of materials available in order to identify gaps in our current knowledge and where possible, to suggest ways of plugging those gaps. We also expect them to suggest areas of further fruitful explanation.

We need to state at the onset that the reader will find that we have preserved the individual contributors' style in order to do justice to their particular discipline of expression rather than provide a uniform style. The discerning reader will nevertheless notice that each contributor has maintained the central theme and this has been no mean feat. It is also worth noting the inconsistency in terminology when referring to black, African, Afro-Caribbean or African Caribbean, West Indian, Afro-American or African American. This is inevitable as the source material on which our contributors rely span several generations and thus reflect the prevailing terminology of the time.

Our own view is that the term black refers to Africans in the Diaspora and not the political black as 'non-white'.

The subjects were selected by the editors from their own understanding of disciplines, which they regard as capable of illuminating this area of psychiatry. These are disciplines that have preoccupied themselves with belief systems, feelings, emotions, thought, politics, language, religion, the law and decision making.

In some areas, there was little material available from literature searches, so the reviewers had to rely on their own understanding of the subject matter rather than existing literature to write their critical essays. What we have discovered is that there is still a long way to go in the exploration of the subject of black people's experiences of psychiatry.

It seemed appropriate to start with the long association of psychiatry with race. Central to the survival of slavery and later imperial colonialism, was the need to differentiate the colonised as inferior races. Apartheid was the last bastion of a socio-political system based on the biology of racism to collapse in recent times. Scientific arguments were marshalled in the justification of the supremacy of the white race over other races and psychiatry has been a useful, if sometimes an unwitting ally, in the way it pathologises uncommon cultural idioms as abnormal or psychiatric manifestations or racial differences.

British psychiatric research has tended to focus on black rather than white immigrants, and on increased rates of psychoses in hospital-based populations rather than on large scale population surveys, which can illuminate the broad spectrum of psychiatric disorders.

To date, very little is known about the prevalence of depression, anxiety disorders, alcohol and drug-related conditions which will be expected to correlate strongly with adverse life events such as racism and socio-economic deprivation.

The western notion of the ideal family as a nuclear entity, comprising of two parents and their children, continues to be celebrated, while the single parent household (commonly found in African Caribbeans), and complex family structure with several generations in the household (commonly found among Asians), are seen as deviations which are used retrospectively to explain psychological disorders in their offspring. Regardless of the socioeconomic circumstances of black children, they become aware at an early age of the negative value placed on their racial group by the predominant white culture. There is thus a strong case to be made for longitudinal studies looking at the effect of child-rearing practices across ethnic groups and the effect of such practices on social exclusion, self-esteem and identity as these are negative correlatives of mental health, both in childhood and in adulthood.

The pernicious effect of immigration laws on the mental health of migrants from the new Commonwealth has received scant attention among academics. These laws tend to focus more on people from Africa, Southeast Asia and the Caribbeans.

The legal system has been more preoccupied in holding the view that by consistently treating every one in the same way, it achieves certain just ends regardless of the cultural context or ethnicity. In practice however, black migrants' experience of the immigration law is discriminatory, wholly unsatisfactory and leads them to feeling powerless, angry and alienated.

The over-representation of African-Caribbeans in the use of the provisions of the Mental Health Act has been consistently demonstrated without any serious attempt at undertaking systematic studies at finding the cause for this anomalous observation. Service providers, academics and policy makers by their inaction, appeared to have accepted this worrying finding as 'normal' for this population. We disagree.

We agree with many of our contributors that social policy in the UK and many western societies have an adverse impact on black people from cradle to grave. We believe that this in turn could explain the younger generation's sense of alienation and a turning away from the traditional values that have not served their parents well. Many black people feel excluded and only have a tenuous stake in the society in which they exist at the margins and are only noticed when they become mad or bad.

Chapter 1

From Enlightenment to Eugenics: Empire, Race, and Medicine 1780–*c*1950

Trevor Turner and Susan Collinson

The race question dominates all other problems of history, that it holds the key to them, and that the inequality of races from whose fusion a people is formed is enough to explain the whole course of its destiny (*Essay on the Inequality of the Human Races*, Comte de Gobineau, 1853).

Introduction

The idea that biology can be used to classify and judge the value of the races of humankind[1] may have formally fallen from grace with the dismantling of the *apartheid* (separation by race) regime in South Africa in the 1990s. Informally however, it is a theory that still holds currency with many extremist groups throughout our early twenty-first century world. In essence, there is the belief that humankind consists of genetically superior and inferior types. It has a long history; and it is a history with which the profession of medicine has had an intimate and influential relationship, to the extent that by the end of the nineteenth century, *race*, which is neither a science nor a disease, had become both. The nineteenth century was the great period of British imperial expansionism, a business involving not just the trade in goods and people, but also the exportation of British institutions and culture. Experienced from within the British Isles, the British acquisition and colonisation of other lands and their peoples were the actions, and responsibility, of a morally enlightened and progressive society, fulfilling its duty towards other, less fortunate 'native' peoples. The morality of Britain's actions could be measured by observing how science, technology, the civil service, religion and the law were being used to improve the dependants. In 1899, a leader in *The Lancet*, discussing overseas medical missions, observed the important role that medicine had played within the great imperial adventure:

> 'The White Man's Burden' [is] a complex as well as a weighty one and its medical constituent is as important as any other ... no other nationality has combined, as has the British, colonial development with civilisation – civilisation of which the inferior races sooner or later feel the benefit and from which they take a new departure in their evolution.[2]

The encounter between European medicine (including 'psychological' medicine) and the societies of the lands colonised by the European powers during the period 1780–*c*1950 contributed to the development of a complex account of race, framed within a language of scientific neutrality. During the first part of this period, at a time when the practice of medicine was still more of an art than a science, the literature on race reflects the late eighteenth century and especially the Victorian delight, in the classification of all phenomena. One has the feeling that the Victorian anthropologists, palaeontologists, biologists, geologists and all the other men of '-isms' could not quite believe their good fortune at the cornucopia of new lands, flora, fauna and peoples being set before them for their indulgence and edification.

While Britain flourished commercially during the first half of the nineteenth century, she was also busily consolidating and confirming her supreme position through the activities and industry of the growing, and increasingly prosperous, professional middle classes. This was a time, for Victorian Britain, of buoyant optimism, and a time when the Victorians confidently regarded themselves as a superior and progressive race, emblematic of the onward march of civilisation, in contrast to many of the 'primitive peoples' whom they had colonised, and whom they believed to be representative of degenerative races, sliding towards extinction. However, by the last quarter of the century, the very fruits of imperialism seemed to be turning rotten. The idea that other races could and would degenerate, which had been used as a powerful justification for British imperial acquisitiveness, appeared suddenly to be true, too, of the British national stock. The once unshakeable belief in the inevitability of progress was degenerating into *fin de siècle* pessimism. Anxieties predicated upon the very taxonomy which had once reassured the white Victorian male of his racially and morally superior position began to manifest themselves in a fatalism which suggested that all of mankind was on the edge of descent as the new century dawned.

'A Tangled Bank, Clothed with Many Plants of Many Kinds'[3]

The theoretical concept of a taxonomy of races, which became known during the nineteenth century as 'scientific racism', is a direct product of a golden age of biology, when the great scientists of the eighteenth century devoted themselves to the classification of all the flora and fauna in the known world. This eighteenth-century equivalent of today's Human Genome Project was begun in an age when mankind was regarded as being set apart from the 'great chain of being' as devised by Linnaeus and Buffon. Mankind was not included within this essentially static and hierarchical arrangement of all living organisms, but was placed at the pinnacle. His role was to observe the beauty and wonder of God's creation.

The orderly, intellectual framework of the eighteenth century, with its tradition of taxonomic organisation based upon the observation of the external features of living organisms was gradually dismantled during the first half of the nineteenth century. The essential stasis of the Great Chain of Being was reorganised according to a concept of organic progression by Lamarck, and then broken down by Cuvier into an immense network in which the species depended upon each other. During the early decades of the nineteenth century, as man was gradually drawn into the arena of biological study, scientists found it useful to retain the classificatory system that had characterised the work of their predecessors. Inevitably, with the publication of the *Origin of Species* (1859), Darwinian arguments in favour of heredity and variation dispatched forever the idea of the fixity of species, but this in turn was replaced by a chronological taxonomy, which included the concept of the plurality of the species of the mankind, and which was constructed according to a formula whereby those races which had evolved furthest would be ranged above those whose development was still judged as being at an early stage of human evolution.

Race: Changes in Meaning and the Development of 'Race Science'

During the period with which we are dealing, it is important to bear in mind that the word 'race' has been the subject of shifting definitions and perceptions. Many of these are with us still today, in the form of race as territory, race as environment and time, race as revolution, and race as class.[4] However, other meanings, and those which are at this moment most interesting, were generated by the major themes of theology, biology and economy which preoccupied European intellectuals from the middle of the eighteenth century. However, three of the essential problems for theologians, scientists and political economists during this period concerned the biblical account of the development of mankind; the position of mankind within the continuous 'chain of being'; and the uneven civilisations of different 'tribes'. Until the end of the eighteenth century, for example, it was commonly held that climate was the ultimate determinant for the state of civilisation of a people. This proposition was further developed by Adam Smith and other Enlightenment philosophers as the 'four stages theory', providing a framework whereby climate, geography and natural circumstances were the influences for the progress, or decay, of civilisations. Climate also seemed to provide an answer to questions of human physical diversity: those living in harsh, hot weather had developed dark skins in response to their environment (thus the term 'Aethiop' from the Greek, meaning 'burnt face'). The European colonisation of Asia, the Far East and Africa went some way to discrediting this theory. It became apparent that despite moving to a colder climate, the darker skin of Indians and African retained their hue.

Authors on 'race' at this time, including the highly influential Johann Friedrich Blumenbach, a professor of anatomy, developed their accounts of racial variation according to a benevolent, monogenist[5] theory, whereby the difference between civilised and savage tribes was judged as analogous to the difference between domesticated and wild animals. Late-eighteenth-century racialism allowed that because cross fertilisation engendering fertile offspring was possible, all humankind belonged to a single species. Although Europeans at this time commonly expressed distaste for blacks, this was based upon a cultural and aesthetic antipathy: many whites simply did not like the features of black men. However, the Enlightenment conviction that change and improvement in the less civilised peoples was both possible and desirable, is strikingly different to the theories of racial separatism and purity which were to dominate racial theory during the later nineteenth century, and led eventually to the social policies for racial improvement implemented in countries such as Sweden, Germany, Canada and the United States of America during the 1920s and 1930s.

Among those who held sympathetic attitudes towards the 'other' races, the Quakers were notable. The Quaker physician, Dr Thomas Hodgkin, founded the Aborigines Protection Society. Hodgkin and his fellow Quakers were firmly monogenist in their approach. In 1843, a group of professional men drawn from the membership of the Aborigines Protection Society founded the Ethnological Society (motto *ab uno sanguine*), 'for the purpose of inquiring into the distinguishing characteristics, physical and moral, of the varieties of Mankind which inhabit, or have inhabited the Earth; and to ascertain the causes of such characteristics'. The Ethnological Society's dominant tone was monogenetic and humanitarian, in accordance with the anti-slavery movement that reached its peak in England during the 1830s, led by reformers such as William Wilberforce. However, these first instances of a more humanitarian approach to the trade in slaves were soon to become eclipsed by a considerable hardening of attitudes towards the 'other' races. By mid-century the growth of the 'scientific' in fields such as medicine was to give birth to 'race science'.

Although the Abolitionists (those who wished to abolish slavery) were very successful during the first half of the nineteenth century[6] this period also marks the beginning of a fundamental change in the approach to the study of humankind, and nowhere is this more apparent than in the language used in relation to man at this time.[7] As man was gradually drawn into a more intimate relationship with the natural world (and with the apes in particular), the eighteenth century use of semi-divine imagery was abandoned in favour of a more scientific vocabulary which relied upon biological and anatomical descriptions. Although these were used initially to describe the physical characteristics of an individual, or race, it was not long before they were extended, not as metaphor but as a true explanation for the culture and civilisation of a race. The anthropologist John Beddoes developed an 'Index of Nigrescence' based on the principle that 'darker types' within any society or population were generally more 'primitive'. This applied to Celts, Iberians and Africans alike.[8] The degree of civilisation of any race was deemed subject to the laws of evolution, and a product of them, while the primary and dominant explanation was biological. While pre-Darwinian ethnologists had attempted to make a connection between the physical and the cultural sophistication of a race, based upon their work in comparative anatomy, Darwin and his colleague Alfred Russel Wallace, despite their apparent omission of the question of man in the *Origin* ('Light will be thrown on the origin of man and his history', wrote Darwin as his final statement in *On the Origin of Species*), had formulated a theory which supplied a biological mechanism which could be used to explain almost anything. For race, it was this more than any other factor that ushered in the 'dawn of biological pessimism'.[9]

Undeniably, a scientific theory of racial taxonomy complemented nineteenth-century British ethnocentrism. It reassured the Victorian that his sense of himself, in relation to the rest of the world had been achieved according to a meritocratic, biological law. Although in the first part of the nineteenth century trade between Britain and Europe slowly fell away, so that by the 1860s only two-fifths of her trade was with the continent, her share of the world market during the same period was 25 per cent.[10] By the middle of the nineteenth century, Britain appeared to be at the height of an industrial golden age that set her apart from, and in advance of the rest of the world, including Europe. Britain's material and intellectual prosperity was there to be seen, in the form of roads, railways, factories and cities; in art and technology; in a nascent democracy, and new professional and middle classes in science, medicine and monotheistic religion. The engine of production for all these was the strength of the mid-century belief in progress and a superior racial stock. With these in sight and in mind, there could be no question for the Englishman of the superiority of his own 'Anglo-Saxon' culture and intellect when compared to that of the African Bushman or the Australian Aboriginal.

'Race is Everything'; 'Race is Nothing'[11]

The close relationship between biology, social science, medicine and politics during the second half of the nineteenth century is rooted in the formulation of those theories of variation and heredity which, from Lamarck onwards, were also applied to the study of man. This relationship was of supreme importance in the forging of the nineteenth century Eurocentric concept of 'race' that was based upon the assumption that all other races of the world possessed lower mental abilities. A critical link for 'race science' within the different scientific specialities was that between biologists and anatomists. The great eighteenth century botanist, Linnaeus, believed in divergence of talent between the races: *Homo Europaeus* (whites) were lively, inventive and ruled by custom; *Homo Asiaticus* (Asians) were stern, haughty and avaricious, while *Homo Afer* (the African) was cunning, slow, phlegmatic, careless and ruled by caprice.[12]

Paul Broca, craniologist and brain surgeon, developed the goniometer, stereograph and occipital crochet for the measurement of the skull, while Ernst Haeckel used comparative anatomy as proof of the superiority of the Northern European whites over all other 'races'.

Notable among the biologists and anatomists of race during the nineteenth century were Dr Robert Knox, the infamous Edinburgh anatomist, Jean-Baptiste Lamarck, Marie François Bichat and Georges Cuvier. However, it took the absolute conviction of the aristocratic Comte de Gobineau to persuade brilliant scientists such as those above that race was not 'nothing', but 'everything'; and that the interpretation of history should be properly seen as conflict between races, characterised by continuing social decadence and disorder.

The scientific study of humankind, eventually to become 'race science', was pursued on the basis of an objective study of human differences. As we have seen, it was carried out in Britain during the first half of the nineteenth century predominantly by ethnologists. Influenced by the work of the comparative anatomists, ethnologists took as their methods of measurement both the 'internal' (intellectual and moral) and 'external' (physiological) characteristics of a race, as manifested by their cultural and social achievements. Although the ethnocentricity of this approach ensured the Victorian his place at the top of the tree, the rise in the fortunes of the rival London Anthropological Society, founded in 1861, can be seen as emblematic of the hardening of racial attitudes during this time. By the middle of the century the older Ethnological Society had gradually fallen into debt and out of favour with current thinking, and the new discipline, or science, of anthropology, arose in opposition to the older and gentler science of ethnology. Significantly in 1871, the year in which Darwin published his *Descent of Man*, the racialist, polygenist Anthropological Society made a hostile but successful takeover bid of the traditionally Christian and humanitarian Ethnological Society, to form the Anthropological Institute. This event, as much as any, is characteristic of the move of science away from the realm of the amateur, the sentimental and the theological, towards a firmly secular, rational and professional domain. The study of race, and racial difference, had truly become 'race science'.

Amongst the membership of the Anthropological Society were physicians such as Dr James Hunt, who had a great contemporary influence on nineteenth century race science, and who used comparative anatomy to support racial theories. Hunt's polygenetic view was that human races were unmodifiable over time. He held in particular very strong views as to the inferior status of the Negro within the taxonomy of race. He stated that the Negro was a distinct species; that the Negro was closer to the ape than to the European races; and that the Negro was intellectually inferior and naturally subordinate to the European. The Negro could only be civilised by the European, although European civilisation was not suited to the Negro's requirements and character. Anthropologists held the fashionable theory that mental growth in the Africans known as the 'Child Races' ceased early; that childhood was never left behind; that they had therefore a very poorly developed moral sense; and that an obsession with sex in the African was responsible for arresting his mental development at puberty.[13] One anatomist described the Hottentots as 'the nearest approximation to the lower animals'. An inner clique of the Anthropological Society, the 'Cannibal Club', were gavelled to order by a mace in the form of a Negro head. Given the contemporary fashion for craniology at this time, which had developed a whole series of measurements of the skull in order to quantify the relationship between physical feature and character, especially intelligence, this may have been judged an appropriate use for a Negro skull. The European skull was used as the standard measurement, and any deviation from this was judged to be degenerative in form, or inferior in development.

The explorer Richard Burton, also a member of the Anthropological Society, wrote in 1860 of the tribesman of East Africa: 'He seems to belong to one of those childish races which, never rising to man's estate, fall like worn-out links from the great chain of animated nature.' He was also 'wilful, lazy and improvident, selfish [and] irreverent'.[14] Most Europeans who came into contact with Africans in particular felt that something sinister lurked behind the childlike simplicity and 'low moral awareness' of the 'savage'. Very little happened to alter these perceptions of the Africans, for these are precisely the characteristics which Buchan uses in his depiction of the Reverend John Laputa and other Africans in his novel *Prester John*, first published in 1910.

The 'Anglo-Saxon' Victorian

The Victorians needed to be assured not only of their superiority over the native races in their colonies, but also over other European races, the figure of the 'Anglo-Saxon' possessing great significance within the history of British imperialism. The 'modern' Anglo-Saxon was to all intents and purposes however created in the 1840s[15] in the works of well-known and popular authors as Scott, Disraeli and Kingsley. The Anglo-Saxon also inhabited the theoretical framework of British scientists of race[16] as a specific and distinct race of humankind, a sophisticated product of the modern reorganisation of Europe into races which were defined as culturally, psychologically and physically distinct. It was part, too, of the process whereby the definition of race, as applied to humankind, shifted from being a genealogical to a physiological concept.[17] The racial and ethnological work carried out in France by de Gobineau, Renan and Michelet, symbolised by ideas of race and national character was readily adopted by the 'educated' classes in England, not least de Gobineau's obsession with the conflict and antithesis which he believed were necessary tensions between the races. De Gobineau predicted a terrible degeneracy of the Aryan race, the inevitable result of the mixing of incompatible racial elements. For his German followers, de Gobineau's theory echoed the Teutonic myths of the downfall of the gods and the death-struggle of the Nibelungs. His influence persisted in Germany and it was from Richard Wagner's circle that the German Gobineau Society sprang.

In Britain, the concept of an Anglo-Saxon history established a common identity which cut across class interests when necessary, by identifying a unique set of qualities which were innate to all the Queen's subjects. These were deemed to have enabled the Victorians to gain an ascendancy over the rest of the world, and thus led to the racially imperialistic visions of 'Saxondom',[18] marching towards a goal of universal world rule, that were popularised by politicians during the ebullient 1860s. The extinction of the cheaper races, a category which included the troublesome Irish, was part of this process which could now, courtesy of evolutionary theory, be attributed to the operation of the law of nature.[19] This ambition to achieve the 'moral directorship of the globe, by ruling mankind through Saxon institutions and the English tongue',[20] helped to set Britain on a course of isolation from her continental neighbours which was to last for the rest of the century.

Race and the Imperial Ideal

At its height, the British Empire encompassed 12.5 million square miles, was inhabited by 450 million people (a quarter of the human race), and was described as 'the empire on which the sun never sets'. The same tools of government, institutions, language and religion were imposed alike on Bengalis and Boers, Malays and Maoris, and the white settlers in Canada, Australia and New Zealand. The era of mid-century imperialism is even now referred to as a 'golden age' of prosperity and optimism, but the imperial ideal, which held that the English were a chosen race entrusted with a duty towards the less fortunate races of mankind really only reached its zenith when Britain's commercial ascendancy had actually begun to wane, in the years between 1880 and 1914. In 1897, an article in the widely read periodical *The Nineteenth Century* proclaimed Great Britain's duty as being: 'To carry light and civilisation in the dark places of the world; to touch the mind of Asia and of Africa with the ethical ideas of Europe.' The profit motive, already suffering from the powerful challenge of neighbours such as Germany, was replaced in the British popular imagination by the assumption of 'the White Man's Burden', which was also understood to be a duty expressly given to the British. As Lord Rosebery said in 1883: 'We have to remember that it is part of our heritage to take care that the world, as far as it can be moulded by us, shall receive an English-speaking complexion, and not that of other nations.'

The Decline of Optimism

During the last quarter of the nineteenth century, Britain's domestic culture and institutions underwent considerable change. Church attendance, and presumably religious belief, declined; there was a flourishing popular press; and a steadily increasing franchise as Britain edged towards a universal franchise. There was also a steadily increasing economic depression; growing trades union membership; Social-Darwinism; the Fabians; right wing social-imperialists and 'fair traders'. The political context had changed greatly since the years of Palmerstonian ebullience and optimism, when imperialism in any form had scarcely stood in need of justification. The last quarter of the century saw a

> ... growing climate of apprehensions and dissolving certainties, especially the fear of being eclipsed economically, navally and in other ways, which in turn affected British imperial policy. The country became more defensive, less willing to take chances, much more suspicious of foreign powers and much less tolerant of indigenous peoples.[21]

The imperialism of the last quarter century was both more conscious, and more reluctant. The African colonies were the difficult and unrewarding fruits of the 'dark continent'.

Despite the grand rhetoric, it is of course true to say that the motive force behind British imperialism was commercial. The ethnocentric convictions of cultural and moral superiority which are such a consistent motif within contemporary thought did not motivate the white races to go out and colonise the non-white; that was the responsibility of the quest for wealth. From the late eighteenth century onwards, Britain had been the imperious centre for the importation and distribution of the unfamiliar and exotic goods brought into port by her huge merchant fleet. Such was the wealth generated by this trade that the great City of London bankers were described by Disraeli as 'mighty moneylenders whose *fiat* sometimes held in balance the destinies of kings and empires'.[22] The justification for imperialism on the grounds of the 'racial responsibility' of the 'superior' for the 'inferior' races is but a side show within the grander, economic and political fairground of empire. However, once the ascendancy of science over superstition validated the idea of a racial taxonomy, it was not difficult to 'endorse the moral view of empire that Britain had an obligation to bring the benefits of civilisation to the backward parts of the world'.[23] This form of justification was, however, an accessory to the fact of acquisition, rather than a primary motive for it.

Public opinion certainly subscribed to a popular racism which offered an unproblematic justification to the British conquest and domination of those other strange and childlike races. Most Victorians had no personal contact with the exotic peoples and places of which their colonies consisted. Their opinions were formed according to the sources of their information, and these sources were for the most part the popular press and literature. The mass medium of the written word reduced the observations and theories of serious research into the sorts of parables of difference and deviance that helped the Victorian reader understand his role, his duty and his superiority. Mass elementary education, the mass production of literature and a popular press appeared to reinforce an ebullient British identity as the island race whose destiny and duty it was to take their superior cultural and social order to the less civilised and socially well-ordered races of the world.[24] The ordinary Victorian man and woman was fascinated by the coloured, and colourful, aliens. Their image of the tropics was essentially one of hostile and untamed lands, inhabited by childlike people who were unable to distinguish between reason and superstition. The existence of 'witch doctors', practising 'native, voodoo medicine' contributed powerfully towards this perception. The magic and ritual of native medical practice were further evidence of the primitive nature of the African and Asian 'civilisations'. The Victorians believed that it was their duty to take European medicine to the 'backward civilisations', in order to improve and ameliorate their health and well being.

Medicine within English Racial Thought

The growing efficacy of western medicine inevitably became one of the tools of imperial expansionism. The 'lower civilisation' of the native peoples of Britain's empire was already manifest by their failure to differentiate between science and religion. Similarly, their medical practices frequently reflected beliefs in illness as punishment for the breaking of taboos, and this was invariably interpreted by the European as evidence that these were people with crude sensibilities and 'lower moral power'. Although 'savage man' suffered from none of the 'diseases of civilisation' such as lack of exercise or over-indulgence in alcohol, the simplicity of his mental and physical state characterised him as being closer to animals than to civilised man. During his first journey in Africa, Dr Livingstone reported that after he had operated on native Africans, the two edges of the incised skin grew together with the extraordinary rapidity that one would expect from a horse or a dog, rather than a human.[25]

The nineteenth century is regarded as having given birth to 'scientific medicine', and medical science is certainly interlaced with the triumphs, both great and small, of Victorian Britain. The nineteenth century also saw medicine's emergence as a more effective and scientific profession, whose superior practitioners became men of influence and authority.

At the beginning of the century, however, the doctor's role was alleviation rather than cure. The aetiology of most disease was still unknown and the doctor was, on the whole, unable to treat the underlying cause of an illness. Anatomical description still depended upon the belief that the body was a single entity, made up of a series of orderly and readily identifiable structures and organs: it was these alone that were affected by disease. If an organ was diseased, this could be detected by palpation whilst the patient was alive (sometimes) and by autopsy after death. Early developments in histology broke away from the concept of organs to formulate a theory of tissues,[26] and this development was soon enhanced by microscopic examination. There was a similar advance in the understanding of the natural history of organic disease, in terms of causal factors, theory of disease origins, and advances in microbiology. The work of Pasteur, Koch and others helped to provide biological understanding of the infectious disease process by isolating pathogens associated with particular diseases. By 1866, Lister had capitalised upon their work by applying antiseptics to wounds after surgery, thus consolidating the 'germ theory of disease'. By the end of the century, these significant advances in medical science and knowledge were reflected in the new specialities of physiology, psychiatry, histology, neurophysiology and comparative anatomy, all of which became a standard part of medical practice, investigation and diagnosis.

Notions of infection were not however confined to physical illness, but were thought also to pertain to both mental and 'moral' contagion. This belief certainly helped to enforce the strict separation that was maintained throughout the Empire between Europeans and natives. Although the mortality rates for whites in the tropics were always high, it was also thought that there were certain diseases which were race specific. For example, in 1892, Dr John Sykes wrote that 'some diseases are peculiar to race just as others are peculiar to individuals ... Negro lethargy is purely a disease of Negroes'.[27] By mid-century European concern about the well being of the white in the tropics was deepening. A network of lunatic asylums was constructed throughout the colonies, especially India, to cope with the burden of mental illness among both the civilian and military expatriate population. There was a high mortality rate from diseases such as malaria and yellow fever, and an antipathy towards the alien flora and fauna. There also appeared to be strong evidence on the side of those who argued for theories based upon racial susceptibility and resistance to disease. The arguments were of course exclusively eurocentric. Little regard was paid to the 'fatal impact' of those diseases imported by the colonisers, such as measles and influenza (or alcohol dependence), upon the native inhabitants of the colonies, though one doctor wrote to *The Lancet* condemning the role of the blanket in the disintegration of such peoples as the Aboriginals in Australasia.[28] White morbidity was, however, the foremost concern of white science, and

> ... the thesis of white degeneration in the tropics gave scientific weight to the importance of maintaining the correct psychological and sexual distance from the very places into which the white race, by its putatively 'natural' vigour, ambition, restlessness, and dominance, was moving.[29]

Degeneration

Darwin's *Descent of Man* was published in 1871. By 1873, Britain was entering the long years of depression which were to last until the end of the century.[30] The mid-century years of buoyant prosperity were drawing to an end, and giving way to a late Victorian imperialism which can now be understood as fearful and uncertain, rather than confident and aggressive.[31] By the mid-nineteenth century, the idea of *degeneracy* had entered medical pathology and psychiatry within the context of the more general theory of 'morbid anthropology'.[32] Any adulteration of race and class was seen as the mechanism for racial degeneration. The medico-racial theory of degeneration was developed to include any and every kind of illness, social pathology, deviance, abnormal psychological states or physical conditions.[33] Even an apparently healthy individual could be harbouring, unknown, some degenerate condition, whether excessive 'nervousness' leading to 'feeble-minded' offspring, or the inherited germ of syphilis and such-like conditions.

Nor was all well at home. The mighty empire appeared to be harbouring a hideous mirror image of the 'degenerate' native in the form of its own lower classes, who thronged the grotesque slums of Britain's great cities. Contemporary observers described the British working class as being characterised by low intelligence coupled with excesses of sexuality and excessive fecundity. The late Victorian belief in the expression of mental disturbance through the physical body reinforced the conviction that the working classes had more in common with the primitive races than with the middle and upper classes of their own race. They shared their somatological and psychic racial stigmata not with contemporary mankind, but with the primitive races. In his story 'The Sign of Four' (1890) Sir Arthur Conan Doyle represents this apparent affinity through the sinister relationship between a white ex-convict and an Andaman Island pigmy:

> that face was enough to give a man a sleepless night. Never have I seen features so deeply marked with all bestiality and cruelty. His small eyes glowed and burned with a sombre light, and his thick lips were writhed back from his teeth, which grinned and chattered at us with half-animal fury I can see the two of them now as they stood: the white man with his legs far apart, shrieking out curses, and the unhallowed dwarf with his hideous face, and his strong yellow teeth gnashing at us in the light of our lantern.

Racial typology was used in tandem with observations upon class and society as a way of understanding all things ominous and unhealthy, and variously covered physical, psychological, moral and intellectual characteristics. Degenerate individuals were regarded as resembling the 'lower' races. They were like children, like savages, and like lunatics: incapable of moral responsibility. The same language was used of them and their vices as was used of the native races of the colonies, particularly when the need was to describe the over-abundant intemperance, hedonism and sexuality which all appeared to have in common. Criminal anthropologists defined white wrongdoers as genetically retarded; they were compared with children, and with adult Africans and Indians. Havelock Ellis made the observation that white criminals, white children and South American Indians were all incapable of blushing; they were too infantile to be able to understand or express shame. Rudyard Kipling, who summed up the onerous side of British imperialism with the phrase 'the white man's burden', referred to the subjugated natives he encountered in India as 'half devil and half child'.

The Victorian urban poor were 'persistent paupers' who formed a degenerate class; they were clear examples of 'race degeneration', spreading like a contagion both the physical and mental stigmata of degeneration through their irresponsible sexual incontinence. The black native too, was seen as sexually immoral and promiscuous. This shared *furor sexualis* was judged to be characteristic of a lower type of brain organisation. Physical and moral degeneration and atavism was invariably associated with an individual's sexual proclivities and appetites. It was especially feared that the black man 'lost sexual control' when he came near a white woman. This was attributed to a relatively defective development of the centres of psychological inhibition, characteristic of a low grade of intellectual development, and one of the Negro's racial handicaps. Another aspect of this apparent 'kinship' between primitive black and low grade white was based upon the observation that both were susceptible to the same types of physical and mental diseases, and that this was especially the case with mental diseases. The lower classes and the primitive races both displayed a high morbidity towards mania and dementia, while the white upper classes tended to suffer from the neuroses and hysteria. Both passed on their uncontrollable taint to their offspring. The task for medical science appeared to be how to contain and cleanse the progeny of racial degeneration.

Miscegenation

Victorian Britain was both fascinated and repelled by the conjunctions of sex and race.[34] This was reflected in the language popularly used to describe the irregular, the unconventional and the socially unacceptable: 'bad blood'; 'black blood'; 'impurity of blood'; 'gone native'. The horror of miscegenation and hybridity created powerful and unacceptable images of social chaos in a world that depended upon a set of clear and careful distinctions as to who was, and who was not, a gentleman. By the 1860s, there was a welter of literature, much of it medical, concerned with inter-racial fertility. It was strongly suggested that racial mongrels, like the mule, were sterile. If this were not immediately the case in the first or second generation, it would certainly be so by the third or fourth. This was a reassuring prospect for those who feared the potential of racial admixture would further blur racial and class distinctions and confuse the national blood.

There was much alarmist debate around the issues of miscegenation and hybridity, as the products of such unions would inevitably possess the most degenerate taints from both races. Those of mixed race descent were viewed with especial mistrust and disfavour. A South African psychiatrist (Duncan Greenlees) wrote of someone of mixed race as 'The Bastard – a mixture of white and black blood [who] morally seems to present all the worst characteristics of both races ...'.[35] Dr Hack Tuke's paper on insanity in Australian Aboriginals, published in 1890, asserted that:

> as might have been expected in a dark-skinned race, the prevailing type of the malady was mania, usually acute, and as a rule accompanied by turbulence and

violence, and this passed away rapidly much more rapidly than in Europeans into dementia, with filthy and degraded habits.[36]

These experiences generated theories of native inferiority that informed the approach of many colonial psychiatrists (see below).

'Race is Everything; There is no other Truth. And Every Race must Fall which Carelessly Suffers its Blood to become Mixed'[37]

In 1883, Francis Galton introduced the word 'eugenics' into the study of humankind. He defined it as the 'study of agencies under social control that may improve or impair the racial qualities of future generations either physically or mentally'. His research had led him to conclude that human progress could only be sustained if the superior races, which now looked in danger of deterioration, were improved through selective breeding. Galton was part of an hereditarian tradition that had persisted within the race biology movement since the early nineteenth century.[38] The environmentalist approach of the public health movement during the middle years of the century had for a while overshadowed hereditarianism, but the social tensions and unease of the last quarter of the century once again gave credence to the belief that intervention was propping up social decay. What he interpreted as the blight of racial degeneration filled the cities in the form of the poor, the criminals, the prostitutes and the insane, sustained by social policy and replenished by waves of alien immigration.

The belief that there was a 'proper place' for each race underlined the conviction that any race which moved from its original 'centre of creation' could expect to degenerate, possibly to the point of extinction. In North America it was widely feared that freed blacks who moved into white geographical and social space would bring with them diseases and depravity which would undermine the white population.[39] Each human race was thought to be anatomically distinct and therefore intellectually and morally unique.[40]

Physical organisation determined mental and moral characteristics. Encroachment by one race upon the territory and the integrity of another would lead inevitably to the debasement of both, but the superior race would suffer the greater detriment. Contemporary nosology included the idea that specific races characteristically nurtured certain diseases. This was well within the older tradition of humoral medicine and the newer trend of medical typology, which classified patients according to the similarity of their conditions.

Individuals were also described in terms of 'type': when a person was described as 'consumptive', 'chlorotic', 'scrofulous', 'pthisical', everybody knew exactly what was meant. A similar typology was applied to race. Negroes were believed to be especially prone to consumption and to venereal disease; a morbidity which was understood to be hereditary. They were however also regarded as a race that was being hastened towards extinction by the abolition of slavery. Once freed, the Negro was at liberty to indulge all his degenerate and self-destructive racial appetites. This process of 'reversion' was Nature's way of 'weeding out the weak' in the struggle for survival.[41] The fear for the white Southerner, as he watched the old order crumbling away, was that the slave's revenge would be to infect the master with his own mortal taint.

Although the folk-devil image of the decadent mulatto took his place within the pantheon of popular villains, alongside the usurious Jew, the pig-tailed Chinaman and the murderous Lascar, eugenics never gained very widespread political support in Britain. Its supporters were mainly members of the 'progressive' middle classes: doctors, lawyers, psychologists and other professionals with an interest in social reform. Galton's early proposition, that heredity dominated over environment,[42] was given encouragement by William Bateson's introduction of the new science of genetics in 1905. However, as Stepan[43] points out, the main concerns of the eugenists were the heritability of behavioural traits, especially mental behaviour, and the measurement of 'intelligence' or 'ability'. Galton was not daunted by the task of measuring these traits. If they were fixed by heredity, then they would be consistently expressed in some obvious form. He selected social and economic standing as his index, and even used professional status as a method of measuring 'genius'. By dismissing as negligible the influence of social environment, supporters of the eugenics movement could present a case for man selecting where nature could not.

Researching Racial Aspects of Mental Illness in a Historical Context

If one considers the technical, psychiatric literature concerning mental illness in different racial groups, one is immediately confronted by a number of difficulties. These include the use of an outdated and often pejorative language (e.g. 'Negro'), the problem of accessing some of the more obscure journals that may no longer be in publication, the lack of a significant research tradition, and the limited quality of the papers available. Research generally has to be direct rather than computerised, given the nature and chronology of the journals involved, particularly those in the period 1850 to 1950. For it is during this period that there is the beginnings of a sufficient psychiatric literature, the dominant publications within the English language tradition being the *Journal of Mental Science* and the *American Journal of Insanity* (later the *American Journal of Psychiatry*). This section attempts an outline review of the literature available in the former journal, and tries to summarise several general themes that inform this resource.

The *Journal of Mental Science* (*JMS*) was first published in 1853, and its fourth volume (1857) included articles on Insanity in Africa, Insanity in China, and The Asylum at Constantinople. In fact reviews of various foreign asylums, especially colonial asylums, become established as a regular feature of the Journal between the nineteenth and early twentieth centuries. Asylums in Bengal, British Guiana, Cuba, Brazil, Egypt, and other parts of Africa are all reviewed, usually with regard to the basic statistics of admissions, recoveries, types of illness and so forth. Although there are a number of qualitative comments, the implicit assumption made by most of the authors of these reports is that they are treating the same illnesses as one would see in Europeans. The roles of alcohol and cannabis (hashish) are often discussed, and there is intermittent comment as to the more 'primitive' psychology of non-Europeans.

Another group of papers is focused on the nature of mental illness amongst specific racial groups. Thus, titles such as 'Insane Negroes in the USA' (Vol. 13), 'Insanity among Africans' (Vol. 26), and 'Insanity in Coloured Races' (Vol. 38) are typical in this regard. Such reports can take on a more technical character, for example those entitled 'Paranoia among Brazilians' (Vol. 50), or 'Mental Degeneracy in Syria' (Vol. 54), or 'Epileptic Reactions in the Negro Race' (Vol. 78), or 'Crime and Insanity in India' (Vol. 79). Particularly in the twentieth century there are attempts at a more specific analysis of illnesses, for example 'Schizophrenia among Parsis' or 'Temperament, Conflict and Psychosis in a Stone Age Population' (both Vol. 76). Studies on witchcraft, syphilis, the use of hashish/ bhang, or other more direct racial characteristics are associated with this literature, but tend to be more anecdotal than quantitative.

In general there are fewer studies discussing particular 'culture-bound' conditions, although 'Amok of the Malays' (Vol. 39) and 'Demoniacal Possession among Primitive Races' (Vol. 76) are of this type. There are also attempts to compare, occasionally, different racial groups, such as in an article on 'Negro and White College Students' (Vol. 76). Some studies of specific psychologies are also included, for example 'The "Character" of American Indians' (Vol. 79), or 'The Psychoanalysis of Primitive Cultural Types' (Vol. 78).

In general therefore this literature is impressionistic, and based largely on a combination of anecdote, travellers' tales, personal experience and rehashed reports from other sources. It often uses asylum populations, which in themselves can be deemed somewhat unusual given the context of colonialism, minimal clinical resources, and a limited professional language. Thus terms such as 'defect', or 'imbeciles', or 'barbarous nations' are scattered widely and used with poor definition. Authors constantly speculate as to the role of 'intemperance' (whether the use of alcohol or hashish), religion, 'primitive' belief systems, and intelligence, and there are many rather poorly organised statistics. If there are any generalisations to emerge from all this, they are that:

a) there is a general acceptance of a reduced incidence of 'insanity' amongst 'primitive races'; and
b) there are no significant attempts to construct separate diagnostic categories.

The flavour of this literature can be obtained by reviewing a selection of these papers.

In a relatively early article entitled 'Does Civilisation Favour the Generation of Mental Disease?' (*JMS*, 4, 1858, pp. 94–110), Daniel H. Tuke quoted from a number of sources and gave an especially eurocentric view of this dilemma. He contrasted the peoples of 'European civilisation' as being in a state of 'continual intoxication' (he was quoting from a Dr Guislain), in contrast to the life of 'a savage' which 'enables them to support pain …'. He also described the use of stimulants in Europe (by which he largely meant alcohol) as being much more 'extensively injurious, both to bodily and mental health' than opium was to the peoples of China and Egypt. He admitted to the lack of reliable data, quotes a Dr Butler of America as having never witnessed 'a well-marked instance of insanity' among the Cherokee Indians, and supports this with comments from travellers in Nubia (Southern Egypt), Abyssinia, and other parts of Africa. He also quotes from an 1856 volume (*Medical Times and Gazette*, 8 November) in which a Dr Cartwright described a form of disease called 'Drapetomania'. This of course is 'an irrestrainable propensity to run away', but Tuke considers that Cartwright must be 'enjoying a joke at the expense of his readers'. He goes on to write, 'in our judgement, the absence of such a propensity would be a melancholy proof of imbecility or incipient dementia'. Tuke is more willing to accept another apparent disease entitled 'Dysaesthesia Aethiopica'. This condition apparently presented with careless movements, destructive behaviour, and wandering about at night while keeping in 'a half nodding state by day'. Such behaviours were apparently due to the 'stupidness of mind and insensibility of the nerves induced by the disease'. Tuke attributed this to physical factors, including a poor diet, and the blood thus becoming 'unfit to stimulate the brain to energy'.

Tuke was in fact rather cutting about this particular condition, and seems to have been fully aware of the particular socioeconomic conditions in which it developed. His overall case, however, was that 'insanity attains its maximum development among civilised nations; remaining at a minimum among barbarous nations, as well as among children, and animals below man'. His distressing (to us) assumptions of 'civilisation' and 'barbarity' according to racial characteristics, are unfortunately typical of his time, and are reflected in much of the subsequent literature. Thus in an article entitled 'Notes on Lunacy in British Guiana' (*JMS*, 1876, Vol. 22, pp. 76–81) a Dr James Donald used the statistics of the Berbice Lunatic Asylum to study insanity 'as exhibited among different races'. He considered that the types of illness were very similar but that there were nevertheless some distinctive features. He avoided trying to compare the prevalence of mental disorder with, for example, that in England, and admitted that 'in many cases national peculiarity is mistaken for mental derangement'. He attributed the high rates of mania, particularly with 'delusions of a religious character' to the strong religious sentiment that 'exists in the mind of the Negro', describing minds haunted and imaginations excited 'by the terrors of the mysterious Obeah', and expressing the hope that with the advance of education such practices (i.e. Obeahism or witchcraft) would 'become gradually extinct'. He also commented on the high rates of epileptic mania amongst the Chinese, possibly due to opium eating, but denied the role of the climate in the aetiology of the insanities he was seeing. Intemperance, particularly amongst 'Creoles and Portuguese' was in his view a much more relevant factor.

Such language and attitudes are further developed in a paper (already quoted) by Dr Duncan Greenlees entitled 'Insanity among the Natives of South Africa' (*JMS*, 1895, Vol. 41, pp. 71–8). He described the 'study of the mental characteristics of savage and semi-savage races' as one of the 'most difficult investigations possible', admitting the need for careful study of 'their mode of life, their normal mental state, and such folklore as is accessible to us'. He was prepared to admit to the 'devastating effects of modern civilisation', but distinguished as to these effects between different native tribes. Using statistics from the Grahamstown Asylum, he looked at the ages of patients admitted, the forms of insanity, the history of the cases and the causes of insanity. He was struck by the rather excessive number of cases of mania over other forms of insanity, considering that this represented a loss of 'the lower developed strata of the mental organism', in contrast to the damage to the 'higher and latest developed strata' associated with melancholia. He thus uses the prevalence of mania amongst 'natives of low developed brain function' to prove his theory. The low levels of General Paralysis of the Insane (GPI) – i.e. tertiary syphilitic infection of the brain, a terminal condition – are noted, while the causes are attributed to excessive drinking, the smoking of dagga (a plant almost identical with cannabis), and, of course, masturbation. His overall view though was that 'the native brain has its analogue in the European child's cerebrum', therefore studying such conditions enabled him to look at an aspect 'not obtainable in any other way'.

Amongst later articles, that on the 'Amok of the Malays', by W. Gilmore Ellis (*JMS*, 1893, Vol. 39, pp. 324–39) is particularly detailed, and gives descriptions of two particular case histories, namely of individuals running amok, and of the British judicial response thereto. He quotes from a medical report written in Singapore about the year 1845, by a Dr Oxley, that suggests that Amok resulted from

> an idiosyncrasy or peculiar temperament common amongst Malays, a temperament which all who have had intercourse with them must have observed, although they cannot account for or thoroughly understand it. It consists in a proneness to chronic disease of feeling, resulting from a want of moral elasticity, which leave the mind a prey to the pain of grief, until it is filled with a malignant gloom and despair, and the whole horizon of existence is overcast with blackness ...

Although looking at the forensic aspects of these cases, Dr Ellis did conclude that 'Amokers' are genuinely insane and 'unable to refrain from obeying their homicidal impulses'. He was especially struck by the lack of recall of the sufferers, and by the subsequent depressive state that often persisted. In particular he related the condition to another form of Malay mental disorder entitled 'Sakit-hati', which apparently meant 'heart sickness'. Such cases were reported to recover quickly, and it is clear that Ellis considered them to have some sort of brain disorder, almost a kind of 'masked epilepsy'.

Such a specific racial characteristic was reflected in another article entitled 'The Insane Jew' (*JMS*, 1900, Vol. 46, pp. 731–77) by Cecil F. Beadles. This considered that Jews became insane at a younger age, that GPI was rare amongst them, but that 'they possess all the worst features, in an exaggerated degree, of the chronic and hopelessly insane'. The author related this to Jews being more prone to mental anxiety and worry, because they are 'all excitable and live excitable lives, being constantly under the high pressure of business in town'. Comments as to how they are 'destructive of clothing' reflect other comments about other races made in this literature, attributing behaviours within asylum confines to specific racial characteristics.

Approaches to treatment also tend to have a particular racial slant, although this again reflects a somewhat variable and poorly quantified approach. Thus in a report on East Indian asylums (*JMS*, 1859, Vol. 5, p. 219) it is suggested that restraint ought to be applied exclusively by European attendants (to the European patients). This was to avoid any impression of humiliation, but was also noted to be related to 'a peculiar condition' among European insanes. The same report considered that to European soldiers and sailors 'manual work is distasteful', by contrast to the apparent benefits that Indian patients obtained from industrial employment in 'the manufacture of jute ropes and mats'. Furthermore, some asylums were roundly criticised for their over-crowded state (e.g. 1860, Vol. 6, p. 162, on the Jamaica Lunatic Asylum), describing up to a dozen people 'disordered in mind and it may be in body also' in a wretched 14ft by 10ft cell in a tropical climate. This article actually called for an inquiry into these circumstances, and for 'a thorough investigation into the state of lunatics' throughout the West Indies. The *JMS* was also quite critical of the 'deep-rooted repulsion which is felt to a black skin in the United States', commenting on the setting up of a separate house for Black patients in an asylum in Ohio (*JMS*, 1867, Vol. 13, pp. 552–868).

The persistent attempts at interracial analyses can also be found in the *JMS* in the first part of the twentieth century. Thus a Dr Nichols (*JMS*, 1944, Vol. 90, pp. 862–8) in an article on 'Neuroses in Native African Troops' suggested that there was an increased proneness to hysteria and suggestibility amongst these soldiers. Although 'more dramatic' in expression than one would expect in Europeans, apparently, there was no difficulty in any kind of differential diagnosis with regards to schizophrenia or manic depressive psychosis. The author commented on these patients 'readiness to respond to kindly forms of treatment and suggestion'. He also pointed out the importance of knowing thoroughly 'their customs, beliefs and modes of living' and bemoaned 'the unknown world, and complete change of environment full of danger' that they were facing. There is comment also on these troops, when at home at least, living in 'an almost animistic stage', with every sickness being attributed to spirits or witchcraft.

In a not dissimilar article entitled 'A Comparative Study of Disease Incidence in Admission to a Base Psychiatric Hospital in the Middle East'

(*JMS*, 1946, Vol. 92, pp. 118–27), a Dr M. Sims compared officers and NCOs of a British background with Africans and Mauritians as well as Cypriots and Italian prisoners of war. The author attempted to look at differential diagnosis, but was aware of social differences. Thus he wrote 'the question the psychiatrist had to answer was "is this man a mentally defective Basuto pioneer"? and not "is this man a mental defective"?'. He felt that hysteria was often confused with manneristic and catatonic schizophrenia, 'especially in non-British personnel', and that the 'influence of race and intelligence has probably some bearing on the size of the proportions of illnesses'.

The author also had a number of comments to make about background factors in the selection of his cohorts. Thus he considered that recruiting of the African troops had been done by the heads of the villages, and therefore 'one cannot help thinking that many a village undesirable was got rid of by a cunning and unscrupulous chief'. He also dismissed the high incidence of hysteria amongst the African cohort, since he felt that the best recruits had been drafted into combatant (as opposed to pioneer) units. He considered that there were very large numbers of African natives who did not develop hysteria 'although subjected to more strain than those admitted'. He also noted that anxiety was rare in this group, and that in fact the highest rates of schizophrenia were amongst the Italian prisoners of war.

Finally, in this context, the most interesting article from the *JMS* is that entitled 'An Investigation concerning Mental Disorders in the Nyasaland Natives' (*JMS*, 1936, Vol. 82. pp. 701–30). This was by Drs H.M. Shelley and W.H. Watson, and looked at the Central Lunatic Asylum in Zomba, capital of Nyasaland (the colonial name for Malawi), to try to consider the incidence and forms of insanity in that country. It contains many tables and details of the nature of illnesses and the various groups, looks at family histories and physical states, and the incidence of crime amongst the mentally disordered. It is of note that the authors divided delusions into 'native and European types', the latter being defined as 'a delusion which could not have occurred before the advent of Europeans to this country' (e.g. 'someone borrowed £200 from him'). There is also discussion on the relationship of European contact to insanity, comparing the communal existence of the natives with the more 'individualistic' European life. The different forms of treatment from missionaries, officials and those engaged in commerce is also considered problematic, and the authors felt that it was 'small wonder that his [the African's] sense of values is confused and often can be distorted'. In general Europeanisation is deemed problematic, and the higher incidence of mental disorder amongst those tribes more in contact with the Europeans was seen as clear evidence of this detrimental effect.

Overall the picture that emerges from this kind of literature is to be contrasted to the approach that is often found in more modern analyses. Thus in his *Imperial Bedlam* (University of California Press, 1999), Jonathan Sadowsky has a much greater discussion about the social construction of diagnoses in the development of British attitudes towards the mentally ill in colonial Nigeria. Likewise the much admired Franz Fanon (e.g. *History of Psychiatry*, Vol. 7, Pt 4, No. 28, December 1996) developed a significant part of his social and anti-colonial critique (for 'The Wretched 26 Main Issues in Mental Health and Race of the Earth') in the context of working in the asylum service in Algeria. There is also no doubt that the assumption amongst the pre-Second World War European medical establishment was of a European superiority in terms of the complexity and intelligence of their 'civilisation' and the effectiveness of their psychiatric approach. Unusual behaviours, in the context of mental illness, displayed by 'native' patients, were very much placed in this context. Apart from the exceptions outlined above (e.g. Amok) however, there seems to have been little systematic attempt to construct an alternative or additional diagnostic categorisation. This may have been a function of the relatively broad psychiatric categories used at the time, but is equally likely to have been a genuine experience of lack of difference. After all, European alienists certainly considered their 'native' charges to be different in some sense in terms of culture and background, so one would have assumed at least a motivation to try to create new diseases. As in the famous Arthur Conan Doyle story of 'The Hound of the Baskervilles', the interesting question is why the dog did not bark.

Much further, systematic work needs to be done on this literature, not only reviewing the attitudes and language used in the context of racial difference, but also perhaps considering differences in the approach of the various European and American writers. There is also an interesting question as to why colonial asylums were built at all, when the general acceptance of much lower rates of insanity (at least amongst the colonial 'races') seems to have been widespread. It is as if the asylum came as part of the standard package of colonialisation, along with the church, governor's mansion and courthouses so typical of European impositions. There also seems to have been a considerable understanding of the deleterious effects of alcohol and syphilis, by contrast to the more ambivalent comments about the roles of hashish/cannabis. Again, much more detailed work will be required to consider these factors, but in general it is difficult not to conclude that, at least in the British colonial literature, there is a general acceptance that overt rates of 'insanity' were increased by the colonial experience. Whether this was due to an altered perception of aberrant behaviour, or the direct effects of European-style cerebropathic habits (i.e. rotting your brain with alcohol), or the more sociological and environmental aspects of racial attitudes remains a fascinating research question.

Conclusion

By the turn of the century science and technology had become extremely powerful social forces. The discoveries of scientific medicine had given doctors a special body of knowledge and expertise which gave them social and political power and status. As the body of medical and psychiatric knowledge grew, doctors began to specialise, and to present themselves as experts in a variety of formal contexts, and to exert authority over the moral, mental and physical management of society. As Mrs Vincy said, 'Why, my dear, doctors must have opinions ... What are they there for else?'[44]

The medicalisation of race coincided with the growing apprehension of the urban poor in Britain's cities as also being a 'race apart'. This synchronous perception of race and class provided a common vocabulary in which words such as 'savage' and 'barbaric' were used interchangeably by expert and lay person alike. It also meant that a common formula could be employed for the treatment of both the 'degenerate' white and the primitive black. Medical pathology still leaned upon classification of 'type', and typology was organised according to the actual or the morbid state. Thus, the medico-racial theory of degeneration could be extended to include every conceivable kind of physical and psychological disease and condition.

The power of western medicine had already been used to underwrite European imperialism. During the second half of the nineteenth century, a great campaign had been waged against tropical disease in order that the European might have a better chance of survival. Contemporary medical theory tended to implicate the alien or exotic environment with European physical and psychological ill-health. Very little attention was paid to the needs of the autochthonous peoples, many of which were equally devastated by the introduction of European disease. These races, whose 'lower' civilisation was characterised by their failure to differentiate between science and religion, and whose medical practice frequently reflected beliefs in illness as punishment for the breaking of taboos, had less refined sensibilities and lower 'moral power'. It was important that a psychological and a social distance be maintained; a conviction readily transferred from the overheated colonies to the dark and lawless rookeries of Britain and their inhabitants. Fear of disease emphasised the need for separation, although so alien had the working classes and their habitat become that a young man called Thomas Cook capitalised on the fascination of the wealthy by offering escorted tours, not to the Far East, but to the East End.

The late nineteenth and early twentieth centuries appeared to experience a proliferation of 'new' chronic, degenerative diseases, both physical and 'moral', the so-called 'diseases of civilisation'. Racial theory perceived them as the products of race deterioration and degeneration; promoted through hereditarianism; damned by eugenics; rising with the birth-rate; characterised by the feeble-minded; exemplified by race suicide; unchecked by the progress of medicine and medical specialism. Whilst the writers of many of these articles were medically qualified, those who were not nevertheless invoked medical evidence on behalf of their argument. The themes that abound in the periodicals are also to be found in scientific and quasi-scientific books of the period. Readers of popular science had available to them a large library of works which also anxiously examined, and proposed solutions to, the same pressing questions, whilst medical textbooks of the time often present ideas drawn from 'race science' as part of the pathology of a particular disease or condition.

From the perspective of the psychiatrist practising in the late twentieth century, we should do well to bear in mind the words of Richard Shryock when trying to come to terms with the role of doctors within the infamous development of 'race science'. As Shryock has said, 'the interaction of ideas, diseases and social developments' fall within the 'interplay of internal and external factors in medicine'.[45] Nor should these influences be assumed to be the products of their own time, for in this assumption lies the danger that 'cultures, periods, or social classes are closed, self-centred entities, an assumption which, in the final analysis, would make historical studies senseless'.[46] The monstrous assumption of the race scientist was, after all, to attempt to show the validity of 'race' science by presenting 'evidence' from biology and medicine, purely in order to pursue a non-scientific, 'moral' objective. Details of the history of psychiatric practice within this context remain relatively obscure, but there is sufficient source material for numerous questions as to this process to be more fully understood.

Notes

1   Although the term 'humankind' is used here, 'man' and 'mankind' are used throughout the rest of the chapter, in keeping with the Victorian meaning.

2   'The Medical Factor in Imperial Expansion', *The Lancet*, 1 (1899), pp. 785–6.

3   Darwin, 1859.

4   Hannaford, c.1996, p. 236.

5   Monogenists believed that all people were the result of the same, single act of creation; polygenists believed in separate origins for the races of humankind.

6   Slavery in the British Empire was abolished in 1833; the 12-year apprenticeship of slaves which followed the abolition of slavery in the British colonies was abolished in 1838.

7   Stepan,1982, p. 77.

8   Beddoe, 1885.

9   Stepan, 1982, p. 87.

10 Kennedy, 1984, pp. 20–38.

11 This phrase is used to sum up the dominant scientific dispute of the first half of the nineteenth century between the monogenists and the polygenists concerning the creation and the origins of the universe.

12 Jones, 1996, p. 172.

13 Kiernan, 1988, p. 232.

14 Burton, 1860.

15 He looms large in the work of early race scientists such as Robert Knox (1862), and is also a key figure in the history of colonisation.

16 See, for example, the work of the physician William Lawrence (1822) and the Bristol alienist James Cowle Prichard (1973). Prichard's work was first published in 1836–41.

17 Stepan, 1982, p. 20.

18 A term introduced by E.H. Dance in *The Victorian Illusion* (1928).

19 Curtis, 1971, p. 46.

20 Dilke, 1869, p. 562.

21 Kennedy, in Eldridge, 1984, p. 33.

22 Quoted by Checkland, 1965, p. 209.

23 Bolt, 1984, p. 14.

24 Eldridge, 1984, p. 186.

25 Collier, 1889, pp. 622–7, on pain in animals and their lowered sensitivity, which was also to be found in the 'savage' races.

26 Virchow's development of cellular pathology in 1858 became the basis for modern medicine. He showed that the body was a 'cell-state in which every cell is a citizen'. The body was no longer one entity, or a collection of tissues, but a mass of cells, rendered visible by the microscope. The process of disease caused normal cells to become distorted, or to proliferate at an abnormal speed. If the disease process depended upon the abnormal behaviour of normal cells, then the cause of disease could be found in the reason why cells were behaving abnormally. Medical investigation began to rely upon the laboratory pathologist.

27 Sykes, 1892, p. 16.

28 '"The Decadence of Races": on the Decline of the Maoris, and the Impact of European Disease', *The Lancet*, 2 (1860), p. 396.

29 Stepan, 1982, p. 25.

30 Kennedy, 1984, pp. 20–38.
31 Eldridge, 1984, p. 11.
32 Morel, 1857.
33 See Stepan, 1982, pp. 119–24.
34 Ibid., p. 93.
35 Greenlees, 1895, pp. 71–8.
36 Tuke, 1890, pp. 71–82.
37 Chamberlain, 1899.
38 Stepan, 1982, p. 112.
39 See Nott and Gliddon, 1854.
40 See the work of Knox, 1862, pp. 2–38.
41 Stepan, 1984, p. 58.
42 Galton, 1874. He proposed that mental ability was inherited differentially by individuals, groups and races. Like height, it followed a normal distribution curve in the population. Ability appeared to run in families (his own being a good example). It was transmitted from generation to generation by biological inheritance. This being so, then humankind would appear to have the opportunity to intervene in the heritable process, to the best advantage of the race.
43 Stepan, 1982, p. 125.
44 Eliot, 1988.
45 Shryock, 1947.
46 *The Historiography of Modern Medicine*, 1971.

References

Beddoe, J. (1885), *The Races of Britain: a Contribution to the Anthropology of Western Europe*, J.W. Arrowsmith, Bristol and Trubner & Co., London.

Bolt, C. (1984) 'Race and the Victorians', in Eldridge, C.C. (ed.), *British Imperialism in the Nineteenth Century*, Palgrave-Macmillan, London, pp. 126–47.

Burton, Sir R.F. (1860), *The Lake Regions of Central Africa. A Picture of Exploration*, Longman & Co., London.

Chamberlain, H.S. (1899), *The Foundations of the Nineteenth Century*.

Checkland, S.G. (1965), *The Rise of Industrial Society in England 1815–1885*, Longmans, London.

Collier, W. (1889), 'Insensitivity of Animals to Pain', *The Nineteenth Century*, Vol. 26.

Curtis, L.P. (1971), *Apes and Angels: the Irishman in Victorian Caricature*, Smithsonian Institute Press, Washington.

Dance, E.H. (1928), *The Victorian Illusion*, Heinemann, London.

Darwin, C. (1859), *On the Origin of Species*, John Murray, London.

Dilke, C. (1869), *Greater Britain*, Macmillan, London.

Eldridge, C.C. (1984), 'Sinews of Empire: Changing Perspectives', in Eldridge, C.C. (ed.), *British Imperialism in the Nineteenth Century*, Palgrave-Macmillan, London, pp. 169–89.

Eliot, G. (1988), *Middlemarch*, ed. with an introduction by David Carroll, Oxford University Press, Oxford (first published 1871–72).

Galton, F. (1874), *Hereditary Genius*, Macmillan, London (facsimile reprint, with introduction by R. Schwartz Cowan, Frank Cass, London, 1970)

Greenlees, T.D. (1895), 'Insanity among the Natives of South Africa', *Journal of Mental Science*, Vol. 41, pp. 71–8.

Hannaford, I. (c.1996), *Race: the History of an Idea in the West*, Woodrow Wilson Center Press,Washington DC.

Jones, S. (1996), *In the Blood*, Harper Collins, London.

Kennedy, P. (1984), 'Continuity and Discontinuity in British Imperialism 1815–1914', in Eldridge, C.C. (ed.), *British Imperialism in the Nineteenth Century*, Palgrave-Macmillan, London.

Kiernan, T.J. (1988), *The Lords of HumanKind*, Century Hutchinson Ltd, London.

Knox, R. (1862), *The Races of Men: a Philosophical Enquiry into the Influences of Race over the Destinies of Nations*, 2nd edn, Henry Renshaw, London (first published in 1850).

Lawrence, W. (1822), *Lectures on Physiology, Zoology and the Natural History of Man. Delivered at the Royal College of Surgeons*, James Smith, London.

Morel, B.A. (1857), *Traité des Dégénéréscences*, Paris (Nancy printed).

Nott, J.C. and Gliddon, G.R.(1854), *Types of Mankind*, Philadelphia (printed).)

Prichard, J.C. (1973), *Researches into the Physical History of Man*, ed. and with an Introductory Essay by George W. Stocking Jr, University of Chicago Press, Chicago/London.

Shryock, R.H. (1947), *The Development of Modern Medicine: an Interpretation of the Social and Scientific Factors Involved*, Knopf, New York.

Stepan, N. (1982), *The Idea of Race in Science*, Macmillan Press, Oxford.

Sykes, J.F.K. (1892), *Public Health Problems*, Scott, London.

The Historiography of Modern Medicine (1971), ed. by Edwin Clarke, Athlone Press, London.

Tuke, H. (1890), 'Insanity in Australian Aboriginals', *Journal of Mental Science*, Vol. 41, pp. 71–82.

Chapter 2

Recovering the Obvious – Race and Mental Health

Valentine Y. Mudimbe

> … to work on a concept is to vary the ways in which it can be extended, to understand and generalize it by incorporating certain exceptional traits, to export it beyond its original context, to take it as a model or, conversely, to seek a model for it – in short, to progressively confer transformations upon it that are regulated by the function of a form (Georges Canguilhem).

One of the best ways for introducing this meditation would be from the outset, to refer to Michel Foucault whom I shall be using as a guide in this reflection that will focus successively on a deconstruction of the notion of 'race', those of 'normality' versus 'abnormality' and concludes in invoking 'styles' of, actualising, mental 'disorders' as systems in their own right.

Two positions might introduce my general argument. The first is at the foundation of the *Order of Things*:

> This book first arose out of a passage in Borges, out of the laughter that shattered, as I read the passage, all the familiar landmarks of my thought – *our* thought, the thought that bears the stamp of our age and our geography – breaking up all the ordered surfaces and all the planes with which we are accustomed to tame the wild profusion of existing things, and continuing long afterwards to disturb and threaten with collapse our age-old distinction between the Same and the Other. This passage quotes a 'certain Chinese encyclopaedia' in which it is written that 'animals are divided into: (a) belonging to the Emperor, (b) embalmed, (c) tame, (d) sucking pigs, (e) sirens, (f) fabulous, (g) stray dogs, (h) included in the present classification, (i) frenzied, (j) innumerable, (k) drawn with a very fine camelhair brush, (l) *et cetera*, (m) having just broken the water pitcher, (n) that from a long way off look like flies'. In the wonderment of this taxonomy, the thing we apprehend in one great leap, the thing that, by means of the fable, is demonstrated as the exotic charm of another system of thought, is the limitation of our own, the stark impossibility of thinking *that* (Foucault, 1973, p. XV).

And, the second is a stimulation: to Michel Foucault stating that with him 'madness' could speak about itself Jacques Derrida responded by a question: in which language could it speak if it is not the language of reason?

Michel Foucault responded to Jacques Derrida's critique (1978) of *Histoire de la folie*. *'Mon corps, ce papier, ce feu'* was first published by Foucault in the Japanese journal *Paideia* and then included as an afterword to the 1972 version of *Histoire de la folie*. The real issue in this debate is about the statute and the role of dream versus that of madness in the Cartesian doubt.

> A dream allows doubting of and about this locus in which I am, of and about this sheet of paper, of and about this hand I am offering; but madness is not an instrument or a step of the doubt; in effect 'as the I who thinks, I cannot be mad' and thus exclusion of folly.

This is the basis of Foucault's counter-argument opposing Jacques Derrida's interpretation of Descartes's text. Echoing for himself an objection from an imaginary opponent questioning his claim that all knowledges originating from the sensible domain can be misleading Descartes asserted, 'I am here and writing and you hear me, I am not and you are not crazy; we are people with their good sense'. This is to say the example of madness might not be revealing the fragility of the idea of the sensible. Thus, any possible opponent could qualify such a position as extravagant, since it refers to mad peoples. Yet, from this extreme comparison, it is not realistic to oppose the concept of madness to that of dream. The latter, indeed may include all incredible possibilities to the point that one could say that, vis-à-vis knowledge, the dreamer is crazier than the mad person.

In brief, let's proceed from contextualising the concept of race in the history of the last centuries in the West to a critical analysis of the notions of 'normality' versus 'abnormality' and then, face concretely the daring thesis of Freud on 'the analogy between the process of civilisation and the path of individual development' (1989, p. 106).

What is in the Concept of Race?

In his 1998 study on Afrocentrism Stephen Howe opens part one by a question: 'Race: What's in a name?' The issue is important as formulated. Apprehended as a name and not as a scientific category, it relativises the more traditional classifications which, about animals, conceives generally the zoological species (e.g. as subdivided into sub-races) characterised by specific hereditary traits (e.g. equine, feline) and, *à propos* humans divides them, firstly into different groups qualified by pigmentation, blood group representations and frequencies; and, secondly, by extension, into ensembles presenting clusters of similar cultural, physical and psychological features. It is from this type of distribution that we have inherited such expressions as 'black', 'red', 'white', 'yellow' races in which the adjectives are, strictly speaking, metaphors of something else, facticities. Moreover, they fuse and confuse the physiological, the psychological and the cultural.

This distribution is a legacy of centuries of Western taxonomies, and we can rigorously follow their progressive development and complexification since the seventeenth century (e.g. Foucault, 1973). In contemporary popular representations, it amalgamates complex tables: the legacies of the past, and the fact well put by Stephen Howe that allows me 'to talk of human difference in terms of "ethnic groups", rather than "races"' and, also, that 'race is not a biologically, genetically, anthropologically or sociologically meaningful concept' (1998, p. 19).

Yet, it is from this historical perspective and its determinations that a web of values concerning races have been articulating, recycling and readapting, impacting transformations observable in a number of disciplinessuch as biology, craniology, history, psychology for instance. Focusing on the last years of the end of the eighteenth century, Michel Foucault, in *The Order of Things* (1973), could hypothesise that a new principle of classification organises itself and its aim. As it was already in the project of Linnaeus, its project

> ... is still to determine the 'character' that groups individuals and species into more general units, that distinguishes those units one from another, and that enables them to fit together, to form a table in which all individuals and all groups, known or unknown, will have their appropriate place (1973, p. 226).

The major principle of this mutation is the concept of organic structure understood 'as a foundation for ordering nature, as a means of defining its space or delimiting its forms', exemplifying and articulating the basis of essential functions of the living being: (a) the interdependence of characters, and thus, the fact that all of them and each individually are just 'the visible point of a complex and hierarchized organic structure'; and more importantly, to quote Foucault referring to Cuvier, 'it is not because a character occurs frequently in the structures observed that it is important; it is because it is functionally important that it is often encountered' (1973, p. 228); (b) to classify is, from now on, to go beyond the visible, the external aspects in two complementary movements: a descending one into a 'hidden architecture' of a natural being and then to come back to the visible organisation and its signs; (c) the order of classification does not coincide any longer with that of naming; in fact,

> in order to discover the fundamental groups into which natural beings can be divided, it has become necessary to explore in depth the space that lies between their superficial organs and their most concealed ones, and between these latter and the broad functions that they perform (Foucault, 1973, p. 230).

In sum, with the prevalence of this general principle of classification, that of organic structure, a discontinuity indicates the possibility of both a biology and a renewed anthropology, as they will begin stammering by the end of the eighteenth century; and, in any case, a radical move from hierarchy to history. This is not to say that the new horizons are radically unprejudiced, as witnessed by the foundations of craniology as a discipline, in their approaches to races but, simply, that their methods open up new ways of classifying human beings. If, by the end of the nineteenth century, anthropology, as a 'science', promotes the concept of alterity as in the case of the highly controverted monumental work of Sir James George Frazer, *The Golden Bough*, first published in 1890 in two volumes, it also displays the most systematic racial preconceptions. Yet, it is important to note the progressive generalisation of a potentiality actualised by the notion of organic structure as what makes characters dependent upon each other according to their specific functions in an ensemble which, ultimately, can be conceived as a system articulating its own rules and norms.

One perceives easily such possible deployment by opposing the methodology of Natural History between 1775 and 1795 and comparing it to that which sustains Carl Linnaeus's *opus magnum* of 1735. Throughout his *Systema Naturae*, whose fundamental preoccupation was to present a general table of flora, it is a universal schema which hierarchises everything: any variety is described and ordered under species, the species under genera, genera under orders and these under classes. As Margaret T. Hodgen (1964) puts it: 'once the system was set up the collector's burden was eased'. From minerals to human beings, through flora and animals, everything is classified in a catalogue witnessing to a universal hierarchy of being. 'To find the appropriate place for a new specimen, or to look up an old one, (the collector) had only to open a correctly ticketed drawer or turn to the right page.' The conceptual tools for the classification are always visible features, physical (e.g. skin colour) or cultural (e.g. political system). The very meaning of the diversity of beings and things is in this way properly negated in what claims to render its manifestations. This gives, among other things, the tension between the following two sets: on the one hand, *Homo Sapiens*, and its hierarchised varieties; on the other, *Homo monstrosus* and its equally hierarchised types.

Homo Sapiens, varying by education and situation, was composed of

- Wild man: four-footed, mute, hairy.
- American: copper-colored, choleric, erect. Paints self. Regulated by customs.
- European: fair, sanguine, brawny. Covered with close vestments. Governed by laws.
- Asiatic: sooty, melancholy, rigid. Covered with loose garments. Governed by opinions.
- African: black, phlegmatic, relaxed. Anoints himself with grease. Governed by caprice.

Homo monstrosus, varying by climate and art, included

- Mountaineers: small, inactive, timid.
- Patagonians: large, indolent.
- Hottentot: less fertile.
- American: beardless.
- Chinese: head conic.
- Canadian: Head flattened (Hodgen, 1964, p. 425).

What these signs express is not really new, if we pay attention to the long history that goes back to the medieval period of naming human differences through the grids of the Chain of Being. The Ancients had their monsters (dog-headed humans who did not have proper names or could not dream etc.), and the Greeks as well as the Roman mythology is full of god-like or man-like animals. The peculiarity of Linnaeus's tables is elsewhere: it visualizes the extreme development of a classifying method initiated in the seventeenth century and, at the same time marks its limits. To know anything, since the period of Descartes on the continent and Locke in England, means to establish procedures for distinguishing identities and differences in terms of strict discriminating techniques that include proof by comparison, an exhaustive enumeration of elements constituting the empiricity, separation of easy connections based on apparent similitudes, analysis and comparison of differences, comparison of the tables representing them, and, finally and most importantly, such a perspective takes place in a radical suspicion for interplays between science and history, positivity and imagination (see, e.g. Foucault, 1973, pp. 50–8). Linnaeus might represent one of the last shining moments of a fabulous ambition. It is in these new prescriptions that resides the madness of Don Quixote: he walks and thinks with categories of bringing together beings and things in an intellectual configuration dominated by principles of ordering in classes. He opposes them to the beautiful rules for reading the book of nature with such concepts as convenience, emulation, analogy and sympathy, to use only a limited number of possible actualisations of similitude as transcendental. As Foucault put it, it was Linnaeus 'who said that *Naturalia* (the naturally observable on earth) – as opposed to *Coelestia* (celestial beings and objects) and *elementa* (that is elements) were intended to be transmitted directly to the senses' (1973, pp. 133–4). The primacy of what is visible and sensible inscribes itself in a vocation: to order and name. But how? By being systematic and reproducing rigorously on a table the seen, observed, discriminated and analysed. Concretely, an example (1973, p. 134):

> when, as Linnaeus wrote, one studies the reproductive organs of a plant, it is sufficient, but indispensable, to enumerate the stamens and pistil (or to record their absence, according to the case), to define the form they assume, according to what geometrical figure they are distributed in the flower (circle, hexagon, triangle), and what their size is in relation to the other organs. These four variables, which can be applied in the same way to the five parts of the plant – roots, stem, leaves, flowers, fruits – specify the extension available to representation well enough for us to articulate it into a description acceptable to everyone: confronted with the same individual entity, everyone will be able to give the same description; and, inversely, given such a description everyone will be able to recognize the individual entities that correspond to it. In this fundamental articulation of the visible, the first confrontation of language and things can now be established in a manner that excludes all uncertainty.

Mineral, flora, animals, humans are just names. In their diversity, they situate themselves vis-à-vis each other on the basis of preconceived categories of form, position or proportion. They have no life. They witness to nothing apart from being named from their outsidedness. They are members of this or that class, situated here and not there, on the basis of a 'light' of reason classifying them, and not on the basis of their internal economy. The scientific or philosophical vocabulary – they are not then well distinguished – convey what existed as a priori before their own systematic articulation in a rigorous language of knowledge.

I have, so far, avoided the notions of normality and abnormality although they spring clear and uncomfortable from the methods analysed.

Let's pause one moment by bringing into discussion a diametrically different horizon. Contemporaneous with the transformation under by the concept of structure, specifically that of organic structure, takes place a major upheaval of political nature. It is well documented, and, concerns the existence of 'two races' and their organic structures in France. Hannah Arendt dwelt on it briefly in her *The Origins of Totalitarianism* (1979) initially published in 1948. More recently, Michel Foucault has revived the complexity of the issue in his posthumous *Il faut défendre la société* (1997).

Let us begin by noting, after Margaret T. Hodgen, that during the European Renaissance, 'the word "race", in its many linguistic forms and cultural applications held little meaning'. More mundanely, one observes that in texts, people are

> differentiated from one another as 'nations', while the term 'race' carried a zoological connotation properly applicable only to animals. As long as man even pigmented man was regarded as monogenetic in origin and homogenous in descent, he could not be submitted to zoological divisions, or to terms used to designate them (1964, p. 214).

The seventeenth century already, but mainly the eighteenth century are periods discovering the diversity of peoples, histories and mores existing in the world. The book of Michèle Duchet, *Anthropologie et histoire au siècle des lumières* (1971) demonstrates the extent of this curiosity and its import on new developing disciplines, particularly anthropology (Buffon, Helvétius, Rousseau, Voltaire etc.). A new approach for understanding the diversity of human beings and cultures vis-à-vis the experience of Western cultures, takes place and indeed, as actualised by the French space, it comments fundamentally on itself. If, one century before, Descartes did not doubt about the permanence and the universality of reason, the eighteenth century would rather tend to valorise Locke's intellectual position and that of his eighteenth-century French equivalent Condillac: some peoples are different as in the case of children, idiots and savages. In any case, to refer to an ill-known treatise in the Anglo-Saxon world, *La pensée française au XVIIIéme siècle* by Daniel Mornet (1969), French intellectuals travel a lot. They are all over Europe: Beaumarchais, Bernardin de Saint-Pierre, Diderot, d'Holbach, Chénier, Condillac, Rousseau, Voltaire, etc. They mark in their writings what is different and particular elsewhere. Thus, to use Mornet's expression, with them, geography meets history (1969, p. 72). There is more, if with the Montesquieu of the *Lettres persanes*, one faces the most explicit challenge about otherness – 'how is it possible to be a Persian?' – such an issue may now be solved in at least two ways. The variety of human societies is linked to general laws of nature, and these depend on climates since these laws are in a relation of necessity with the nature of things. Supposedly, they are created by generations of peoples submitted to a given climate, and as a consequence, they cannot be reasonably be the same in France, Holland or Italy. Hence, for each people 'the best laws are those based on (climatic) differences and not on what could be found, through reasoning, as being common between a Chinese, a French, a Hollander and an Italian' (Mornet, 1969, p. 76). Another way of facing the challenge incarnated by the diversity of 'nationalities' and cultural variations: anthropology is, then, constituting itself as a science of non-Western peoples and spaces vis-à-vis the West, and, in France, Buffon's *Histoire naturelle* marks in 1749 a foundation. It incorporates everything that can be known in Natural history on varieties of humans, animals and things (Duchet, 1971). Very concretely, reading Duchet, one sees it: a history of political administration in France with its extension (a politics of colonisation) can be related to a history of ideas concerning the expansion of the West and its missions. They are even linked to the usefulness and pertinence of a new discipline, anthropology. Its observations should and do constitute an inventory of exotic spaces, their inhabitants and customs.

In sum, the two entries used thanks to the works of Duchet and Mornet – on the one hand, anthropology and history and, on the other, geography and history – are simply conceptual tools for a new intellectual configuration in which the visibility of otherness demands an understanding in order to be classified on a general table. Hannah Arendt rightly notes that this 'rising interest' in exoticism ('Chinese paintings', 'simplicity of savage and uncivilized peoples', 'the content of culture that lay far beyond European boundaries') culminated in the (French Revolution) message of fraternity, because it was inspired by the desire to prove in every new and 'surprising specimen of mankind 'the old saying of La Bruyère: 'la raison est de tous les climats [reason can be found under all climates]' (1979, p. 162). Yet, it is in this context that one faces adverse and complementary theses to a unifying project of egalitarian liberation (with, indeed, their own classificatory principles and preconceptions). Let us call it a counter-discourse on an organic structural and historical inequality between two 'French races'. One could argue on the ambiguities of this new spirit. After all, did not such a revolutionary as Condorcet write that 'some humans are more equal than others' (Badinter, 1988). In itself such a statement, but in its context, might open a fruitful debate. But that is a different issue and strictly speaking, it should not be confused with Hannah Arendt and Foucault's *Il faut défendre la société* (1997) perspectives on the eighteenth-century paradox of a race-thinking theory conceived from a so-called organic and hereditary structure of being French. Its general theme is simple: France would be composed of 'two nations' as Count de Boulainvilliers, a disciple of Spinoza and a strong believer in the 'might' thesis, put it in the first part of the eighteenth century. There are two races in France: a superior one of Germanic origin whose original roots were in Friesland, and an inferior one constituted by the Gallics, a mixed blood populace enslaved and colonised in the past by Romans. A right of conquest would justify an 'eternal distinction' between the two and, thus, found the principle of 'obedience always due to the strongest'. As noted by Arendt, for Boulainvilliers the French aristocracy was 'a separate ruling caste which might have much more in common with foreign people of the same society and condition than with its compatriots' (1979, p. 163). Towards the end of the century, in his *Les origines, de ou, l'ancien gouvernement de la France, de l'Allemagne et l'Italie* (1789), another Count, Du Bbuat-Nançay, promotes the idea of bringing the French nobility in an aristocratic *Internationale* of blood:

> the true origin of the French nation was supposed to be identical with that of the Germans and the French lower classes, though no longer slaves, were free by birth but by 'affranchaissement', but by the grace of those who were free by birth of the nobility (1979, pp. 163–4).

The aristocrats organised effectively. For them, the French Revolution with its principle of equality and fraternity was an aberration. Arendt writes that 'Count de Montlosier openly expressed his contempt for this new people risen from slaves ... [a mixture] of all races and all times'. As a matter of fact, at least politically, it seems clear that the aristocracy was then opposing the 'Roman Republicanism'. With its theme of an organic blood Germanism and its absolute superiority, it explicitly confused two notions, *class* and *race*. Another aristocrat, Count de Rémuzat, ratiocinated on it. Finally, Count Arthur de Gobineau with his *Essai sur l'inégalite des races humaines* (1853) crowns this type of thinking enterprise and makes it move from 'race-thinking' 'scientific racism': 'Instead of princes, he proposed a race of princes, the Aryans, who he said were in danger by being submerged by the lower non-Aryan classes through democracy' (Arendt, 1979, p. 173). De Gobineau is, as Arendt says it well, 'the last heir of Boulainvilliers and the French exiled nobility who, without psychological complications, simply (and rightly) feared for the fate of aristocracy as a caste' (1979, pp. 171–2). He is also the father of two scientific hypotheses: the first links the degeneration of a race and the decay of a civilization; the second promulgates the thesis that, in all mixtures of races, the lower race becomes dominant. The new grid integrates all the presuppositions concerning the Chain of Being. New tables of varieties of human beings include the new discoveries in 'craniology' and their socio-cultural impact, and at a political level, claim to demonstrate scientifically absolute essential differences and inequalities between 'races'. Africa and peoples of African descent, along with a number of other non-western peoples, could but constitute a question mark. Are not they 'essentially abnormal'?

What's Abnormal? What's Normal?

It is in reading Georges Canguilhem's classical treatise on *The Normal and the Pathological* (1991), originally presented as a doctoral dissertation in medicine in 1943 at the School of Medicine in Strasbourg, France, and first published in Paris by the Presses Universitaires de France in 1966, that I was confronted with a puzzling issue concerning the meanings of such important concepts for mental health as *anomaly, abnormal, norm* and *normal*. Referring to André Lalande's *Vocabulaire technique et critique de la philosophie* (1962), Canguilhem emphasises a French curiosity: '*Anomaly* is a substantive with no corresponding adjective at present; *abnormal* on the other hand, is an adjective with no substantive, so that [French] usage has coupled them, making *abnormal* the adjective of *anomaly*' (1991, p. 131). On the other hand, the English language witnesses a perfect parallelism between *anomaly* versus *anomalous, abnormality* versus *abnormal* and *normality* versus *normal*. It is true, as Canguilhem notes, there was a French equivalent for *anomalous, anomal*, but it went out of usage in the mid-nineteenth century. The theoretical implications of this difference are important for cultural and medical taxonomies. Thus, for instance, in English to be *anomalous* does not necessarily mean to be *abnormal* although they can in some cases combine. In French, to the substantive *anomaly*, the only corresponding adjective is *abnormal* with all its weighty semantic, sociological and psychiatric deductions.

Lalande defines *anomaly* (German: *abnormität*; French: *anomalie*; Italian: *anomalia*) as any phenomenon that, in general, seems unusual as in the particular case of an organic or a functional alteration. Thus, the term is, in accordance with its Greek etymology, indicative of an irregularity or, more significantly, an unevenness. Canguilhem makes an addition and, after Louis Boisse quoted in a footnote by Lalande (1962, p. 60), insists on the fact that 'a mistake is often made with the etymology of '*anomaly*'", by deriving it not from (the Greek) *omalos* but from *nomos*, hence the compound *a-nomos*. This etymological error is found right in Littré's dictionary and Robin's *Dictionnaire de médecine*. The Greek *nomos* and the Latin *norma* have closely related meanings, law and rule tending to become confused. Hence, in a strictly semantic sense 'anomaly' points to a fact, and is a descriptive term, while 'abnormal' implies reference to a value and is an evaluative, normative term; but the switching of good grammatical methods has meant a confusion of the respective meanings of anomaly and abnormal. "'*Abnormal*' has become a descriptive concept and '*anomaly*', a normative one" (Canguilhem, 1991, pp. 131–2).

Canguilhem's note should lead to a reformulation of the relationship between anomaly and disease, normal, norm and pathological. I shall come back to this after a brief detour that, from Lalande's entries, will focus on the semantic questions concerning the rapport between *norm* and *normal*. A norm from Latin *norma* (German: *norm*; French: *norme*; Italian: *norma*) is, strictly speaking, the equivalent of the canonical, that is a model or an abstract formula witnessing what should be or exist according to specific requirements, concretely, an ideal, a rule, an objective. Thus, the normative (German: *normativ*; French: *normatif*; Italian: *normativo*) is what constitutes, spells out, or concerns rules in the sense of expressions such as a 'normative judgment', 'normative disciplines'. Yet, as indicates Lalande, 'normative' is not synonymous with 'imperative' since a norm is not necessarily a law, nor a commandment but rather an ideal. Thus, to use the quoted phrase from Simmel's *Einleitung in die Moralwissenschaft* (I, 321), one would agree that 'a normative science normalizes nothing; it only presents (or explains) norms and links that they can have between them'. Hence, it becomes clear as pointed out by Lalande (1962, pp. 690–91) that, taking into account the philosophical tradition, 'the three fundamental classes of norms are that of logical thought (the idea of truth), that of voluntary action (the idea of good) and that of free representation or, as some think, that of sentiment (the idea of beauty)'.

As to *normal* (German: *normal*; French: *normal*; Italian: *normale*) the most striking thing is its semantic ambiguity. The concept may mean: (a) what is straight (German: *senkrecht, gewöhnlich*; French: *normal*; Italian: *solito*). By extension, it might have other values: firstly, (b) what is correct, good, just, proper (German: *richtig*; French: *bon et juste*; Italian: *retto*); and, finally, (c) what in a given population presents the highest statistical frequency, and, as such it often includes the idea of average as in usual expressions such as 'the normal American is this or that; the normal child should experience this or that'. We should finally mention that in English the value presented under (a) – what is 'straight' – tends to include also the meaning of customary. In this sense, one could think that it is 'normal' to have an annual rate of x suicides, rapes, assassinations in a given city; or that, everything being equal, it is 'normal' that the death rate of young Blacks in the US should be higher than that of their white counterparts.

In the critique of the concept, Lalande (pp. 689–90) emphasises the ambiguity of the notion. In effect, *normal* may designate a fact that can be observed and evaluated scientifically and universally; but, it can also signify a value that the analyst or the speaker bestows on the fact (e.g. 'a normal woman should have such behaviour'). Even in technical debates, *normal* is, semantically, in a relationship of partial inclusion with the significance of *norm* and *normative*. The *Vocabulaire* addresses also the delicate issue present in the realist philosophical tradition in which the usage of *normal* is often confusing: if an observable generality witnesses to an idea, then should not one conclude that the normal is expressed by the (c) meaning – the statistical average represented by the Gaussian Curve – and which would unveil the essence of a particular species or population?

Lalande moves on to show how this confusion is well present in the medical language. Concretely, for example, does the expression 'normal state' mean the usual physical balance of an individual or the recovery of his balance after a disease? What do they have in common the 'normal state' of a 25-year-old young man without major health problems versus that of a 75-year-old person with a heart condition? What's a normal state for a haemophiliac versus that of a young baby dying of cancer in an intensive care unit? It is here that we should return to Canguilhem's analysis (1991, pp. 125–49) and note some of his affirmations that warrant further reflections and, literally, to use his own expression, make one tremble (1991, p. 289):

- Anomaly is a fact of individual variation which prevents two beings from being able to take the place of each other completely.
- The *anomalous* is not the pathological. Pathological implies *pathos*, the direct and concrete feeling of suffering and impotence.
- There is one way to consider the pathological normal, and that is by defining normal and abnormal in terms of relative statistical frequency. In a sense, one could say that continual perfect health is abnormal.
- Another reason for avoiding confusion between anomaly and disease is that human attention is not sensitized to each (concepts of sick, pathological and abnormal) as being divergences of the same kind.

- An anomaly manifests itself in spatial multiplicity, disease, in chronological succession. It is characteristic of disease that it interrupts a course ... . Hence, we are sick in relation not only to others but also to ourselves.
- When an anomaly is interpreted in terms of its effects in relation to the individual's activity and, hence, to the representation which develops from its value and destiny, an anomaly is an *infirmity*. Infirmity is a vulgar but instructive notion.
- The problem of distinguishing between an anomaly ... and the pathological state is not at all a clear one; but it is nevertheless, quite important from the biological point of view because, in the end, it leads us to nothing less than the general problem of the variability of organisms and the scope and significance of this variability.
- The pathological is not the absence of a biological norm; it is another norm but one which is, comparatively speaking, pushed aside by life.

All this might seem highly abstract. Let us bring it back to the dimension of individualities and reflect on Louis A. Sass's commentary (1994) about the International Pilot Study of Schizophrenia and the determinants of Outcome Study, a research sponsored by the World Health Organisation (WHO). Sass begins by clearly distinguishing pathogenic factors as a concept which is determined in the disease from pathoplastic factors that are essentially cultural and, in this sense, enculturate a disease. If we accept this hypothesis, then, it becomes obvious that a psychiatrist could state that: 'cultural relativism is of no value in explaining (a) psychosis; for the culture of a group can determine the content but not the forms of a psychosis' (1994, p. 358). Indeed, here, the organization of symptoms and their interpretation could be marked and reduced to technical grids, say, internet games for highly sophisticated psychologists or psychiatrists with a mathematical background, foundational sagas of a history involving gods or theology, even the combination of the two. But let us follow carefully Sass. First, his presentation of the WHO project:

> The International Pilot Study investigated psychotic individuals who were admitted to psychiatric centers in nine cities: Aarhus (Denmark), Agra (India), Cali (Colombia), Ibadan (Nigeria), Taipei (Taiwan), Prague, London, Moscow, and Washington, D.C. It was found that patients who manifested schizophrenic symptoms – in particular, a nuclear set of features that included Schneider's First Rank Symptoms – showed up in all the locales and did not seem to be especially rare in any of them. Since the International Pilot Study offered no way of estimating the overall frequency of schizophrenia in its various settings (it simply studied the characteristics of patients who had schizophrenialike symptoms), this objective was attempted in the subsequent Determinants

of Outcome Study, which found that patients with certain clinical features of schizophrenia did in fact seem to be as common in the developing as in the developed societies. Although these findings, have often been taken to undermine the significance of sociocultural factors in the etiology of schizophrenia, such a conclusion is unwarranted (Sass, 1994, p. 359).

What do we deduce from this? Indeed one could think of the provocative indictment of capitalism by Deleuze and Guattari in *Anti-Oedipus: Capitalism and Schizophrenia* (1977). For example, they write (p. 245):

> [Capitalism] produces schizos the same way it produces Prell shampoo or Ford cars, the only difference being that the schizos are not saleable. How then does one explain the fact that capitalist production is constantly arresting the schizophrenic process and transforming the subject of the process into a confined clinical entity as though it saw in this process the image of its own death coming from within? Why does it make the schizophrenic into a sick person – not only nominally but in reality? Why does it confine its madmen and madwomen instead of seeing in them its own heros and heroines, its own fulfillment?

The statement might seem excessive and it is. But it demands a rigorous reflection when facing Sass's analysis. Sass notes a number of things. First, a question: how to understand, from subtype diagnoses qualifying methodically acute schizophrenia, the 'difference' between the Western context and the Third World, more specifically,

> ... the fact that 40 per cent of the 'schizophrenics 'in the developing countries versus only 11 per cent of those in the developed countries were given the subtype label 'acute schizophrenic episode' (also called 'oneirophrenia' and 'schizophreniform attack' or 'schizophreniform psychosis, confusional type' ... is certainly not one of the core or prototypical forms of schizophrenia (1994, p. 360).

It goes without saying, as Sass himself puts it,

> ... various studies have indicated also that Schneiderian First Rank Symptoms (delusions and hallucinations observed in the absence of evidence of coarse brain disease) are less commonly found in schizophrenics from developing countries than in those from Western Cultures (1994, p. 360).

Two things should be noted: first, the silent omnipresence of the relation normality versus schizophrenia; secondly, the fact that the WHO studies are about averages, which led Sass to a question full of implications:

> the Third World settings that were examined were all in developing societies, where the allied forces of modernization, Westernization, and industrialization had already been able to have a significant degree of influence (1994, p. 361).

Should one deduce that the capitalist mode of production, which converted Africa, would mainly account for the extension of schizophrenia, and thus, conclude that the colonization of Africa was what allowed it? There is something of a paradox here. Africa was colonized on the pretence that she was diseased and needed to be lifted up psychologically. Sass has a telling case:

> A particularly interesting report comes from the anthropologist Meyers Forte and his wife, the psychiatrist Doris Mayer. Fortes first lived among the Tallensi of northern Ghana for two and a half years in the mid-1930s when they were still a traditional, farming people, hardly touched by technology, Western education, or a money economy; at that time Fortes encountered only one clearly psychotic person in a population of five thousand. When he returned with his wife in 1963, the society had changed considerably, largely due to the fact that many of the young men spent long periods of time in southern Ghana where they could earn wages. They had brought back with them a money economy that was now firmly fixed atop the communal, subsistence patterns of the traditional Tallensi way of life. This time Fortes and Mayer found at least thirteen obviously psychotic people, of whom ten appeared to be schizophrenic – a rise far greater than the modest population increase in the intervening years, and involving blatantly psychotic cases of a kind Fortes could not have missed during his earlier stay. Fortes and Mayer attributed the rise to the economic and social changes that had taken place, noting that most of the psychotics had become ill while in the south. ('They travel South and are brought back mad', as the tribal elders of some of the northern tribes would say.) (Sass, 1994, p. 362).

Inscribed in the archeology of its own history, the conceptual debate on normal and abnormal is more complicated and confused than one might think. For illustration purpose, I shall refer to only three significant enterprises. The first, *Seeing the Insane* (Gilman, 1996), 'a cultural history of madness and art in the Western world' is fundamentally about a difference, and the way it is perceived as abnormality and thus object of prejudice. Thomas S. Szasz's book on *The Manufacture of Madness* (1977) narrates simply but brilliantly an awful history about how abnormality has been conceptualized and intellectually and politically manipulated. Just one example that should be more known: it is the Christian Church which long before Hitler, invented a distinctive sign for the Jew in order to qualify him as different and abnormal. In effect among many other things, the fourth Lateran Council, ordered by Pope Innocent III in 1215, decreed that 'all Jews were to wear a distinctive garment or a special badge to set them apart from other men' (Szasz, 1977, p. 294). With his *Histoire de la folie à l'âge classique* (Foucault, 1961), Michel Foucault focuses on an impossible challenge: how to make madness speak about its difference and abnormality within conflicting intellectual interpretations? In the introduction (1978) to the series on *The History of Sexuality*, he indicts the power of a number of normalising centres. They include eighteenth and nineteenth century medical discourses on sex, along with psychiatry 'when it set out to discover the etiology of mental illnesses', criminal justice with its focus on interpretations about 'heinous' crimes and 'crimes against nature'; and finally the politics of social control (Foucault, 1978, p. 30). But it is in his description of the 'domain' of sexuality and its deployment that Foucault touches an essential point about the gradual constitution of a science of sexuality (normal and abnormal) and its strategies. He names and comments on four of them: (a) a hysterisation of women's bodies; (b) a pedagogisation of children's sex; (c) a socialisation of procreative behaviour; and (d) a psychiatrisation of perverse pleasure (1978, pp. 104–5).

Instead of repeating arguments well made by these three scholars, I would like to bring them together to a symbol which works and exhausts them even when it is not explicitly invoked: the cultural representation of the woman as the basic paradigm of an abnormality inscribed on her body. To illustrate this point, I shall use a little-known and paradoxical text, that of Josse Bade (1500), which reacting to negative representations wants explicitly to celebrate 'Eva' (Eve), and in doing so damns her beautifully by bringing about her exceptionality: she would be both the incarnation and the actualisation of an excess that could be conceived also as a supplement. Madness as an excess or a supplement of a way of existing would be actualised in an exemplary manner in 'Eva, our first mother'. Her sin would have fully involved the five senses and they all contributed to the folly signified by a false promise 'you will become eternal and like gods you will know the good and the bad'. She heard and explicitly accepted the invitation, for a closure. Then, there is the sight which contemplated the fruit and judged it as good and beautiful; her feeling it in her own hands, the smell which convinced her to taste and enjoy it. Thus, when Eva and Adam were eating the apple the source and absolute origin of madness come to life. In her message of complaint to the human race, Eva states:

> Listen, mortals, the lamentations of your unhappy mother and orient your boat far from my ship. The woman I was, untouched by corruption, who could not experience evil nor face death and who immaculate was to give birth to a beautiful descendency ... Me, I say, who was such, since I dared to crunch with my own teeth the forbidden fruit, I find myself carried away into a long exile. The first, in effect, I am entering the ship of fools whose course is uncertain and will be exposed to deadly perils. And I am the mother of madness. Because in my immense folly, I wanted to acquire divine thought, here I am now with my posterity demned to death (Josse Bade, 1500).

The demonstration is didactic. It brings together the Renaissance humanist domain, its heavy Greco-Latin knowledge with Christian beliefs and unveils successively five 'nefs', in actuality, frameworks symbolised by the five senses. Depending on Sebastian Brant's *Das Narrenschiff* (1497), as to its structure and aim, Bade's book presents itself as a *fabula* intended to teach while pleasing, and explicitly situates itself in a tradition going back to Aesopus. Each 'nef' is divided into two parts of unequal length: the first, in prose, elaborates a theory of the specific sense chosen, and supports it with biblical or classical maxims and *exempla* illustrating potential and possible excesses; the second part, in verses, tries to manifest visibly the road to sin, thus reflecting concrete, yet symbolic, representations of senses gone wry: the wild sight, mirrors itself in a woman doing her own hair; the wild hearing, a singing woman; the wild smell, a woman accepting unguents and perfumes; the wild taste, a group of women eating and drinking; finally, the wild feeling, represented by a woman receiving a kiss from a man. The misogyny is obvious. It goes well with the general cultural configuration of this period with its debate known as 'la querelle des femmes' (the quarrel about women). It accounts for example, for both the pro-women stances represented by Symphorien Champier's *La Nef des femmes vertueuses* (1503) and François de Billon's *Le fort inexpugnable de l'honneur du sexe féminin* (1555); and, on the other hand, Erasmus's ambiguous description of the woman which in his *Praise of Folly* symbolises a natural unreason: Woman is 'admittedly a stupid and foolish sort of creature'.

> But since man was born to manage affairs he had to be given a modicum, just a sprinkling, of reason; and in order to do her best for him in this matter Nature called on me for counsel here as she had on other occasions. I was ready with

a piece of advice worthy of myself: she should give him a woman, admittedly a stupid and foolish sort of creature but amusing and pleasant company all the same, and she could share his life, and season and sweeten his harsh nature by her folly. For Plato's apparent doubt whether to place a woman in the category of rational animal or brute beast is intended to point out the remarkable folly of her sex. If ever a woman wanted to be thought wise she only succeeded in being doubly foolish, just as if one enters an ox for a wrestling match, they say, one cannot hope for the approval and support of Minerva. The defect is multiplied when anyone tries to lay on a veneer of virtue and deflect a character from its natural bent. As the Greek proverb puts it, an ape is always an ape even if clad in purple: and a woman is always a woman, that is, a fool, whatever mask she wears (Erasmus, 1993, pp. 30–31).

In the 1971 and 1993 editions of *Praise of Folly*, A.H.T. Levi notes that

Folly's reference to Plato's doubts about whether women were human or animal (*Timaeus*, 90e) does not give a fair idea of what either Plato or Erasmus thought. Rabelais borrows this reference for *Tiers livre* (chapter 32). The two proverbs in this paragraph are both commented on in the *Adages*. That concerning Minerva refers to the attempt to teach something to someone who cannot understand. The idea that women's folly sweetens the harsh nature of men comes from Aulus Gellus (15, 25, 2) (Radice and Levi, 1971, pp. 30–31).

In any case, such ideas exemplify Erasmus's paradigm that opposes human to divine madness; and, more concretely, illustrate a contemporary debate on women's soul. It becomes clearer that from Brant (1494) to Bade (1500) and then to Erasmus (1515), what is most striking is the progressive solidification of the equation, madness is sin (and indeed, sin is madness) and its inscription on the woman's body. Of the five senses, let us comment briefly on that of the sight of 'Eva'. It is presented as subtle, of a quasi-immaterial nature, this sense, as postulated in its Greek etymology (*theon*, the one who observes; *theoreo*, I see; *theoremia* or *theoria*, contemplation) would be almost a divine function by its potentiality for reaching the real and the truth. Two orders of reference reduce the sight to its objective limitation: on the one hand, Ancients' theories (e.g. Plato's and Stoicians's conception of perception as an emission of rays, Epicurian theory of simulacre: the seen is not the real, etc.) and on the other hand Paul's masterful statement – 1.Cor. 13, 12: 'For now we see through a glass, darkly; but then face to face: now I know in part; but then shall I know even as also I am known.' In what it allows, human sight reflects a mirage. And, in the conclusion of the *Nef*, the invitation of the wild sight 'towards the fields of Venus where beautiful bodies meet tender young girls' sanctions the sheer madness of a sight perceiving and naming irreality and its dubious images. Dubious, indeed, the image or the discourse reflects an empiricity it cannot render; and it is there that resides abnormality, that is a lack of coincidence between the represented and its representations.

I have suggested the slippery aspects of the concepts of normality and abnormality and, after Canguilhem the nightmarish issues they bring about; the synthesis on the WHO research has shown, I would hope, the complex intercultural problems in time or in space one faces when referring blindly, let's say, to a 'psychiatric bible', to an ideology or pre-conceived paradigms worked out overtime by intellectual configurations that make possible individual or collective differences. Finally, my brief commentary on Josse Bade's text celebrating Eve as a symbol of womanhood indicates how even generous intellectual intentions can backfire in precepts, reduce individualities to a presupposed essence, and in this way confuse nature and styles of being different. They should not. Let us tackle the problem.

A Style, not an Essence

Sass's analysis on the prevalence of schizophrenia from the cross-cultural dimension is an excellent summary. Competent, brief and clear, it indicates the main points of ambiguities. First, that the evaluation in terms of averages (about schizophrenia or other mental diseases) seem to be locked up in a semantic confusion well described by George Canguilhem in his *The Normal and the Pathological* (1991). Secondly, this predicament inscribes itself in a configuration that goes back to the eighteenth and nineteenth century, and which womanised and made Africa the paradigm of abnormality. Both have been supporting each other in the literature justifying colonisation (Hammond and Jablow, 1977) and, in the interpretation of symbolism of colours at the foundation of both psychiatry and psychoanalysis. On the one hand, there is the stereotyping of a whole continent even in the most learned knowledges or simply the negation of the pertinence of its difference as actualising other ways of existing. On the other hand, in the name of science, cultural inscriptions reduce the black symbolically or effectively to the margins of normality.

It would be significant to go back to Freud or Jung and read their references to the concept 'Black'. Let us begin by emphasising Freud's reduction of the symbols of black to issues of identity concerning the Jew. Freud says Sander Gilman (1993, p. 19) 'wanted to believe' that 'Jews [are] really "white"'. The issue is a major one since the 'blackness' of the Jew went along with associations concerning the body and particularly the 'syphilitic body': 'Jews are black because they are different, because their sexuality is different, because their sexual pathology is written on their skin' (Gilman, 1993, p. 153; Szasz, 1977, pp. 168–9). Such a qualification illustrates more than what it says explicitly: the Jew is, in the Western context, 'the marginal one', close to the Black who is present in an absence magnified by a colour. Importantly enough, the Jew is generally pathologised as an 'Uranist' or homosexual. Gilman puts it squarely:

> The question is not whether there are homosexual Jews. Indeed, there is debate whether there is the same proportion of homosexuals among the Jews as 'among other races.' The image of the Jew and the image of the homosexual were parallel in the *fin de siècle* medical culture. But within the gay culture in Germany, Jews were seen essentially as when they were also identified as gay. They were given Jewish nicknames (such as Sarah or Rebecca) even when their given names were in no way identifiably Jewish (1993, p. 165).

What is presented here as a stigma is linked to a 'race', and, witnessing to its perversion. As Gilman notes, 'this assumption is internalized, often in the complex manner, by those stereotyped'. Freud himself gives signs of such a rendering. Gilman comments on his 'romanticisation of "darkness" [as] an acknowledgment of the "blackness" of the Jews and its glorification' (1993, p. 33) but also insists on a curious case. In a letter to Wilhelm Fliess in 1898, Freud qualifies his own brother-in-law Moritz Freud as a 'half-Asian' suffering from '*pseudologica fantastica*' (pathological swindling), a technical term for a preconception going on then with the image of the Jew. It is interesting, when one moves from Freud to Jung, to see the latter systematically linking the Black to the terrors and sin of Genesis. Blackness means the unconscious and should be related to the Earth Mother (e.g. 1980, p. 301), and conceived as 'what acts as a counterbalance to woman's conventional innocuousness' (1980, p. 185), as it is actualised in metaphors of the 'raven' and its mother at the foundation of Egyptian culture (1989, p. 511), as well as in the mythological narratives about the 'bird of Hermes ... a restless, unsleeping spirit [... who] is the "heaven" and at the same time the "scum of the sea"' (1989, p. 510). Indeed, there is more: the reference to the biblical Shulamite woman. She incarnates the perfect metaphor: black outside, white inside. This 'inner beauty' is opposed to her external blackness which has a history, one of damnation: 'By the sin of Eve, says Jung, she is plunged, as it were, in ink, in the "tincture", and blackened, just as in Islamic legend the precious stone that Allah gave Adam was blackened by his sin' (1989, p. 423).

The point to be made is that Freud and Jung are elaborating interpretations in a configuration already charged with signs situating the woman, the Jew and the Black in relations of exclusion which are also supposed to illustrate abnormality. Their status is varied and their positioning as their individual or collective known reactions in the unfolding history have been different. What they share is a reduction perspective, a radical essentialisation from a dominant mainstream legitimate culture and its classifications. Yesterday, as today, one thus, could think, after Thomas Szasz, that 'when man is faced with important mass-beliefs ... he is more interested in preserving popular explanations which tend to consolidate the group than in making accurate observations which tend to divide it' (1977, p. 187). The real issue becomes then one of the universal beliefs and behaviours versus the particular ones, and here, in the history we are considering, we have to recognize that the situations of the woman, the Jew and the Black diverge and meet. Some references might make it obvious even though they do suscitate more problems than they resolve. When in *Poetics*, Aristotle writes that 'both a woman and slave can be good; but a woman is perhaps an inferior being – and a slave utterly worthless' (15, 1454a, pp. 20–22), he is advancing a number of things. They suppose a background in which the *oikos* (the inside, the house, the feminine) is opposed to the *politikon* (the outside, the public place, the masculine), and an overall organisation of gender relations carefully stipulating duties and obligations on ethical and legal basis, (see e.g. Gordon, 1982; de Beauvoir, 1974). More recently when, introducing Léopold Sédar Senghor's anthology of Francophone black writers, Jean-Paul Sartre writes that:

> For our black poets, to the contrary, being comes from non-being as a rising phallus. Creation is an enormous and perpetual coition; the world is flesh and son of flesh. On the sea and in the sky, on the stands, on the rocks, in the wind, the Negro rediscovers the velvetness of the human skin; he is 'flesh of the flesh of the world'; he is 'porous to its every breath', to all its pollen. He is by turn the female of nature and its male; and when he makes love with a woman of his race, the sex act seems to him the celebration of the Mystery of being. This spermatic religion is like a tension of the soul balancing two complementary tendencies; the dynamic emotion of being a rising phallus, and that softer, more patient and feminine, of being a plant which grows. Thus negritude, in its most profound origin, is androgyny (Sartre, 1976, pp. 46–7).

Sartre simply underlines here an amazing yet ordinary fact: for centuries, the differences signified by sex or ethnicity were observed and, when necessary, could be integrated in technical grids as signs of abnormality, morphology and its facticities thus reflecting symptoms represented by symbols (e.g. Gilman, 1982). The paradigmatic type would be the reference which in the Western world, from the insane incarcerated in the Bethlem Royal Hospital (1247–1676) possibly 'the oldest' with its 'continuous history of caring for the mentally disordered' (Allderidge, 1995, p. 2), through the spaces made possible by Samuel Tuke's *Description of the Retreat, An Institution near York for Insane Persons* (1813) which is still haunting contemporary psychiatric spaces. They comment in their institutionalisation on the geography of abnormality, thus name, for example, mental disease and, in this sense, a face. As Gilman writes:

> the structuring of madness was both a way of dealing with 'real' mental illness in its historical context as well as the creation of categories that had political and ideological significance. Madness existed in the world and could be measured by psychic pain; madness could also be used as a metaphor for other states of difference (1982, p. 225).

To illustrate the point, we could simply bring back into the discussion Foucault's masterful work on madness during the classical age (1979). The 'abnormal' ones imprisoned within the walls of L'hôpital général include certainly some sick or deranged peoples but also criminals, prostitutes, unemployed persons. This invocation is important. Yes, there is, culturally, a preconceptual a priori about so-called abnormality. Yet, this does not indicate necessarily a disease in the person even when stereotypes had been internalized. There is not such a predetermined essence in a Black, a Jew, a woman, which would make him or her act out automatically an already existing fatality; and symptoms cannot in an absolute way unveil transparently the significance of a disease, and much less an existing nature dependent on an essence. Since the constitution of the 'clinic' as we know it – that is specifically since the last part of the eighteenth century (e.g. Foucault, 1973) – one can surely say that:

> There is no longer a pathological essence beyond the symptoms: everything in the disease is itself a phenomenon; in that respect, the symptoms play a simple role, primary in nature: 'Their collection forms what is known as the disease'. They are nothing more than a truth wholly given to the gaze; their link and status do not refer to an essence, but indicate a natural totality that has only its principles of composition and its more or less regular forms of duration: 'A disease is a whole, because one can assign it its elements; it has an aim, because one can calculate its results; it is therefore a whole placed between the limits of invasion and termination'. The symptom has therefore

lost its role of sovereign indicator, being merely a phenomenon of the law of appearance; it is on the same level as nature.

Yet not entirely so: something, in the immediacy of the symptom, signifies the pathological, which distinguishes it from a phenomenon belonging purely and simply to organic life. 'By phenomenon I mean any notable change in the healthy or sick body; hence the division into those that belong to health and those that designate disease: the latter are easily confused with the symptoms or sensible appearance of the disease'. By this simple opposition to the forms of health, the symptom abandons its passivity as a natural phenomenon and becomes a signifier of the disease, that is, of itself taken as a whole, since the disease is simply a collection of symptoms (Foucault, 1973, pp. 91–2).

Then, what do physicians do? Face some basics: one, is there an organ which is sick or reorganising itself? Two, are there ways of explaining the transformation? Three, how to normalise? The procedures, in method, are fundamentally the same in physiology as well as in psychology. Thus we should be, once more, going back to Canguilhem and keeping in mind his written admonition: 'Medicine', says Sigerist, 'is the most closely linked to the whole of culture, every transformation in medical conceptions being conditions by transformations in the ideas of the epoch' (1989, p. 103). One might be anomalous because of a cultural configuration and seems sick. But should not we remember that

> ... it is a characteristic of a disease that it interrupts a course; in fact it is critical. Even when the disease becomes chronic, after being critical, there is a past for which the patient or those around him remain nostalgic. Hence we are sick in relation not only to others but also to ourselves (1989, p. 138).

Here are two African case studies: one novelised and the other a scholarly geography. In collapsing them I would like to illustrate a fabulous intuition of Freud.

> The analogy between the process of civilization and the path of individual development may be extended in an important respect. It can be asserted that the community, too, evolves a super-ego under whose influence cultural development proceeds. It would be a tempting task for anyone who has a knowledge of human civilizations to follow out this analogy in detail. I will confine myself to bringing forward a few striking points. The super-ego of an epoch of civilization has an origin similar to that of an individual (Freud, 1989, p. 106).

In an individual neurosis we take as our starting point the contrast that distinguishes the patient from his environment, which is assumed to be 'normal'. For a group all of whose members are affected by one and the same disorder no such background could exist; it would have to be found elsewhere. And as regards the therapeutic application of our knowledge, what would be the use of the most correct analysis of social neuroses, since no one possesses authority to impose such a therapy upon the group? (Freud, 1989, p. 110).

Here are two cases: an individual expos lived by an African woman, Ken Bugul, and the second, a magnificent rendering by the American social scientist, John Janzen, of an institution meant to protect the 'well being' of a central African community. Both in their own right, are challenging since they imply on the one hand the possibility of conceptualising an epidemiology of representations; and on the other the fact of culturally constructed (dis-)ordered systems.

The Abandoned Baobab by Ken Bugul (alias Marietou M'Baye) (1991) is supposedly 'the Autobiography of a Senegalese Woman' (subtitle of the American version). The narrative collapses a life into a drama reducible to a descent into a hell actualised by an European sojourn. The before and the after speak of an unhappy 'home' perhaps but significant for the well-being of the character. The whole story comments on a rupture and an 'exotic' fundamental root, a 'baobab tree that had been witness to and accomplice in the mother's departure, the first morning of a dawn without dusk' (1991, p. 159). From an African village to Brussels and back, the narrative is basically about a cross-cultural crisis. Two different worlds, two conflicting horizons: on the one hand, a reference 'Oh god, that village where I was born' (1991, p. 21) and the symbolic solidity of a healthy baobab; on the other, what seems to be a complete relativist and nihilist gray, and intimidating universe. This young woman goes through all the unimaginables: sexual preconceptions, racism, *ménage à trois*, prostitution, drugs and suicide temptation. And yet, for her sanity, she keeps alive in her memory fantasies about 'the sweet realities of my race and my people' (1991, p. 62). Even her doubts about her psychological balance do not seem to have points of certainties.

Colonialism had shattered everything. And consciousness had drowned itself in the alienation of a third dimension, both fascinating and hideous. But I didn't want to be aware of all that and have to react. I refuse to believe that colonialism was its only cause (1991, p. 51).

Her predicament can easily be reduced to two strange statements redefining her as a determined being-for-others and, around which, one could understand the whole 'biography'. Once, she confesses to her bisexual lover (and she knows her competitor): 'You know, Jean, I suffer from a void created by the absence of what is familiar' (1991, p. 102). Some pages later, thinking about her difference in the all white Brussels *milieu* of leftists and other hippies, she brings to her own consciousness a judgment: 'The white man and the Black woman, life, a jumble of history and meta-history' (1991, p. 106). Yet this critical retraction is presented as a reaction to an apparent compliment: 'Hello, you're very beautiful. You're from Africa?' (1991, p. 106). It was already supported some pages earlier by a very offensive remark from a white woman: 'Men like you, Ken. You are a Black woman, you could make yourself a fortune' (1991, p. 104).

Is Ken sick and how sick? Let's note at least three things: first, the pen name – Ken Bugul – chosen by the author who supposedly is writing about her life; it means in the Wolof language 'the person no one wants'; secondly, the original title of the book, *Le baobab fou* (1984) translates literally as the 'mad or crazy baobab'. It indicates explicitly that the author meant to narrate a story as her own. Should we believe her? The narrative makes any reader uncomfortable because of its violent content. The third remark is a question. Why and how could anyone want to identify with this woman? That might not be the major point. We can, in effect, reflect on what the story symbolizes about being a Black woman back in the 1960s or 1970s in Belgium and positing oneself as both 'anomalous' and 'mad'.

The geography of scholarly researches on African health and its problems which could, perhaps, contribute to a good understanding of the paradox of *Le baobab fou* (1984), is rich with important and varied contributions. Let us focus on an exemplary work and then suggest a table with areas of questions. John M. Janzen's work on *Lemba, 1650–1930*, a narrative of a social order, witnesses a difference on how to handle health and harmony situating individualities as integrated part of a 'we' inscribed in a temporality and intentionality which simultaneously account for them and that, in return, they actualise and justify in their behaviour.

This research is a remarkable contribution to Central African anthropology; not only because it is the result of canonical exploration which integrates the best of both historical and anthropological approaches, but also for its particular features: its thorough analytical style of description and categorisation, the general pragmatic competence of the author and his intellectual prudence in theoretical generalisation and extrapolation. On the whole, there is no doubt that Janzen is very successful in describing and analysing 'a seventeenth-century "cure for capitalism", created by insightful Congo coast people who perceived that the great trade was destroying their society' (1982, p. 13). Yet one might note that there are some methodological hesitations to face. They may, curiously, find an explanation in an opening statement of the author. He claims to have avoided 'the faddish language of contemporary social analysis, both of the value-neutral school and of the critical Marxist' in order 'to show how one segment of coastal African society tried ... to cope with a force that transformed African society' (1982, p. 13). All critical students of African affairs would admit that the mediocre and pretentious jargon of some Marxists generates virtually nothing of value. But can this imply, as Janzen's statement suggests, an inherent incapacity of Marxist language to marshal in a clear and understandable idiom needed evidence on *Lemba*?

Lemba is, to define it simply, a cult and a social institution which from the seventeenth century onwards, controlled the trade, routes, markets and processes of exchange between Malebo Pool and the Loango coast in Central Africa. Janzen studies it in three complementary parts.

Part 1, entitled 'The Public Setting of *Lemba*. Management of Society and its Resources', explores the history of the *Lemba* region as defined by natural boundaries, the Zaire and Kuilu-Nyari River systems on the south and north, respectively, and by the ocean on the west (1982, p. 27). Janzen's focus bears, first, on the socio-political institutions of some coastal kingdoms (Loango, Kakongo, Ngoyo, Vungu) and Yombe chiefdoms; second, on the Teke federation and the Nsundi region; finally, on 'the life between the Kingdoms, where *Lemba* took on its most sophisticated form as "government of medicine"' (1982, p. 45). Though at first sight the political structure of this region does not seem different front the Kongo region in general, its character is discreetly but essentially distinctive.

On the one hand, the chiefs are attached 'either to descent or residential com munities and markets' (1982, p. 71). Thus, one can follow and accept Janzen's distinctions about the organisation of power: (a) a variety of local leaders comprising the lineage or clan chiefs; (b) a variety of ceremonial *minkisi*, including *Lemba*, which have explicit and socially accepted authority; (c) the pervasive power of market laws, that is, 'a set of prohibitions and practices that spelled out the rules of peaceable trading, and regulated adjudication and punishment for their violation' (1982, p. 70). On the other hand, the presence of these laws of the market in one region and their absence in others.

The 'laws of the market' (*minsiku mla nzandu*) and supporting roles, functions, and ceremonials, reflect a unique political system. The market system in north-

bank society operated around the four-day week .... . Each market, located on
an open plain between several villages, was ruled by a market committee of
chiefs or judges from these surrounding communities. While the notion of a
sovereign was absent in this system of acephalous governance of markets,
the functions of large scale government were very evident. The market was
regarded as 'court', with the right to impose capital punishment. The market
committee and its constituent communities constituted a 'market area', which
could combine with neighboring market committees to solve larger-scale
disputes. Often village or clan chiefs would have tenure in two markets for
more effective regulation of disputes. The 'laws of the market' thus regulated
both trade in the markets as well as the fabric of society that kept the markets
open and viable (1982, p. 72).

One dreams of what a rigorous test of, say, some of P. Ph. Rey's propositions
in *Colonialisme, néo-colonialisme et transition au capitalisme* (1971) could
have brought about à propos the confrontation of modes of production, and,
particularly, the political mediation of the laws of the market in both lineage,
mode of production and capitalism. In effect, the biographical sketches of
some *Lemba* leaders at the beginning of the colonial era (1982, pp. 81–91)
illustrate the complexity of this confrontation: *Lemba* leaders are forced to
use the fabric of their organisation in order to provide capitalism with labour,
assist the programme of colonialism and, thus, essentially, contribute to the
destruction of their 'mode of production' and to a rearticulation of class
alliances. But Janzen has chosen to emphasise the political behaviour over
the economic. His penetrating sketches are excellent and convincingly show
'how colonial collaboration was now necessary to preserve one's influence,
although it destroyed one's authority through taxation abuse' (1982, p. 82).
On the other hand, why this ambiguous integration in the new organisation
of power and production led ultimately some leaders, such as Kimbangu, to
question the colonial ideology and actualise themselves as anomalous vis-à-
vis the new power-structure, remains a question mark.

    The second part of the book deals with rituals of *Lemba* as signs and means
of managing reality. How real is real? It consists of five descriptive analyses
of variants of *Lemba* in different settings: the Northern Kongo (Kamba and
Yaa), the Eastern (Lari), the South-Central (Nsundi and Bwende), the Western
(Yombe, Woyo and Vili), the New World (Brazil and Haiti). Janzen, in general,
begins each section by producing his 'source of evidence on the *Lemba* rituals',
that is 'unpublished indigenous texts, with supporting evidence coming from
ethnographies and the mute records of museum artifacts' (1982, p. 95). He
proceeds with the analysis of what he calls 'the expressive domains and their

codes', specifying four axes: (a) the spatial and temporal dimension of rites and institutional events, and their meaning; (b) the role of the economic structure and the significance of procedures of exchange which take place during or along the rituals (the exchange structure of a *Lemba* séance is described as composed of goods, service, symbols and persons); (c) the relationship existing in *Lemba* between medicine, social context and symbols; (d) the lyrical component, which expresses symbolic linkage between the *Lemba* world and the kingdom of ancestors and spirits or, as in the case of a Western Kongo variant, unveils an interpretation of the mythical origins of *Lemba* itself through the grid of a trickster's adventures. The publication of local narratives on *Lemba* is per se a substantive event.

Their very terms bring about important issues: first, on the significance of the corpus; second, on the nature and the authenticity of texts themselves. We learn, for example, about the sources of the northern version, that '*Lemba* texts are a small portion of the overall catechists' corpus of 23,000 pages' (1982, . 105), but not, exactly, how small they are, nor their composition. We are, à propos the Eastern variant, introduced to the existence of a series of versions (e.g., Kimbembe, Stenström, Anderson, Malonga), but, there is no formulation, no discussion of the relationships that these versions have with the text chosen for publication (1982, pp. 158–63), nor even an interrogation of the authenticity of manipulated versions. In the same vein, what could have been the basis for a technical and stimulating debate on the textual credibility of the South Central variant seems too easily reduced to anecdotal details of a competition involving the author and two of his Kongo friends. Finally, reading the introduction to the *Lemba* sources in the New World, one understands that, in fact, the major problem of this Part II of the book is one of philological demands for establishing and publishing oral texts. That is a pity, because, as a consequence, one can question both the solidity of this part of the book and its generous metaphorical transpositions.

The last part of the essay deals with *Lemba* therapeutics in two highly and magnificently cohesive chapters: the first, on modes of *Lemba* thought; and, the second on the ideology of Lemba therapeutics. For Janzen, *Lemba* thought should be understood from the structuration of a mythic charter.

> The structure of a mythic charter, whether of an *n'kisi*, a ruling dynasty, a prophetic or clan Genealogy, has three stages of reference, reflecting a temporal, spatial, social, and cosmological sequence: first, the original 'anchoring' Figure; second, the mediator, last, the human here-and-now. An attempt is made, to relate the fragmentary, multiple, dispersed, or confused state of present human

society to the unitary, idealized, and orderly condition 'in the beginning.' The charter myth's sequence of names, priests, officeholders, or places inhabited, and conditions met and dealt with, thus refer to the structure of society and the universe or to recollected human events and individuals. Frequently Kongo aetiology myths have been confused with history, or with pure legend, because of the parallel (metonymic) series of persons, roles, legendary figures, animals, colors, or cosmological categories which inhabit them. An effort to resolve this problem of history in myth is pertinent to understanding *Lemba*, whose lyrics contain, as the last section shows, a combined view of human and non-human structures (1982, p. 297).

In order to demonstrate this point, Janzen uses three paradigms: (a) the successional and relational mode of authority which, in Kongo region, unites two radically different discourses, the mythical and the historical, to the point that transference becomes the rule, and actualises 'the resolution of human and cosmic dilemmas' (1982, p. 304); (b) the conjunctive and disjunctive mediation exemplified by the *Lemba* lyrics, which present heroes reflecting on ways of integrating opposite virtues, qualities, and choices; (c) finally, the complementary dialectic of humanisation and naturalisation of the discourse. If something can be said about this analytical orientation, it is its prudence. I only regret the emphasis that Janzen puts on therapeutic virtues of *Lemba* rituals. He knows as well as I do that most of the so-called traditional 'healers' were, or are, often a nuisance.

I do not wish to argue for or against the manner Janzen chooses to deal with the problem of History in Kongo narratives. But there is in his argument some lack of clarity that I shall note. He is critical of Frobenius's theory of spiritization of human figures and its recent adaptation and application by Bittremieux and Thiel. He writes that

> ... the problem with this approach is the partiality introduced by the historical bias. Some of the figures of *Lemba* charters may very well have been historic persons of prominence ... Yet, at the other end of the continuum there are those charters whose figures are typological male/female, androgynous beings, or some other characterization of a social role or relationship (1982, p. 298).

Thus, one can perceive two complementary processes: the mythologization of history and the historicization of mythical narratives. How does one read and interpret these procedures of metaphorization? Janzen refers to Lévi-Strauss's concept of mythic mediation and then decides to rely on Burridge's notion of *true contradiction* ('only occurs in dramatic situations in recognizable historic events') which, according to him, 'injects into the analysis of myth structure the concrete terms of given historic moments as well as the structure of ideology' (1982, p. 315).

This seems like a historicist *parti-pris*. I suspect that a more fruitful application of Lévi-Strauss's proposition referred to (1981, pp. 561–624) would have been more illuminating. Lévi-Strauss clearly indicates three easily applicable guidelines. (1) Stories, myths are always *already* altered by internal development of a society; (2) the social system, assumes its mythology which

> may be causally linked to history in each of its parts, but which taken in its entirety, resists the course of history and constantly readjusts its own mythological grid so that this grid offers the least resistance to the flow of events (1981, p. 610);

(3) 'even in history itself, certain elements persist, and provide a solid anchorage to which the myths can attach themselves' (1981, p. 610). One may not like de Heusch's structuralist exercises in the Bantu field (see e.g., 1982). At least, they show that the method works. Thus, rather than relying on Burridge's confusing concept of *true contradiction*, it is possible to use Lévi-Strauss's invitation and clarify the question of the existing gap between mythical narratives and history, and then that of existential contradictions metaphorised and categorised in mythical discourses.

As to the ideology of *Lemba*, it should, according to Janzen, be understood as based on the fact that '*Lemba* was a "drum of affliction". It was spoken of as an *n'kisi* whose rituals were drummed up' (1982, p. 315). *Lemba* affliction as well as therapeutics, on the other hand, deal with 'vulnerability and marginality among the influential in a society with a normative ideology emphasizing egalitarian authority and redistributive economics' (1982, p. 318). As a therapy it would impose itself as a psycho-social process of awareness. In effect, symbolisms of therapeutic procedures as well as those of initiation duplicate mythical and aetiological narratives. In sum, for Janzen, *Lemba* is a theory of social order and, more specifically, a model for a 'virtuous and balanced society'.

> Whether a given "drum of affliction" in the Central-African setting is then a dependent or an independent variable of social change and all its forces of contradiction can only be answered once the questions which become the grounds for at tempted solutions are elucidated, including a variety of rituals that pour answers into the questions as well as a variety of efforts to impose

new orders of institutions such as the centralized state. In Greek antiquity such questions had to do with the freedom of the individual in the face of impersonal fate. In Kongo during at least part of the era of the great trade such questions had to do with the accumulation of wealth and influence in a society of egalitarian expectations, the protection of the individual engaged in commerce, his relationship to his kin, and the creation of a regional institution alongside local clans and dependants. Greek society thought out its alternatives and their consequences in the tragic theater and acted on them through a form of participatory democracy. Kongo society thought out its alternatives in legends, dreams, and in affliction etiologies and acted on them in a therapeutic-alliance-trading association. There is no doubt that *Lemba* shaped the public order, although by no means all medicines did so or may be expected to (1982, p. 326).

Should not we confront the fact that there is a kind of categorical difference between explanation in terms of comparison of social choices and explanation in terms of structural reasons, causes and organisation?

This is an excellent research. It illustrates convincingly a Freudian hypothesis on the connections between individual and collective super egos; that both have a similar origin and actualise them in specific and interacting styles, which through the procedures of legitimate mainstream cultural arguments and negotiations stipulate the definitions of normality and abnormality. If my comments of Janzen's book have been critical to the point of seemingly contradicting this, it might be that, because of the exceptional quality of his research, I have been referring to a book only he could have written. This said, let there be no misunderstanding. Janzen's book is one of the best in a very confusing field in which individualities are posited as elements of a 'We', which in return, cannot exist without its components. The question of the health of individualities and all empiricists seems thus linked to the well being of an organic yet abstract 'We' and vice-versa. It is from this reference that one sees the demand of a balance between the two poles and their interaction witnessing to the unbelievable: individualities inhabit their bodies in the same manner that they inhabit their cultures.

Conclusion

The two African case studies teach us a number of lessons. The first one might be the evidence of the connection between individualities and a cultural background. Freud put it correctly when he noted that 'just as a planet revolves around a central body as well as rotating on its own axis, so the human individual takes part in the course of development of mankind at the same time as he pursues his own path in life' (1989, p. 106). The path is indeed marked by the existence of others who unveil his/her being in its objectness as unknown appraisal. It is in this relation that one should situate the existential style of being this or that. As Freud says:

> the analogy between the process of civilization and the path of individual development may be extended in an important respect. It can be asserted that the community, too, evolves a super-ego under whose influence cultural development proceeds (1989, p. 106).

The upsurge of any consciousness, even the most 'pathological' vis-à-vis the mainstream norm is in its own right a perfect totality: an awareness of being itself that cannot be deduced from its outsidedness, but can be understood clinically as a system in its own right ruled by its own norms. It is thus questionable to reduce the rationality of individual systems to the classificatory systems of dominant knowledges.

When Frantz Fanon in the introduction to his *Black Skin, White Masks* asks 'what does the black man want' (1967, p. 8), I think of the predicament of Ken Bugul or of the complexity of *Lemba*. The Dakar School of African 'Psycho-pathology' has published in its journal numerous studies analysing African styles of actualising mental problems. In any case, the library on this issue is already so complex that it could lend itself to a sociology of important trends in research. It would distinguish: (a) anthropological studies on particular cultures; (b) interpretative researches on well localised visions of the world and their influence on everyday life practices; (c) position analyses on differences incarnated by *weltanschaungen* as in the now classical studies by Mary Douglas, *Purity and Danger* (1966); Fortes Meyer and Edward Evans-Pritchard, *Oedipus and Job in West African Religion* (1959); Victor Turner, *The Forest of Symbols: Aspects of Ndembu Ritual* (1967); or M.C. and E. Ortigues, *Oedipe Africain* (1973); (d) comparative historical attentions so well illustrated by Philip Curtin's *Disease and Empire* (1998) and Meghan Vaughan's *Curing their Ills: Colonial Power and African Illness* (1991); (e) there is, also, the well specified domain by *African Psycho-Pathology* journal and its difference illustrated in convincing punctual studies such as those of John Janzen on *Lemba* (1982), *The Quest of Therapy* (1978), and the volume he co-edited with Steven Feierman on *The Social Basis of Health and Healing in Africa* (1992); (f) there is finally a last and dangerous domain, that of witnesses and no one can tell and less know for sure if they are referring to the spirituality of a cultural or an intellectual configuration or to a medical practice and its sociological consequences. To name just three examples: Gérard Buakassa T.K.M., *L'impensé du discours* (1973); Eric de Rosny's *Les yeux de ma chèvre* (1981), Traoré's treatise on *Médecine et magie africaine* (1965).

In sum, one could affirm simply that a pathology or an infirmity is a fact in its own right. Neuroses, for example, might occur in all human beings and they are witness to a rupture and a transformation of an economy which, strictly speaking, actualize then new regulations and norms. They might signify mortality, but they are structured, organised and witness to a system, biological or psychological, transforming itself. In this sense, they are, to refer to Canguilhem, new laws ruling the organism or the psyche. As a matter of fact, I am understanding 'neurotic styles' in a specific sense well delineated by Dr David Shapiro (1965) and that allows him to comment on the 'obsessive-compulsive', the 'paranoid', the 'hysterical', the 'impulsive'. And after Shapiro, I would say that:

> By 'neurotic styles', I mean those modes of functioning that seem characteristic, respectively, of the various neurotic conditions, ways of thinking and perceiving, ways of experiencing emotion, modes of subjective experience in general, and modes of activity that are associated with various pathologies (Shapiro, 1965, p. 1).

More precisely there is a lesson and a perspective.

> I first became interested in the forms or styles of functioning – particularly of thinking and perceiving – characteristic of various sorts of psychopathology through working with psychological tests. In tests, particularly in the Rorschach test, ways of thinking and perceiving are (or at least, should be) the primary material from which inferences concerning diagnosis, defence mechanisms and character traits are drawn. It seems to me that these ways of thinking – ordinarily used to identify defence mechanisms, traits and diagnostic syndromes and, in general, to draw a picture of psychological makeup – must in represent psychological structures of importance and these structures might be of a more general type than the specific traits or mechanisms that could be inferred from them. If, for example, it is possible to identify certain defence mechanisms and specific symptomatic characteristics of an obsessional kind in a given style of thinking and perception, that style can be conceived as representing a psychological structure in its own right. If, as is often the case, minor variations of the same style of thinking suggest other, sometimes adaptive features and traits as well, then perhaps this general style of thinking may be considered

a matrix from which the various traits, symptoms and defence mechanisms crystallise. It seemed plausible, in other words, that mode of thinking might be one factor that determines the shape or form of symptom, defence mechanism and adaptive trait as well (Shapiro, 1965, p. 2).

It is thus just a question of 'style' and this is nothing to do with the vague, controversial and controverted notion of 'race'. Instead, any 'style' might be analysed and understood from the background of an historical arbitrariness determined and overdetermined by economic and cultural configurations.

References

Allderidge, P. (1995), *The Bethlem Royal Hospital*, The Bethlem and Maudsley NHS Trust, London.

Arendt, H. (1979), *The Origins of Totalitarianism*, Harcourt Brace and Company, New York.

Aristotle (1996), *Poetics*, Penguin Books, London.

Badinter, E. and R. (1988), *Condorcet: un intellectuel en politique*, Fayard, Paris.

Beauvoir, S. de (1974), *The Second Sex*, Vintage Books, New York.

Billon, F. de (1555), *Le fort inexpugnable de l'honneur du sexe féminin*, Paris, J. d'Allyer.

Brant, S. (1872), *Das Narrenschiff*, F.A. Brockkaus, Leipzig.

Buakasa, G.T.K.M. (1973), *L'impens du discours*, Presses Universitaires du Zaire, Kinshasa-Bruxelles.

Buffon, G.-L.-L., Comte de (1833–34), *Oeuvres Completes*, Editions du Museum, Paris.

Bugul, K. (1991), *The Abandoned Baobab*, Lawrence Hill Books, New York.

Canguilhem, G. (1991), *The Normal and the Pathological*, Zone Books, New York.

Champier, S. (1503), *La nef des femmes vertueuses*.

Curtin, P. (1998), *Disease and Empire: The Health of European Troops in the Conquest of Africa*, Cambridge University Press, Cambridge.

Deleuze, G. and Guattari, F. (1977), *Anti-Oedipus: Capitalism and Schizophrenia*, University of Minnesota Press, Minneapolis.

Douglas, M. (1966), *Purity and Danger*, Penguin, London/New York.

Douglas, M. (1979), *The World of Goods*, Basic Books, New York.

Du Buat-Nan AY, Count L.G. (1789), *Les origines, ou, l'ancien gouvernement de la France, de l'Allemagne et de l'Italie*, S.L.

Duchet, M. (1971), *Anthropologie et histoire au siècle des lumières*, Maspero, Paris.

Erasmus, D. (1993), *The Praise of Folly*, Penguin Books, London.

Fanon, F. (1967), *Black Skin, White Masks*, Grove Press, New York.

Foucault, M. (1973), *The Order of Things*, Vintage, New York.

Foucault, M. (1975), *The Birth of the Clinic*, Vintage Books, New York.

Foucault, M. (1978), *The History of Sexuality, an Introduction*, Vintage Books, New York.

Foucault, M. (1979), *Histoire de la folie à l'age classique*, Gallimard, Paris.

Foucault, M. (1997), *Il faut défendre la société*, Gallimard, Seuil, Paris.

Frazer, Sir J.G. (1981), *The Golden Bough. The Roots of Religion and Folklore*, Random, New York.

Freud, S. (1989), *Civilization and Its Discontents*, W.W. Norton & Company, London.

Gilman, S.L. (1982), *Seeing the Insane*, John Wiley/University of Nebraska Press, New York.

Gilman, S.L. (1993), *Freud, Race and Gender*, Princeton University Press, Princeton.

Gilman, S.L. (1996), *Seeing the Insane*, University of Nebraska Press, New York.

Gobineau, Comte J.-A. de (1933?), *Essai sur légalité des races humaines*, Firmin-Didot, Paris.

Gordon, R.L. (ed.) (1982), *Myth, Religion and Society*, Cambridge University Press, Cambridge.

Hammond, I. and Jablow, A. (1977), *The Myth of Africa*, The Library of Social Science, New York.

Heusch, L. de (1982), *The Drunken King*, Indiana University Press, Bloomington.

Hodgen, M.T. (1964), *Early Anthropology in the Sixteenth and Seventeenth Centuries*, University of Pennsylvania Press, Philadelphia.

Howe, S. (1998), *Afrocentrisme Mythical Pasts and Imagined Homes*, London, Verso.

Janzen, J.M. (1978), *The Quest of Therapy: Medical Pluralism in Lower Zaire*, California.

Janzen, J.M. (1982), *Lemba, 1650–1930, A Drum of Affliction in Africa and the New World*, Garland, New York and London.

Janzen, J.M. and Feierman, S. (1992), *The Social Basis of Health and Healing in Africa*, California.

Jung, C.G. (1980), *The Archetypes and the Collective Unconscious*, Princeton University Press, Princeton.

Jung, C.G. (1989), *Mysterium Coniunctionis*, Princeton, Princeton University Press.

Lalande, A. (1962), *Vocabulaire technique et critique de la philosophie*, Presses Universitaires de France, Paris.

Lévi-Strauss, C. (1981), *The Naked Man*, Harper and Row, New York.

Meyer, F. and Evans-Pritchard, E. (1959), *Oedipus and Job in West African Religion*, Cambridge University Press, Cambridge.

Montesquieu, C.L. de S. de (1997), *Lettres persanes*, Bookking International – Classiques français, Paris.

Mornet, D. (1969), *La pensée française au XVIIIéme siècle*, Colin, Paris.

Ortigues, M.C. and E. (1973), *Oedipe Africain*, U.G.E., Paris.

Rey, P.-P. (1971), *Colonialisme, néo-colonialisme et transition au capitalisme. Exemple de la comilog au Congo-Brazzaville*, Maspero, Paris.

Rosny, E. de (1981), *Les Yeux de ma chêvre*, Paris, Plon.

Sass, L.A. (1994), *Madness and Modernism*, Harvard University Press, Cambridge, MA.

Shapiro, D. (1965), *Neurotic Styles*, Basic Books, New York.

Simmel, G. (1989–91), *Einleitung in die Moralwissenschaft*, Suhrkamp, Frankfurt.

Szasz, T.S. (1977), *The Manufacture of Madness*, Harper & Row, New York.

Traoré, D. (1965), *Médecine et magie africaine*, Presence Africaine, Paris.

Tuke, S. (1813), *Description of the Retreat, An Institution Near York for Insane Persons*, Printed for W. Alexander and Sold by Him, London.

Turner, V. (1967), *The Forests of Symbols: Aspects of Ndembu Ritual*, Cornell University Press, Ithaca.

Vaughan, M. (1991), *Curing their Ills: Colonial Power and African Illness*, Stanford University Press, Stanford.

Chapter 3

Identity and Psychopathology

David Barker

Introduction

Generations of thinkers have grappled with the problem of racial and ethnic identity. The black scholar, W.E.B. du Bois, highlighted the dilemma within his most famous work, *The Souls of Black Folk* (1903).

> The Negro is a sort of seventh son, born with a veil, and gifted with second-sight in this American world – a world which yields him no true self-consciousness, but only lets him see himself through the revelation of the other world. It is a peculiar sensation, this double consciousness, this sense of always looking at one's self through the eyes of others, of measuring one's soul by the tape of a world that looks on in amused contempt and pity. One ever feels his twoness – an American, a Negro; two souls, two thoughts, two unreconciled strivings; two warring ideals in one dark body, whose dogged strength alone keeps it from being torn asunder. The history of the American Negro is the history of this strife – this longing to attain self-conscious manhood, to merge his double self into a better and truer self. In his merging he wishes neither of his older selves to be lost. He would not Africanize America, for America has too much to teach the world and Africa. He would not bleach his Negro soul in a flood of White Americanism, for he knows that Negro blood has a message for the world. He simply wishes to make it possible for a man to be both a Negro and an American, without being cursed and spit upon by his fellows, without having the doors of Opportunity closed roughly in his face (W.E.B. du Bois; cited in Harris et al., 1995).

These words encapsulate what du Bois felt to be the core issue for African-Americans. This concept of 'double consciousness' conceived by W.E.B. du Bois inspired a wide range of recent publications devoted to the theme of ethnocultural identity and have included its prominence in a variety of domains and disciplines. From the media of books, films and popular music to its transcendence as a major topic in the arenas of psychology, social anthropology, literature, theology, philosophy, linguistics, political science and so forth. For example, *Lure and Loathing: Essays on Race, Identity, and the Ambivalence of Assimilation* by Earley (1993) consists of essays by scholars from a diverse number of fields such as law, theology, literature and the social sciences. They provide a multidimensional overview of the experience of identity at the level of race (Harris et al., 1995).

In returning to the above oft-quoted statement of W.E.B. du Bois one can reconcile how it may be relevant to those members of minority groups within any one dominant culture. How it would apply to those peoples who in their minority status experience the alienation, disempowerment and disenfranchisement within their society. Psychiatrists have long known that stability of self and identity plays a central part in determining individual vulnerability to mental illness, how it may be central in its genesis, presentation and course. Also, of how its impact may at a number of levels, all, or some operating according to known and unconscious rules, to produce psychological breakdown and social and occupational compromise.

In the black Caribbean diaspora within Europe these issues seem particularly relevant. Within the last 200 years these peoples have undergone two major dislocations from Africa to the Caribbean thence to Britain, France and Holland. Whatever their setting they have looked within, towards black America and black Africa for inspiration, hope and identity. A sense of legacy, destiny and brotherhood has resulted, concomitant with feelings of distrust, fear, bewilderment and even ignorance towards these sources of inspiration. This diaspora, particularly those born in Europe have a confused sense of belonging, impacted upon by the institutionalised prejudiced attitudes of the dominant society, within which they have found themselves. These children grow up with the same expectations as their white counterparts, but are denied the same opportunities. They are not seen as children of immigrants but as immigrants, even though some have yet to visit the land of their parents let alone the land of their ancestors. The subcultural identification of London and Parisian black Caribbean (as well as black African) youth to the black urban street culture of America, is central in maintaining some sense of social esteem and purpose, as well as personal sense of self.

The complexities of these issues, whilst attended to both academically at a historical and socio-political level, and in terms of creative expression through the arts, literature, music and films, have been seriously neglected in the field of health and disease. In the United Kingdom black Caribbean people are disproportionately diagnosed as having a psychotic illness, particularly schizophrenia. Similar findings have been noted in Holland. The methodological issues alone require searching analysis, let alone all the other impingements, real or imagined. Nevertheless, placing all that aside, black Caribbean people are being over-represented in mental institutions and are experiencing adverse pathways into such institutions. This is a tragedy for such a vulnerable group and a major public health exercise is needed to address the issue.

My objective in this chapter is to discuss and analyse issues of ethnocultural identity and associated concepts, and how it is brought to bear in the abnormal psychology in black Caribbean people, particularly in the schizophrenic-like psychoses within the context of racial discrimination and disempowerment. The main body of this work will consist of the following.

First, I will look at the wider issues of white-on-black stereotyping through imagery with its powerfully racist connotations, illustrating its role in shaping black identity and esteem at many levels from the subliminal to obvious. In the next part, ethnic identity is tentatively explored, as it refers to the young black community in the UK, and how it may relate to severe psychic compromise. The following part leading on from issues of ethnocultural identity, is an examination of 'double consciousness', paranoia and persecution, hinting at their involvement in the excess 'diagnosis' of schizophrenia in the black community. The conclusion will attempt to coalesce all those elements previously discussed, to construct a model for understanding the aetiology of this 'excess', concentrating on meaning within the context of observed, informed and theoretical phenomena.

Black Stereotyping through Imagery

Central to the perception of human groups and their differences is the process of stereotyping. In cognitive psychology stereotypes are taken to be schemas (cognitive structures that represents an organised knowledge about a given concept or type of stimulus) or sets which play a part in cognition, perception, memory and communication (Fiske and Taylor, 1984). Stereotypes are based on 'simplification and generalisation', or denial of individuality. They can be positive or negative, but are usually the former. They may have no basis in reality at all and thus be the result of 'fallacious thinking' (Milner, 1983). Nevertheless stereotyping has real and sometimes seriously adverse social consequences, particularly in the assignment of the stereotyped to certain social roles. They tend to function as self-fulfilling prophecies, as the targets of stereotyping are jostled into particular roles that seemed to be endorsed by the society thus setting up a perpetual cycle of social allocation, social reality, and subsequent social fulfilment of roles. Or, social representation echoes social realities, which are in turn modelled upon social representation (Moscovici, 1981).

This section is concerned with those visualised prejudices prevalent in the West that create and perpetuate myth and stereotype concerning Africans and blacks. Stereotypes such as 'closer to nature', more violent, more emotional, childlike, superior athletes, musical and so forth. The power of images through advertising have in their representations, serious social ramifications on a global scale. Black liberation movements are not only concerned with changing social realities but also representations. Thus black freedom movements are not only concerned with achieving equality at a legal and practical level, but they also oppose with vigour social stereotypes that accompany and sanction inequality whether explicitly or subliminally. The ideology that resists emancipation usually include notions that the distribution of social roles are appropriate based on particular stereotypical characteristics that are inherent; and rejection of any criticism of stereotyping through reference to the social realities that confirm them.

Sometimes the existence of a certain prejudice or particular stereotype exists, but often concomitantly there is the denial that they are widespread, have any real effect, or ascribed to oneself. In addition, the existence of stereotypes is refuted with the sentiment that they are 'facts' that are based in reality with which there is an abundance of evidence. Thus particularly in mainstream society the appearance of stereotypes is 'normal' with opposition to them being 'abnormal'. In this case stereotypes become part of the fabric of the psychology and culture of mainstream society, with any resistance to such misconceptions and prejudices in danger of undermining the comfort of society as a whole. From the perspective of the mainstream such denial usually affords little challenge within the ranks, as they do not concern them or very often is a challenge to their ascendancy. However for those stereotyped the situations is very different. The prevalence and pervasiveness of stereotyping undoubtedly affects black people at a very psychological level as well as socially and practically. This will be discussed later.

As hinted earlier some stereotypes are taken to be true, and in fact seen as a sort of primal image or archetype. In other words, not as an expression of prejudice but as a reflection of the heritable characteristics of the group in question. A fact that is inherent in the constitution of the population that are usually based on erroneous assumptions. Occasionally stereotypes appear positive, may arise from 'sympathy' from the mainstream, or may be transformed by the recipients of prejudice. Classic examples of this in the case of black people are their associations with music and athletics. However explanations for such abilities are usually speculative and often based on those very assumptions that create the negative stereotypes. For example at the turn of the last century in America black people were viewed as musical because of their 'cheerful and childlike disposition and emotionality', and much later, as fast runners because of being 'closer to nature'. Nevertheless such stereotypes are still stereotypes, based on simplification and generalisation and often detract from other abilities, thus 'keeping the black man in his place'. American and European images of Africa through history have undergone numerous changes, but are characterised by the, at times aggressive, nature of their negativity and racist misconceptions. In their multiplicity where is the archetype? Is it the Ethiopian Eunuch or the Golliwog? The King of the Moors or Uncle Tom?

Such social representations have a historicity in their configurement. They are as stated earlier, subject to constant modifications and reparations, usually to suit the times and confirm those premises of the prevailing racist ideologies. Thus, like racism, stereotype imagery is socially constructed to provide a 'social purpose'. Such images by virtue of their ubiquity and pervasiveness are surprisingly durable over time, even in the face of 'facts' that contradict them. Once they have a certain history through the generational embedding in the hearts and minds of people (even including at times those prejudiced), and the accompanying sentimentality, stereotypes can be hard to shift. The following is an account of the power of racist imagery through Western advertising. I believe it is appropriate to touch on this, particularly focusing on the historical aspects, as such influence from the past continues and current stereotyping of black people in commercial advertising has not abated, only become more subtle.

Towards the end of the nineteenth century the development of modern advertising in Europe and America was associated with the onset of extensive industrialisation and mass production, as well as the integration of the colonies into the Western economies. Many of the popular trademarks originated at around this time and their inception coincided with the advent of mass packaging, poster campaigns and magazine ads (Werkman, 1974). This was also a time of significant social and political upheavals particularly concerning black people, from the zenith of the onslaught of European colonialism in Africa, to the civil war and the end of slavery in America. European hegemony, then at its height, was reflected in advertising that affirmed the race, class and gender hierarchies. American advertisement served as a display for white supremacy.

In the consumption of colonial products, with its packaging and advertisements that depicted blacks in a racist light, Westerners were also assimilating and affirming the subjection and oppression of blacks. In their depiction black people continued to be established in the lower reaches of the cultural pecking order. As the colonies continued to be subjected to political integration imperially and economically through the exploitation of their labour, the cultural incorporation of the non-Western world often took the form of 'exoticism'. In advertising, ethnic features were utilised as 'product-image elements'. 'The racial elements have been mainly included to imbue the image of the product with the romantic atmosphere evoked by these (non-western) peoples' (Ross Barnett). The connotations with the term romantic here, include subjugation under European imperialism.

In Europe, blacks did not figure significantly in the everyday life of the people and were seen as more external and therefore as 'exotic' as stated above. However, in the United States blacks were a familiar sight, particularly in the 'Deep South'. Blacks were segregated and subjected to the terrible Jim Crow laws in the American South. Thus images of blacks abounded within the realms of advertising, with their position in society encoded within these images, to reflect the prevailing political and economic conditions at the time. Implicit in these representations was not only the drive to sell products, but to establish the status quo with blacks at the bottom and the confirmation of white supremacy, through infantilising, ridiculing and racist stereotyping (Ross Barnett). The following examination commences with some earlier commercial representations of blacks in products, especially tobacco, rum and other products where the use of black labour was central to production, either in the American South or the European colonies, in particular the Caribbean. It ends with contemporary trends and modes in commercial imagery.

During the seventeenth century when the tobacco industry started to distance itself from the shops and outlets of apothecaries, the first insignia the industry used to identify itself came to be known as the 'Tobacco Indian'. This was often a Negroid figure in a 'feather headdress' and a 'skirt of tobacco leaves'. This image, also termed 'the Virginian', became common in England during the seventeenth century, and in the United States in the eighteenth. It was a composition of those involved in the production of tobacco, i.e. the black slave who toiled in the fields, the 'Virginian' who owned the plantations, and the Indians who originally introduced the white settlers and colonialists to the smoking and cultivation of tobacco (Reno, 1986). The 'southern myth' of black people was reflected in American advertising with images of blacks as happy-go-lucky and contented with their lot on the 'old-time plantations'. Interestingly blacks were often shown as consumers of tobacco as well as *producers* as recognition of the wide potential market of the black community.

Sugar, rum, tobacco, coffee and cocoa were all formerly the products of slave labour in the Americas and previously seen as luxury items, originally only available to the elite (except for tobacco and the sailor's drink rum). Rum labels have depicted black dock workers carrying casks (e.g. Lemon Hart Rum), but above all, is the constant imagery, including up to this day of 'Creole' beauties serving rum. In the eighteenth century chocolate was a highly valued commodity in the economy of Spanish America. But since the late nineteenth century most of the cocoa imported into Europe has come from Africa. Chocolate was often shown being served up by a black servant, similarly with the serving of coffee, whereas in chocolate the sense of black labour in the production of a luxury item for whites was carried through. Over the years the role of blacks in the advertising and packaging of rum has hardly changed (Reno, 1986). The range of black 'tropical' products has been expanded with tropical soft drinks such as 'Kia-ora', only a few years ago being allowed to advertise on British terrestrial television, a frankly offensive and stereotypical cartoon depicting young black boys in a jungle setting.

The washing of blacks white has been a popular motif in the advertising of soaps such as Pears (Everett, 1978). This of course is a classic reflection of symbolic racist thinking, playing on the dichotomy of black/white and comparing this to dirty/clean. By implication it would seem that at the time racist whites wished to communicate to their own populations, the assumption that blacks aspired to be like them, in conjunction of course with the notion that the cleaning product was so powerful it turned even black skin to white. The important issue here is the inability for one group to except the differences of another and to attempt to eliminate this by symbolic transformation. In a social-cognitive perspective in which 'clean', 'white', 'light' and 'good go together as the foundations of civilisation and aesthetics, it is clear that 'dirty', 'black', 'dark' and 'evil' will be lumped together as well. This is of course the context in which the presence of black people in the advertising of soap and hygiene enters the fray (Reynolds, 1974). As implied earlier the white desire to wash blacks in some way expressed the whites' projection that blacks wish to be white. There has been the notion, including within black communities of America, Europe, and Brazil as well as Africa, that the use of skin bleaches and hair straighteners by blacks occurs as a reflection of those who wish to pass as white in societies where 'white' values predominate and associated with prestige and glamour. Fanon (1968) in his book *Black Skin, White Masks*, a classic piece of black liberationist writing, lends us the thought that if blacks have to wear a mask, then it may as well be a white mask. In Brazil there is a saying that 'money bleaches'. I will discuss this issue further in the section exploring identity more specifically.

Traditionally Europeans believed that the natural fertility of the soil in the tropics made the cultivation and growing of food easy, even suggesting that cultivation was unnecessary. Africans, it was surmised, needed only to consume what was around them in abundance. This fantasy was extended particularly to the West Indies, when Thomas Carlyle in 1849 was quoted to say, 'by working about half an hour a day [the 'Negro'] can supply himself, by aid of sun and soil, with as much as will suffice' (Alatas, 1977). The West Indian Negro, reported Anthony Trollope after a tour of the West Indies in 1858,

> is idle, unambitious as to worldly position, sensual and content with little … He lies under the mango-tree, and eats the luscious fruit in the sun; he sends his black urchin up for breakfast and behold the family table is spread. He pierces a cocoa-nut and lo! there is his beverage. He lies on the grass surrounded by oranges, bananas and pine-apples (Walvin, 1982).

This notion of natural tropical plenty and abundance was used as an argument and excuse to justify slavery or other forms of coercive labour. Because it was thought that by nature and constitution, blacks were idle and indolent, they along with a number of other native peoples needed to be disciplined by those who knew better. This of course was part of the racist rhetoric of colonialism and Christendom affirming that blacks and other 'savage' peoples must be civilised lest they regress into chaos. Indeed by enforcing such controls Europeans were doing Africans a favour and that in good time blacks and other natives would be grateful of such 'honourable' European interventions. Of course this was absolute nonsense and blacks were never for one moment grateful for being in bondage or having to be subservient. Fruit was a classic symbol of plenty and used up to this day to denote the natural fertility of the tropics. And hence in the colonial days symbolised black laziness. In American folklore blacks were seen to be overwhelmed by the desire to eat watermelons. Bananas and coconuts have also been associated with blacks, reflected in many of the images of fruit advertisements in the past century.

In recent years the overall pattern of the manipulation of exotic attributes and ethnic characteristics in advertising has not changed, but its complexity and ambiguity have increased. Ambiguity and subliminal messages with the accompanying variety of possible interpretations are intrinsic in some advertising, deliberately carried out to appeal to a wide audience, where only one message can be conveyed. In an increasingly image-saturated world, advertising has to be more innovative to 'capture' its audience. This increases the difficulties of ensuring political correctness. There is not much room for manoeuvre, although this will very much depend on the cultural context. In the United States there has been a significant reduction in negative black imagery in stereotyping since the Civil Rights movement and the 'Black is Beautiful' era of the late 1960s and early 1970s (Ross Barnett). However in the major former European colonial countries such as Britain, France and the Netherlands, and even more so in those European countries without such a significant association with Africa (e.g. Germany), even to this day stereotyping still persists, although there has been some improvement.

Throughout history the roles commonly assigned to black people have been the depiction of them as cooks, servants, entertainers, shoeshine boys, washerwomen, athletes etc. Women are sexualised and men desexualised (at least in earlier imagery to make them less threatening) and criminalised, depending on the intent of the message and/or the times. Virulent negative stereotyping of black people existed up until quite recently in Japan. Black dolls with huge eyes called Sambo and Hannah, and a black doll with thick lips and big earrings, Bibinda, were quite popular in Japan, until protests from the United States ended their production (*Time*, 1988). Only a few years ago Japanese politicians, such as Yasuhiro Nakasone and Michio Watanabe made clearly racist overtures about American blacks. In more recent years the spectrum of black images in advertisement has broadened and there has been significant improvement. For example, more black models are being used in fashion magazines and television commercials in America and Europe are starting to represent blacks in contexts where ethnicity plays no general part, or where white sociocultural norms are set aside. A striking example of the former in British advertising, was the use of a black (non-celebrity) in an Ariel washing-powder advert, and of a black mother and her daughter in a Fairy washing-up liquid commercial. However the general pattern appears to be a reproduction of the familiar old themes only far less obvious with a gradual broadening of the repertoire.

My focus on a discourse on the stereotyping through images exemplifies how symbols exert their effect and become embedded in the consciousness of dominant cultures and hints at how the projections of white (and others) misconceptions of black people affects the identity formation within the black diaspora.

Black Identity in British Caribbean Youth

Identity is an extremely elusive and abstract concept, and as yet there is no acceptable model of it. Anthropology has on the whole rejected the notion that the Western concept of the self is universal, backed by a wealth of ethnographic data. Unfortunately the discipline seems exceptionally reluctant to partake in the heated debate on theories of the self and person that seems central to its construction. As Henrietta Moore (1994) points out, this relative silence has been in the face of 'recent post-structuralist and deconstructionist critiques of the unified, rational subject of Western humanist discourse'. She notes that 'the ambivalent relations between empiricism and social constructionism apparent in anthropological writing and theorising are partly the product of the political liberalism which historically has informed much anthropological thinking'. However, instead of attempting to deconstruct the term I shall merely touch upon black identity in the British people of Caribbean origin, its formation hinting how it may cause and shape the mental morbidity peculiar to this group. Thus leading to the section that continues on the theme of causation on a more phenomenological level incorporating the concept of racial persecution as well as identity confusion. Ken Pryce in his book *Endless Pressure*, a sociological study of West Indian lifestyles in Bristol, states in his chapter 'Racial Alienation and the Problem of Identity':

> The question is of crucial existential relevance to the disadvantaged 'teenybopper' [a term he uses to refer to a young West Indian who is either already a delinquent or in danger of becoming one] because of his own Negro roots, which he despises, and the white bourgeois values which he had been indoctrinated to venerate as culturally and morally superior. He is asked to see himself in terms of the very same values which have rejected him and consigned him to an inferior position in society. But having been brought up to regard his own origins as something to be ashamed of, the teenybopper is left with nothing comforting to fall back on or to help him rationalise his dilemma and thus alleviate – in psychological terms – the shattering and disorientating effects of white prejudice and hostility. He comes from a group that lacks both economic and cultural strength. Unlike his counterpart in the Asian community, whose alien and encircling cultural world affords automatic protection against the worst demoralising consequences of racism and discrimination, the teenybopper finds himself in a veritable state of crisis, shock, dismay and humiliation. In the long run he responds to the closure against him by a wholesale rejection of all that is white, responding to rejection with rejection (Pryce, 1979).

'The need for roots and the attendant quest for identity are said to be natural to peoples everywhere. The phenomena may be said to inhere in a people's need to collate and codify their past collective experience as well as to lay foundations for the realisation of future aspirations' (Nettleford, 1970). This is particularly applicable to those peoples who are in a minority within a dominant culture where they feel disempowered. For black people in Britain the search for a sense of is central in the quest for a sense of self. As mentioned much earlier on in this account, black Caribbean people in Europe with their ancestry in Africa have undergone two major dislocations and have arrived at their current destination via the Caribbean. Along the way, age-old African traditions, and other vital constituents of their original culture such as language, religions, customs, folklore etc. have been decimated, transformed or even disappeared. Much of the culture brought to Britain by those first Jamaican immigrants on the *Windrush* in 1948, derived from Britain. This included fundamental aspects such as basic language and religion. Although of course such cultural components were 'West Indianised' and powerful remnants of West African (and others) heritage existed, not to mention the genesis of new customs and traditions. But that sense of history and heritage afforded to many other ethnic minorities was not there. In addition many Caribbean peoples felt ashamed of the past, characterised as it was by subservience, bondage and suffering. Although there was also much to be proud of, including a history of brave resistance against the Europeans at times in Jamaica (the Maroon wars) and the Windward Islands (the Carib wars), this was underplayed. West Indian immigrants looked up to Britain as the 'Mother Country'. So it came as quite a shock to experience the rabid racial discrimination and prejudice that was confronted on first arrival.

Much of black identity has its historical roots in the 'negritude' movement developed in Africa and the United States in the 1920s and 1930s (particularly in the 'Harlem Renaissance') and in the African–American civil rights and Black Power movements in the 1960s (Milner, 1983). In Britain, according to Sivanandan (1981) it signifies the collective identity of people of African and Asian ancestry in their struggle against English racism. Therefore in this context, black becomes a colour of resistance and an alternative to definitions and identities assigned to them by the racist dominant culture. Thus, Stuart Hall points out, the struggle for black identity is also linked to socioeconomic circumstances.

Sometimes, the class struggle in language occurred between two different terms: the struggle, for example, to replace the term 'immigrant' with the term 'black'. But often, the struggle took the form of a different accenting of the same term: eg. the process by means of which the derogatory colour 'black' became the enhanced value 'black' (as in 'black is beautiful')... It [identity politics] had become part of an organised practice of struggles requiring the building up of black resistances as well as the development of new forms of black consciousness (Hall, 1982).

However numerous writers are critical of this rather unidimensional political definition of black identity. In particular, there has been a debate on the legitimacy of including 'Asian' as well as 'African' and 'African-Caribbean' origin within the above all-inclusive black definition (Banton, 1987). For me, how one defines the concept is up to that person, as long as justification can be made for the definition within the context in which it is used. Clearly, in this context, black identity must include a number of dimensions as it refers to the black Caribbeans. Not because I wish to ignore the plight of Asians, but because their struggles deserve analysis in their own right and are thus beyond the remit of this account. I think the political dimension is important, but not the whole, as clearly the constructs of identity involve psychological, social, cultural and spiritual components that are difficult to separate out. Moreover, specific notions such as a 'sense of belonging' are also thrown into the equation, as we shall see later.

Identity, whilst it has stable aspects, must also adapt to changing circumstances across space and time. Thus, it is a dynamic concept always transforming itself (in some more than others) to adapt and fit in with the surroundings. In microsituations, such as everyday changes from the home to work, to the theatre for example, roles change, along with, to some extent, our identity. Indeed, much of this depends on personal and social expectations. I feel that in the black position such fluctuations in everyday roles and the subtle changes in identity that must accompany them, becomes less predictable. At one level discrimination and prejudices are institutional and all too predictable, but in those everyday transactions and personal interactions, in the High Street, in the pub, with police, situations can easily become loaded (more so than would be the case if you were an indigenous person), particularly those situations where there may be danger (e.g. the police). I hypothesise that this is due to the huge variety in reactions that may not be patent, but that are 'sensed' at a personal level, when somebody of race confronts someone of the dominant culture. Such sensations may be conscious or unconscious, but have a cumulative effect. *Endless Pressure* is a most apt title for Ken Pryce's book. Integration including interpersonal contact and mixing are essential for improving race relations. However, in an ethnic minority group who are vastly outnumbered by the dominant culture, who look very different (and so can experience prejudice from a 'distance'), who perhaps most importantly (and paradoxically) have surprisingly similar cultural values, those who assimilate and are willing to mix, appear to be suffering seriously adverse mental health. I believe, as Ken Pryce suggests, (following informant accounts in his study of Caribbean youth in Bristol in the 1970s) that much of the problem is related to confusion with identity and belonging. If a British-born black male/female of Jamaican origin visits Shropshire, he/she is seen and perceives him/herself as a 'foreigner', 'immigrant' or whatever (even though he/she strictly is not). He/she is certainly seen as 'black' and all that entails (NB: the previous section touching on black stereotyping). If the same person travels to visit relatives in Jamaica, he/she will be instantly noticed as foreign by his/her clothes, manner and demeanour, as well as accent and perhaps his/her outlook. He/she is thankfully perceived as black, but not in the way those in Shropshire see his/her 'blackness'. This must (and does) imbue a confused sense of belonging as well as identity. The identity issue is not that of being 'black' so much, but of being black in Britain. It is easier for the above man/woman to be 'black' in Jamaica than in Shropshire, but due to a lifetime experience of growing up in Britain he/she will have strong attachments to England as with anyone born and brought up in a particular country (though of course this is not universal). It is after all his/her home, but he/she does not quite fit in. Neither does he/she feel fully at home in Jamaica because he/she is not Jamaican, at least at a legal level, although he/she may feel so in other ways, culturally or politically for example. Essentially he/she has a confused sense of belonging that at its most pathological may lead to a distorted sense of self.

Moving on I will now focus on tactics young black Caribbean people utilise to reconcile this confusion, leading to the formation of new identities. My concentration on black youth here is appropriate as the onset of psychosis typically occurs (especially in males) in late adolescence and twenties. These are of course, precisely the times that young people in general, independent of background, undergo identity formation and crises as they find their place in the modern world.

Music and language cultures appear central to how young people in Britain express their 'blackness'. The operation of black linguistic codes helps to connect with blacks in the Caribbean and North America and identify both with black peers and with the others in their world, including young whites (many of whom share their tastes in music and fashion). A number of Creole languages of Caribbean origin are spoken in London, dominant of which are those that originate from Jamaica (Back, 1986). The Creole spoken by the parents is of course very different to that spoken by their children in the inner cities. Black Caribbean youth will often slip into hybrid forms of Creole, 'switching codes' between regional English and Creole (Hewitt, 1986). A variety of 'triggers' have been identified that lead to these switches from the regional vernacular to Creole. These include, during the expression of happiness or anger or greeting friends, when being assertive, when referring to sexual relationships and in the definition of black group identity (Hewitt, 1986). In addition, urban black American vernacular, predominantly through the hip hop culture of music and films, has entered the speech of British urban black youth, particularly the males. Black youth in Britain have for years looked to black America for esteem and inspiration, perhaps more so than the Caribbean in recent years. Indeed, black American culture has influenced youth culture globally, as far away as Japan, where there is a thriving hip hop scene. This is a source of great pride and affirmation for the black diaspora, not least in the United Kingdom.

Black identity in England, it seems, is defined not only through the Caribbean, but through connections with the black diaspora, particularly America. Paul Gilroy (1987) believes (and I would strongly agree) the prime medium involved in this diasporic connectedness is the black musical culture. Black people in England appear to see a common link in the genesis of black American and black Caribbean music. This concept of 'roots' is very important in black musical cultures found in London (Back, 1986). As Gilroy reminds us:

> All these musics announce themselves as 'roots', a complex term which combines the obvious organic similes of Garveyism – 'A nation without its past history is like a tree without root' – with a belief in philosophical and political archaeology for which Alex Haley's book stands as both an example and a paradigm: 'I was drifting away from reality, so far away from the roots in me' (Gilroy, 1987).

Les Back (1986) following the interview of a black youth from South London comments, '... we can clearly see how this young man separates the phenotypic notion of blackness from a cultural notion of "roots". He continues by stating how the black youth he encounters 'connects African origins with both a Caribbean experience and the political legacy of slavery'. He suggests that the notion of 'dread' borrowed from Rastafarianism may be utilised as a 'substitute for blackness ... a tag signifying commonness'.

'Dread' is a rasta notion that means the essence of the black experience. Thus it conveys the highest form of status and the most terrible experiences of exploitation. There are similarities between this notion and the idea of 'soul' in the black American context ... Although it is a core concept within rasta philosophy, it also signifies a condition of collective belonging ... Rasta ethics and maxims are widely available and can form the basis of a metaphorical identification with Africa. Young black people plot the historical connectedness of black people throughout the new world by developing a 'dread ontology' that provides the philosophical and practical matrix in which links are made within the diaspora (Back, 1986).

Les Back also found in his interviews some interesting and varied notions expressed by young black Londoners, concerning attitudes towards being British or English. Many of his respondents saw themselves as British at the level of citizenship. One respondent distanced herself from Englishness, by characterising herself as a 'different kind of English'. Another detached himself completely from the concept of Britishness, preferring to see himself as a 'black person of West Indian parentage'. Back concludes, 'clearly they are in the process of working out this relationship in a syncretic culture that is both black and British'. It would seem to me, and evidenced by a comment made from one of his young informants, that how young black Caribbean conceptualise their (black) identity, sense of self and belonging, is highly influenced by how the dominant white culture perceives them. The 16-year-old woman interviewed by Back states:

It's like you identify yourself as a black person coming from – with West Indian parents. It's like we – they like to know that they are coming from elsewhere. A lot of black people don't see themselves as English. I think you should be aware of that. It is the way the country puts them down already. It makes you feel like you don't want to be from here. It's like when times are good, us – the people who are born here – are considered English, just like everybody else. But when things are bad, jobs are hard to get, we become black! (Back, 1986).

Many blacks will comment how the British take great pride in proclaiming outstanding black sportsmen and sportswomen such as Linford Christie, Sol Campbell and Tessa Sanderson as their own and very much 'British'. However many will not feel as readily accepted as 'British' in their own everyday life (e.g. see above). This societal double blindness echoes almost exactly those psychological conditions postulated at one stage to be a psychogenic cause of schizophrenia (Bateson et al., 1956).

These conditions at the microcosmic level included a parent (usually the mother according to the original theory) having to convey two or more conflicting and incompatible messages at the same time; the child feels he or she must understand and respond appropriately; the child cannot comment on the inconsistency and if the child does respond meets with disapproval. These conditions were said to lead to withdrawal, irrational behaviour, ambiguity and finally schizophrenia. Nevertheless because of the dominance of the medical model over the years, along with 'soft' medical evidence, and the lack of controlled methodology, the theory did not persist. Could however, persisting societal contradictions regarding (national) identity be relevant in the more psychogenic presentations of apparently psychotic behaviour? I am very aware that I have explored only certain dimensions of ethnic identity and its formation, particularly at the political level. For example, I have not explored religion or spirituality, marriage or traditional dress. I certainly acknowledge the importance of these parameters, but I do not include them for three main reasons. Firstly, I wanted to briefly contextualise and analyse those factors that seemed most relevant to urban British black youth. Secondly, following on from this it appears such issues as religion, traditional dress (but not fashion) etc. in general, take less precedence in importance amongst black youth (although not in their parents) in London, compared to for example in the Indian, Pakistani and Bangladeshi communities. To the question 'religion is very important to how I live my life' only 17 per cent of black Caribbean answered 'yes' to this (cf. 55 per cent of those who entered Britain after the age of 16). However within the Indian, Pakistani and Bangladeshi communities, 32 per cent, 57 per cent and 59 per cent respectively of those born in Britain, stated 'yes' to the question (cf. 57 per cent, 83 per cent and 81 per cent respectively in those who entered Britain after the age of 16 per cent) (Modood et al., 1997). Though the question does not explore the level of commitment or meaning religion has in the lives of the respondents, it does lend interesting markers and leads for further investigation, understanding, and explanation. Finally, and most relevantly, I am unable to do justice to all the issues in the space provided. I do acknowledge their importance for a more overall and comprehensive analysis.

I end this section on identity with a passage from Paul Gilroy's book *The Black Atlantic: Modernity and Double Consciousness*, that merges well with the next section, as its theme contextualises my phenomenological (in clinical psychiatric terms) examination of double consciousness (particularly regarding colour) and its association with paranoia, persecution and the subsequent genesis of mental disorder and psychosis.

Striving to be both European and black requires some specific forms of double consciousness. By saying this I do not mean to suggest that taking on either or both of these unfinished identities necessarily exhausts the subjective resources of any particular individual. However, where racist, nationalist, or ethnically absolutist discourses orchestrate political relationships so that these identities appear to be mutually exclusive, occupying the space between them or trying to demonstrate their continuity has been viewed as a provocative and even oppositional act of political insubordination.

The contemporary black English, like the Anglo-Africans of earlier generations and perhaps, like all blacks in the West, stand between (at least) two great cultural assemblages, both of which have mutated through the course of the modern world that formed them and assumed new configurations. At present, they remain locked symbiotically in an antagonistic relationship marked out by the symbolism of colours which adds to the conspicuous cultural power of their central Manichean – black and white. These colours support a special rhetoric that has grown to be associated with a language of nationality and national belonging as well as the languages of 'race' and ethnic identity (Gilroy, 1993).

Double Consciousness, Paranoia and Persecution

And then the occasion arose when I had to meet the white man's eyes. An unfamiliar weight burdened me. The real world challenged my claims. In the white world the man of color encounters difficulties in the development of his bodily schema. Consciousness of the body is solely a negating activity. It is a third-person consciousness. The body is surrounded by an atmosphere of certain uncertainty (Frantz Fanon, 1968).

The above statement is an example of the 'pathological' consciousness experienced by those of colour in the United Kingdom. Before outlining my theory of this 'pathological' consciousness and how phenomenologically it relates to paranoia and the 'mimicry' of schizophrenia, I will refer to the ideas of the great existentialist French philosopher Jean-Paul Sartre. In one of his earlier books, *The Transcendence of the Ego*, published in 1937 (Cumming, 1972), Sartre uses the phenomenological method pioneered by the German philosopher Edmund Husserl to examine consciousness. His starting point was the division of consciousness into 'unreflected' and 'reflected' (he did not believe in Freud's unconscious). Unreflected consciousness is the consciousness of everyday life, of walking down a street, of seeing autumn leaves fall from a tree, etc. There is no 'I' in this unreflected consciousness. However, something untoward may happen that refers to the self, for example, one is in a hurry and runs to catch a bus which is missed. One becomes angry with oneself, and one enters the domain of reflected consciousness as there is now an 'I' in one's thinking. Sartre thought that only in reflected consciousness could the be found in 'self' consciousness. The moment one slips back into unreflected consciousness, one is no longer aware of the self. In perhaps Sartre's most famous work, the enormous *Being and Nothingness*, published in 1943 (Cumming, 1972), he believes 'the self' is not a substantive entity that continues unchanged through time, nor can its absolute certainty be deduced from consciousness (as Descartes believed could be done with his famous saying, 'I think, therefore I am'). Sartre believed that there was a disturbing and troubling side of selfhood, that is uncovered in the confrontation with other people. If one is alone the sudden confrontation with an 'Other' forces one to reinterpret one's surroundings. Previously everything in the surroundings were there 'for me'. Now they are there 'for the Other'. Sartre stated, 'hell is other people'. This was because in the above example the 'Other' freedom destabilises your own. You objectify the 'Other', but cannot do it fully because the 'Other's' gaze objectifies you, turns you into a thing (a typical notion of existentialism). Sartre felt that to see the 'Other' is to understand the 'permanent possibility of being seen by the "Other"'. You may feel this actuality, happening or confrontation as shame, (if, for example you were caught doing something wrong), or as fear (if the 'Other' was in some way a threat to you).

I postulate that the black experience in Britain, along with the experience of a political 'double (identity) consciousness' and all the other 'identity-confusion' issues previously discussed, leads to in many, a heightened awarenesss of 'the Other'. Here I conceptualise the 'Other' as both the ('dominant' indigenous white) individual and the dominant collective people. This hypothesis stems from the experience a white friend and colleague of mine shared with me several years ago. She described to me that, during a multidisciplinary community health team meeting that she was chairing, she had suddenly noticed everyone else was black. Even though these colleagues were perfectly polite and friendly, their very number (about 10) heightened the awareness of herself and the awareness of herself through those around her. She became more 'self-conscious' and 'self-referential'. I think that when this happens in conjunction with the confusion or 'twoness' (see the earlier quote from du Bois) of being black and British, you may experience my phenomenological concept of 'double consciousness'. This is not exactly the 'heightened reflective consciousness' in the sense of Sartre (though this is central), nor is it the same as the political 'double consciousness' in the sense of W.E.B. du Bois and Paul Gilroy (although this too is an essential part of the formula). Rather it is the 'actual experience', the everyday 'essence of being', that is part of the black British experience. This experience hypothetically may contribute significantly to this so-called excess of 'diagnosed' schizophrenia and other psychoses in black people in the UK (and perhaps the Netherlands). But it is not the whole story. I think that another factor is needed, a variable that is inextricably linked with the notion of 'double consciousness'. That is, paranoia and persecution.

> In 1974, when the Cold War was still very much palpable, I drove through Bulgaria with my wife and two small children. One noticeable difference on Bulgarian roads was the absence of the colorful advertisements and neon signs typical in much of the western world. Instead, there was an abundance of huge billboards illustrated with figures whose fingers pointed at passers-by. Although the Bulgarian alphabet was foreign to me, I knew the billboards exalted the virtues of the communist system and 'ordered' people to behave correctly. Outside of Sofia, our progress was brought to a standstill by a policeman stopping traffic. But he was not like the traffic police I was accustomed to in the U.S. or other places who typically used the flashing lights of their patrol cars, bright orange cones, and large signs to stop the flow of cars. The Bulgarian policeman instead held a small cardboard sign that reminded me more of a lollipop which he moved up and down in slow motion. I perceived this policeman as a cartoon character; he seemed more a caricature of a traffic cop, but his power was nonetheless enormous. He was laughable but also scary.
>
> Earlier that same day, as we crossed into Bulgaria, we encountered one of the customs officers, a mean-looking and unsmiling official. He checked our car thoroughly, looking under the hood and bending down to inspect the underside of our car. We had nothing to hide, but as we continued our drive through Bulgaria, the events of that day caused me to develop a fear of being stopped by a Bulgarian policeman, not unlike the cartoon-like traffic cop, and accused of some unknown crime. The unfamiliar external world was stimulating fearful responses in my internal world, making me very worried of sinister external powers. When we left Bulgaria and returned to the 'free world' my paranoia ended, though the memory of it remained (Volkan, 1998).

This lengthy passage written by Vamik Volkan, an American Professor of Psychiatry, is taken from the foreword of the book *Even Paranoids Have Enemies: New Perspectives on Paranoia and Persecution* (Berke et al., 1998). His experience in communist Bulgaria with its 'culture of paranoia' parallels to some extent the experiences of black (or Asian) youth in the inner cities of Britain. That is, a paranoia which has a basis in reality or an external persecution.

The word *paranoia* originates from the Greek language (*para*: out of, beside; *noos*: reason, mind) and refers to a state of 'being out of, or beside, one's mind' in the sense of a disorder of the mind. The word *persecution* comes from the Latin *persequi* (*per*: continually; *sequi*: to follow, pursue), refers to harassment, oppression, suppression, subjugation, tyranny and torture, especially on political, racial and religious grounds (Berke et al., 1998). In psychoanalysis paranoia is a pathological state that arises through the Freudian defence mechanism of 'projection'. This is where unwanted thoughts, wishes and desires that finally lead to an 'internal persecution' of an individual and accompanying anxiety, are dealt with not by repression, but by 'projection' on to others who now act as 'external persecutors'. Freud, who felt that libido was the primary psychic drive, thought these unwanted urges were homosexual and that it was the denial of these feelings through projection that led to 'paranoia'. In 1921 Kraepelin, one of the forefathers of modern clinical psychiatry and the classification of psychoses, incorporated the term into his classification to denote 'a group of psychoses characterised by the insidious development of a permanent and unshakeable delusional system resulting from internal causes, which is accompanied by perfect preservation of clear and orderly thinking, willing and acting (and no hallucinations)' (as distinct from schizophrenia, although of course paranoid features are commonly seen in schizophrenia) (Kendell, 1992). In modern psychiatry the word *paranoid* means 'self-referent' and is not limited to *persecutory*. Delusional beliefs concerned with *grandiosity, love* and *jealousy* are all subsumed under paranoid ideation as they are all self-referential. The fact that abnormal persecutory notions are the most common and notorious ideas of self-reference, explains why the terms *persecution* and *paranoia* have become synonymous.

There is often a thin line between paranoia (internal persecution) and real external persecution. Or fantasy and reality. Indeed paranoia and persecution may coexist, and it is clear that persecution can induce paranoid phenomena. In the case of black people in Britain who have been shown anecdotally and statistically to suffer police harassment (Cashmore and McLaughlin, 1991), the police, courts and other agents of 'social control' (including psychiatry) are the external persecutors. Calvin Hernton a black American poet, writer, social scientist and Professor of African American studies in the USA, in a disturbing account of his experience of persecution at the hands of racist white police in the American South comments:

> Thus, despite having lived where the police are not a menace, whenever white policeman enter the space where I am, I experience anxiety and fear. I can be

rational and control this 'pathology'. Yet, similarly to black people everywhere in the United States, particularly the youth in their own neighbourhoods, I too live with a measured sense of being persecuted by the police. And I strive to negotiate my fear and paranoia in ways that help me survive both the imagined and very real animosity and brutality of the police toward all people whose complexion and status in the eyes of the world are similar to mine (Hernton, 1998).

A number of black writers are convinced that racist oppression and persecution can induce 'psychotic reactions'. Frantz Fanon, a black psychiatrist, working in French-occupied Algeria had first-hand experience of the prolonged oppression of Algerian people engaged in the freedom struggle against their French colonisers. Fanon describes his personal experience of the prolonged oppression of Algerian people engaged in the freedom struggle against their French colonisers. He notes 'reactionary psychosis' with 'events giving rise to the disorder' that included 'the sum total of harmful nervous stimuli', such as the brutality, torture and other atrocities perpetrated by the police. 'Mental pathology ... is the direct product of oppression' (Frantz Fanon, 1967). Richard Wright, an African-American writer before Fanon (1940), wrote in his novel *Native Son*, that in American blacks, in a culture of oppression stretching back centuries, the 'reality of whiteness' has become an almost omnipotent force that creates paranoid feelings, with many blacks promoting the idea of themselves as an 'endangered species'.

Conclusion

There appear to be significant similarities between the phenomenology of double consciousness and the psychopathology of schizophrenia as defined by the medical hierarchy. Whether or not schizophrenia exists within the paradigms used in its operationalisation is open to conjecture and further analysis. However double consciousness does exist and appears adaptive as well as constraining. To see yourself from the eyes of others as well as from within, seems a sensible way to be when confronted with hostility, real or imagined. To place oneself into the consciousness of your foe is to predict what he may do to you and to be one step ahead. With this doubling of awareness is a doubling of arousal seen in acute psychotic states. Within the context of stress, disaffection and hopelessness, that results from a hostile inner-city environment, one may decompensate and crash into a malignant anxiety, characterised by suspiciousness, agitation, inappropriateness etc. This double consciousness, instead of being adaptive, becomes pathological. There is an overwhelming 'sense of self', as the unfortunate cannot reconcile where the real danger is, so it may be attributed to a specific individual or oppressive organisation and become a 'delusion'. Senses become further heightened and even mix. There is dissociation as the psyche attempts to come to terms with the storm. Cultural metaphors of distress invest themselves into the presentation confusing the Western-trained psychiatrist, who may not be culturally sensitive, and the sufferer is labelled. He/she is brought to the clinic by police, family or health service agent for a variety of reasons, but for the same thing. Inappropriate behaviour. The police or health service agent may be quick to see the behaviour as madness, the family are just bewildered. 'First rank' symptoms may be 'elicited' that include passivity phenomena and thought interference. Such psychopathology may nearly be experienced by people who feel disenfranchised and not in control of their lives and may even be appropriate. However if presented in an exaggerated and colourful form, as is likely in severe psychic distress, such phenomena may be misconstrued and seen within the boundaries of a psychosis rather than in a wider context. Thus confirming the assumptions of the psychiatrist. To concentrate on content as well as form of phenomenology is vital here in understanding rather than just categorising. Because the latter involves the diagnostic process, it has real implications for black people, who are more likely to receive adverse diagnoses (especially schizophrenia) and treatments. This is where the whole subject becomes political and sensitive, and shades of McCarthyism and the treatment of Soviet dissidents in psychiatry are evoked.

Such an explanation for a remarkably common scenario makes some sense, and may at least partly explain the overrepresentation of black Caribbeans in psychiatry. Black peoples' vulnerability to psychological compromise, caused by poverty and discrimination and heightened by their social environment in combination with often profound and peculiar life events, will inevitably lead to breakdown in many, manifesting itself through a 'psychosis', with the nature of the presentation representing metaphorically, feelings of alienation, fear, and disempowerment, often expressed through the themes of racism, belonging and identity. There may be no family history of psychiatric disorder, and recovery may be rapid if services are sensitive and appropriate, but they are usually not. The ill will inevitably return to the same social environment and relapse, because the truth is, it is the culture and society that appears to be the major problem and services can only firefight. The outcome is uncertain.

References

Alatas, S.H. (1977), *The Myth of the Lazy Native*, London.

Back, L. (1986), *New Ethnicities and Urban Culture*, UCL Press, London.

Banton, M. (1987), *Racial Theories*, Cambridge University Press, Cambridge.

Berke, J.H. et al. (eds) (1998), *Even Paranoids have Enemies: New Perspectives on Paranoia and Persecution*, Routledge, London.

Cashmore, E. and McLaughlin, E. (1991), *Out of Order: Policing Black People*, Routledge, London.

Cumming, R.D. (1972), *The Philosophy of Jean-Paul Sartre*, Vintage Books, New York.

Everett, S. (1978), *History of Slavery*, Magna, Leicester.

Fanon, F. (1967), *The Wretched of the Earth*, Penguin, London.

Fanon, F. (1968), *Black Skin, White Masks*, Pluto, London.

Fiske, S.T. and Taylor, S.E. (1984), *Social Cognition*, New York.

Gilroy, P. (1993), *The Black Atlantic: Modernity and Double Consciousness*, Verso, London.

Hall, S. (1982), 'The Rediscovery of Ideology: Return of the Repressed in Media Studies', in Gurevitch, M. et al, (eds), *Culture, Society and the Media*, Methuen, London.

Harris, H.W. et al. (1995), *Racial and Ethnic Identity*, Routledge, New York.

Hernton, C.C. (1998), Between History and Me: Persecution, Paranoia and the Police', in Berke, J.H. et al. (eds), *Even Paranoids have Enemies: New Perspectives on Paranoia and Persecution*, Routledge, London.

Hewitt, R. (1986), *White Talk, Black Talk: Inter-racial Friendship and Communication amongst Adolescents*, Cambridge University Press, London.

Kendell, R.E. and Zealley, A.K. (1973), *Companion to Psychiatric Studies*, Churchill Livingsone, London.

Littlewood, R. and Lipsedge, M. (1989), *Aliens and Alienists*, Routledge, London.

Milner, D. (1983), *Children and Race: Ten Years On*, Ward Sussex, East Grinstead.

Modood, T. et al. (1997), *Ethnic Minorities in Britain*, Policy Studies Institute, London.

Moore, H. (1994), 'Gendered Persons: Dialogues between Anthropology and Psychoanalysis', in Heald, S. and Deluz, A. (eds), *Anthropology and Psychoanalysis*, Routledge, London.

Moscovici, S. (1981), 'On Social Representations', in Forgas, J.P. (ed.), *Social Cognition: Perspectives on Everyday Understanding*, London.

Nettleford, R. (1970), *Mirror Mirror: Identity, Race and Protest in Jamaica*, Jamaica.

Pryce, K. (1979), *Endless Pressure*, London, Classical, Bristol.

Reno, D.E. (1986), *Collecting Black Americana*, New York.

Reynolds, R. (1974), *Cleanliness and Godliness*, New York.

Ross Barnett, M. (n.d.), 'Negative Stereotypes of African-Americans in American popular culture', *Distorted Images*, Brooklyn.

Sivanandan, A. (1981), 'From the Resistance to Rebellion: Asian and Afro-Caribbean Struggles in Britain', *Race and Class*, 23, pp. 111–51.

Volkan, V.D. (1998), 'Foreword', in Berke, J.H. et al. (eds), *Even Paranoids have Enemies: New Perspectives on Paranoia and Persecution*, Routledge, London.

Walvin, J. (1982), 'Black Caricature: the Roots of Racialism', in Husband, C. (ed.), *'Race' in Britain*, London.

Werkman, C.J. (1974), *Trademarks: their Creation, Psychology and Perception*, Amsterdam.

Chapter 4

Cultural Studies, Ethnicity and Mental Health

Gargi Bhattacharyya and John Gabriel

Introduction

Despite the blurred boundaries between academic disciplines and the difficulties of disentangling one from another, the organisation of this book nevertheless requires us to make explicit what is distinctive about cultural studies. Without wishing to suggest what follows is the exclusive domain of cultural studies our aim, at least, is to represent some important strands of cultural studies thinking. The chapter will therefore be organised around the themes of: deconstructing mental illness; qualitative versus quantitative research and grass roots mobilisations of subordinate groups. Running throughout will be what has arguably become the debate within cultural studies over the last decade, that is, around questions of identity.

It is also worth emphasising at the outset that, with some notable individual exceptions, cultural studies has *not* made mental health and ethnicity one of its main areas of concern and we shall suggest why this might be the case below. Rather, it has contributed a set of questions, concepts and analytical approaches which are potentially applicable to the field of mental health and ethnicity. In exploring these themes, as well as omissions, we will argue against the idea of cultural studies as a key to unlocking questions of ethnic difference and at the same time to argue for a more politically grounded approach to research in this area. In view of this, we will conclude the chapter by examining some documentary material on the role of grass-roots organisations concerned with mental health and their significance in mobilising communities around ideas of ethnicity and identity.

It will surprise some to learn that cultural studies is *not* concerned with the purportedly neutral study of cultural differences and/or the disclosure of the essential characteristics of different ethnic groups. On the whole, cultural studies has not satisfied those demands on it to encapsulate the values and meanings associated with different ethnic cultures. It follows that cultural studies have also frustrated those who look to it to explain mental illness in terms of ethnic differences. If anything, cultural studies has challenged such taken-for-granted notions of knowledge and culture, a challenge which had its origins in the 1960s. Then, academics like Richard Hoggart, Raymond Williams and Stuart Hall and others challenged the view that culture meant high-literary culture to the exclusion of everyday-lived culture. From the outset such cultural forms and practices as television, popular music, romance novels, drugs, fashion, etc. and the lifestyles associated with them were a legitimate object of study as much as, if not more so than the works of Chaucer, Shakespeare and Milton. Social relations at work, in schools, within families and on the street, brought some interests within cultural studies close to the terrain of sociology, whilst others remained biased towards the humanities, with the emphasis on literary criticism and cultural history.

Cultural studies has thus given rise to research traditions which have focused on such themes as: working class cultures/subcultures; popular media, and theories of culture and ideology, gender and ethnicity. In terms of empirical research methods, the emphasis has been on ethnographic studies in which researchers explore the everyday meanings which help to shape peoples lives and through which people make sense of themselves and others. This body of research has been furthered by use of techniques of participant observation, informal interviews, research diaries and life histories. In more theoretically-oriented work, cultural studies has drawn on diverse bodies of thought from philosophy, literary theory, discourse analysis, psychoanalysis, sociology, Marxism, and several new 'isms' invariably with a common prefix; *post*-modernism, *post*-colonialism, etc. When it is remembered that each of the above traditions, even the more recent ones, has spawned its own sub-traditions, then it becomes possible to grasp the density and heterogeneity of the field as a whole. Despite its breadth, cultural studies has paid little attention to questions of mental health and ethnicity, an absence not unrelated to the historical peculiarities of British cultural studies. Mental health has been widely seen within social science as a social problem which has provoked a set of policy, legal and institutional responses. Since cultural studies has viewed social policies generally as mechanisms of social control imposed by the state from above, and designed to define and regulate subordinate groups, then its avoidance of this particular field of social policy is not so surprising. Moreover, whilst cultural studies has focused some of its research on the perspectives of subordinate groups, the mentally ill, or those defined as such, have not been proved popular within cultural studies. This state of affairs has undoubtedly been exacerbated by problems of access, linked to which has been the agenda-setting role played by the medical establishment, police and social services, not to mention the fraught ethical dilemmas raised by research in this area. It is also arguably true that cultural studies has tended to focus on the celebratory and subversive aspects of youth culture (whilst simultaneously raising questions of gender, ethnicity and class) to the near-exclusion of questions of age, mental and physical illness and able-bodiedness.

Deconstructing Mental Illness

The idea of critiquing orthodoxies is evident in the deconstruction of discourses historically concerned with defining, treating and moralising about mental illness. Michel Foucault's work is pivotal both because it has become such an important canon within cultural studies as a whole and, particularly in this context, through his genealogy of mental illness (1967). Foucault's wide-ranging studies of cultural, including 'scientific' developments, has encouraged us to re-think common sense notions of what it means to punish and to desire, as well as to be mad. In each case, Foucault's method sought to show how understandings changed according to dominant perceptions of the time. In the case of madness he explored the ways in which knowledge was produced and acted on through religious, philanthropic and subsequently medical discourses. These discourses shaped the ways in which madness was understood as well as how people were perceived and treated and perceived themselves. In other words, religion, medicine etc. were knowledges which provided the means by which power was exercised over those labelled and objectified as mentally ill. The asylum became the institutional site on which such knowledge/power was expressed (ibid., 241ff).

Arguably, a historical perspective makes it easier to grasp the political motives which drove definitions of, and policies on the 'insane'. The creation of mental illnesses to support the social structure of the time is no better illustrated than in the case of drapetomania, an 'illness' peculiar to slaves and whose classic symptom was the 'irresistible urge to run away from the plantation' (cited in Torkington, 1991, p. 119). The strategic use of mental health legislation and asylums and the discipline of psychiatry not only had a racial but a class dimension too and was linked to the idea of a lack of self-control on the part of the lower classes (ibid., p. 117). Control invariably meant the regulation of sexuality and female sexuality in particular. In this context, it is remembering the ten thousand young women who were committed to asylums in England in the early twentieth century for having sex before marriage under the 1913 Mental Defectives Act, including one Edna Higginbottom, who was given electric shock treatment and incarcerated for 20 years before she was released in 1959 (cited ibid., p. 113).

The application of Foucault's ideas to contemporary issues and practices surrounding mental health and ethnicity has enabled us to question existing research, for example to ask how some discourses have come to dominate our understanding of mental health and ethnicity and how these relate to institutional practices and questions of identity. One of the strengths of cultural studies has been its interrogative nature including the capacity to critique disciplines which appear to fall outside of its own realm of expertise. In this sense, cultural studies is not the study of different cultures as much as the way we come to understand culture and how those understandings form the basis of political (with a small and a big p) action.

The assumption that mental illness and ethnicity are universal givens (i.e. that there are hard and fast ways of defining them) is not confined to orthodox psychiatry and/or biology. Those who emphasise the significance of migration argue that the trauma associated with the move from an agricultural (primitive?) to industrial (civilised?) society cause higher rates of breakdown amongst immigrant groups (cited ibid.). Such generalisations are always prey to contrary findings. For example, Cochrane found an under-representation of south Asian ethnic groups in mental health statistics despite the fact that many of these groups had migrated from rural backgrounds similar to those from the Caribbean (ibid.). Moreover, such accounts are often underpinned or at least imply notions of 'backwardness' or pathological traits associated with immigrant/racialised groups. Another example would be the suggestion that immigrants suffer from 'delusions of persecution' or 'paranoid psychosis', an idea that might also conveniently serve to undermine accounts of racist experiences.

Accounts which attribute mental illness to the flawed culture of subordinate ethnic groups has been purportedly challenged by the principles of transcultural psychiatry to be found in the work of Philip Rack amongst others. This field was based on the idea that psychiatry was guilty of misdiagnosis of mental illness and called instead for diagnosis rooted in an understanding of ethnic/cultural differences. However, whilst promoting the idea of ethnically diverse teams of professionals, transcultural psychiatry tends to promote the idea of ethnic groups as homogenous and fixed, a cardboard caricature at odds with the idea of ethnic groups engaged in a dynamic interaction with their British surroundings. This is the case for all ethnic groups but no more so than for those fourth and fifth generation immigrants in Britain's port cities, e.g.

Cardiff, Bristol and Liverpool. Stereotypes based on the possibility of distilling the essential characteristics of different ethnic groups enable transcultural psychiatry to distinguish psychiatry for 'them' and 'us'. In the case of the former, specialists need to pull down the cultural veil to get at the heart of the psychiatric problem. For the ethnic white English there is no veil. In other words transcultural psychiatry normalises treatment for the dominant ethnic group whilst it simultaneously problematises it for others.

Questioning White Normality

While cultural studies evades serious consideration of many troubling policy issues, at a broader level cultural studies attempts to unpack the processes which form institutional knowledge and practice. As part of this project, mental health issues are categorised with a range of processes in which power is consolidated through the creation of others. Cultural studies recognises itself as a discipline in part through its problematic and critical relation to other forms of knowledge-making. In particular the more orthodox and institutionally recognised modes of social inquiry provide a focus for a critique of institutional knowledge as a facet of wider unpleasant power structures and it is this mode of critique which characterises much of the work which can be described as cultural studies. In relation to our understanding of issues of race, this critique has entailed an ongoing battle against the common-sense assumptions of much of the sociology of race and its offshoot, the so-called race relations industry. Formative work in cultural studies has charged this industry with propagating a false system of knowledge which pathologises black communities under the pretence of examining and understanding them. In a now widely known and acknowledged account, these writers charge mainstream accounts of the circumstances of black communities with an old-style blaming of the victim. Although much of this work tries to identify deprivation and suggest challenges to its causes, the analyses too often assume that the extra problems of migrants stem from themselves, be this from their unsettled newly migrated status or from their more general failure to adjust to the cultural norms of their new home. It is almost impossible to name racism from these starting assumptions – instead black lives will improve as black people learn to adjust to the normality of white culture and power.

Although little of the critique mounted from cultural studies referred directly to health issues, the criticism of academic work which both veiled and contributed to institutional racism could easily be extended to include discussions of mental health and racialised communities. The lesson of cultural studies is that the pathologisation of certain communities, particularly black communities, is another abusive exercise of power, and that this power is exercised through the use of culture in its widest senses.

More recently, much work in cultural studies has sought to explore the formation of this culture of power. The development of a substantial body of work studying whiteness is an indication of this broader trend towards scrutinising the powerful, rather than further contributing to the pathologisation of the less powerful. This work has tried to identify the various methods by which whiteness presents itself as unracial and the norm for all human behaviour and achievement. A number of writers have suggested that whiteness is constructed as a concept with no content, and that, instead, what is white is marked as no more than the normal and human in relation to racialised others who represent undesirable deviations from the norm of whiteness. In relation to health issues and to mental health in particular, this analysis offers the benefit of exposing the extent to which health is itself defined as an approximation to a powerful norm. What is missing from this evaluation of white normativity is the network of social and institutional structures which enforce whiteness as norm and ensure that race is the identity through which others fail to meet the required norms and are punished accordingly.

While cultural studies has little or nothing to say about the alleviation of suffering, the insights of work in this field can suggest a means of understanding the peculiar dynamics which give rise to suffering, including mental distress. As well as making visible the powerful normativity of whiteness and the institutional sustenance given to this norm, writing in cultural studies has suggested that the creation and maintenance of power, including and perhaps most particularly, the racialised power of whiteness, is itself a pathological mode of behaviour. A range of work reveals that the creation of white identity has required an excessive and vindictive violence against other peoples of the world. While some have argued that this is no more than the pragmatic and purely instrumental violence of the powerful and conquering throughout history, students of whiteness have pointed out the excessive and seemingly endless character of this aggression. Rather than accepting that mental distress and disorder are responses to powerlessness, this work suggests that white power has given rise to its own distressing disorders.

The more interesting developments stemming from writers working broadly in the field of cultural studies, begin to unpack the extent to which the paranoia of white culture impacts on the life experience of other communities. This work builds on the analysis of whiteness as a defensive and unstable construct which must constantly reconstitute itself through a variety of violent strategies and suggests that it is this violence which shapes the suffering of black people. This movement allows space to acknowledge the real pains of mental distress which are suffered among black people, and even to recognise that some forms of distress may be more prevalent among black communities than white. However, the interesting contribution of this work is the suggestion that this distress is a (rational?) reaction to the excesses of a culture of whiteness which is out of control and dangerously unwell. bell hooks writes of the phenomenon of black rage as a potentially transformative state, if it can be acknowledged as a transitory response to black experience in a white supremacist culture. She writes,

> The rage of the oppressed is never the same as the rage of the privileged. One group can change their lot only by changing the system; the other hopes to be rewarded within the system. Public focus in black rage, the attempt to trivialize and dismiss it, must be subverted by public discourse about the pathology of white supremacy, the madness it creates. We need to talk seriously about ending racism if we want to see an end to rage. White supremacy is frightening. It promotes mental illness and various dysfunctional behaviors on the part of whites and non-whites. It is the real and present danger, not black rage (hooks, 1996, p. 30).

hooks is commenting on the outrage expressed on the rare occasions that black people attack whites and the extent to which the fear of this retaliation permeates white culture. hooks argues that whites are haunted by the spectre of this expected violence and that their own sense of well-being is damaged by the anticipation of an understandable and justifiable fighting back by black people. Of course, the irony is that black people are not hitting back in any consistent manner. Instead, hooks suggests, black rage is turned inward to become another source of black distress.

> Collective failure to address adequately the psychic wounds inflicted by racist aggression is the breeding ground for a psychology of victimhood wherein learned helplessness, uncontrollable rage, and/or feelings of overwhelming powerlessness and despair abound in the psyches of black folks yet are not attended to in ways that empower and promote holistic states of well-being (hooks, 1996, p. 137).

hooks argues that black communities have learned survival strategies of dissimulation and evasion that are now damaging their psychic well-being. She argues that black rage must be acknowledged and encountered, not as a route to violent attack, but as a stage of politicisation and a necessary prerequisite for transformation at both individual and societal levels. Without this, hooks suggests, black people can never emerge into the healthy and productive state of 'loving blackness as political resistance'. In many ways, hooks builds on the earlier work of Franz Fanon. The work of Fanon has been celebrated in cultural studies as a method of analysing the effects of colonial structures on the subjectivity of those involved. Fanon's clinical background has been largely ignored, in favour of a reading which stresses the insights of his social analysis. To cultural studies, Fanon offers a way of comprehending the psychology of racism and colonial experience. However, the interest has been less in the individual symptoms of this illness and far more in the collective outcomes of this shared sickness. This echoes the idea that white culture is dangerously neurotic, but also attempts to account for the painful ways in which black peoples may internalise this neurosis. While much of Fanon's work, and most notably *The Wretched of the Earth*, documents the particular pathologies of colonial regimes for both coloniser and colonised, it is the suggestions of *Black Skin White Masks* which have had the most enduring legacy. This work has been taken as a method of understanding the painful subject formation of all racially subjugated peoples and the core insight that the experience of racism may change your sense of who you are remains invaluable to analysis across a range of settings. Fanon's work suggests that the cultures of racism pervade the deepest recesses of subject formation and that the violence and supremacism of white colonising cultures have given rise to dangerous neurosis around race, a neurosis in which we all take part. Fanon suggests that the excessive phobia of blackness which can be seen in many aspects of white culture and in many white individuals is, in fact, an indication of an unrealisable desire for blackness as a sign of the sexual. Even when they wield real and dangerous social power, racists reveal that they themselves are unhappy, fixated upon those they hate in irresolvable ways. More importantly still, for Fanon and for cultural studies, the continuing encounter with racism scars the psyche of black people. In a culture of racism black people come to regard themselves as objects of an unfriendly white gaze.

> And then the occasion arose when I had to meet the white man's eyes. An unfamiliar weight burdened me. The real world challenged my claims. In the white world the man of color encounters difficulties in the development of his bodily schema. Consciousness of the body is a solely negating activity. It is a third-person consciousness. The body is surrounded by an atmosphere of certain uncertainty (Fanon, 1986, p. 110).

Fanon suggests that the exercise of neurotic white power constitutes black people as no more than their burdensome black bodies, in which the ever-present danger of irrational rage resides as a threat to the black self, never the white other.

Cultural studies has thus played a strategic role in problematising the conventional understandings of mental illness and ethnicity. We have already questioned the idea of restricting ethnicity to a common ancestry or sense of belonging associated with language, religion and other cultural traits. The complex differences between ethnic groups, their different historical patterns of settlement as well as class and gender differences make generalisations highly suspect when it comes to ethnic mapping. We have also noted how ethnicity has become a coded world for the racial other, and hence the ethnic characteristics and pathologies of dominant white ethnicity remain hidden.

The tendency to equate ethnicity with skin colour has had another effect, which has been to ignore the racialisation of subordinate white ethnicities. In the case of the Irish, Liam Greenslade has argued that mental illness amongst the Irish can in part be explained in terms of what Fanon referred to as the internalisation of racism. Others have traced the allegedly high rates of mental illness both to the potato famine and repression brought about by English colonialism and Roman Catholicism. Ni Nullain has argued that mental illness is no higher in Ireland than in Britain. The difference is attributed to the different criteria used to diagnose schizophrenia which results in apparently higher rates in Ireland. Moreover, the Irish figure also needed disaggregating since it was also found that illness occurred disproportionately in relatively isolated geographical pockets (Clarke, 1998, pp. 314–15). This still leaves open the question of higher rates of illness amongst the Irish in Britain, a statistic which could be explained in part in terms of the age distribution of the Irish population on the mainland and which in turn might weaken the kind of cohesion which might offer protection against mental breakdown (ibid., p. 315).

Quantitative versus Qualitative Research

Given both its disciplinary background and critique of all forms of elite culture, it is not particularly surprising to find that in terms of research, philosophy and method, cultural studies has traditionally located itself in opposition to positivistic approaches to knowledge (Johnson). There is a strong tendency amongst both cultural theorists and those more reliant on field research to be highly suspicious of quantitative data and the techniques used to collect it. Indeed, in the critiques of such approaches, cultural studies academics have questioned how statistical categories are produced, who produces them, how they get used and whose interests do they serve, the assumption being most data are used to monitor, regulate and objectify, rather than empower subordinate groups. The view is thus widely held that all knowledges including and particularly those which purport to exemplify neutral science have very definite political origins and effects (McNeil).

We shall explore this dominant view within cultural studies with reference to both quantitative and qualitative approaches to the study of mental health and ethnicity. A recent, relatively sophisticated, quantitatively-informed study carried out by James Nazroo and colleagues at the Policy Studies Institute (1996, 1997) will serve to illustrate a number of points of debate with respect to this kind of research. The aim of the study was to measure levels of psychosis and depression across a range of ethnically defined populations. The research did not just take ethnic differences into account but also subdivided groups by gender, country of origin and age, thus providing a more complex picture than many previous studies. The survey revealed, for example, that whilst Bangladeshi men and women were *less* likely to be depressed than white men, Indian and African-Asian men were *as* likely to be depressed as their white counterparts. African men and women, on the other hand, were found to have a higher rate of depression (1996, p. 318). Likewise, in the case of psychosis, Caribbean women were at the highest risk, twice that of white women, who themselves had higher rates than white men (ibid.).

Although the PSI study avoided simplistic and static notions of ethnicity, other questions remain. According to Armstrong, even in their most benign form, population surveys of this kind only serve as instruments of mapping and surveillance (1983, p. 29). Despite the researchers' best efforts to subdivide ethnicity by national origin, gender etc., cultural studies requires us to ask whether these sub-divisions merely represent yet more ways of inscribing and hence objectifying the body in terms of illness and ethnicity. The fact that the study qualifies ethnicity in terms of country of origin, gender etc. does not get around the problematic notion of fixed, essential ethnic differences. You just end up increasing the number of such divisions.

The processes by which people come to see themselves and how they are perceived by others (including both researchers and powerful institutions like medicine, social work or the police) are significant because they shape social relations and inequalities. Research which generates quantitative data is always in danger of imposing identity labels on people along with a battery of policies to match, rather than enabling people to define themselves. Few within cultural studies would endorse the idea of some predefined identity or subjectivity. More commonly held is Judith Butler's view of subjectivity as nothing more than an accumulation of contested versions of self and other.

There is another way of thinking about quantitative research which is arguably in keeping with the spirit of cultural studies if not prevailing tendencies within the field. Rather than assuming that all quantitative data will inevitably lead to labelling and disempowerment as the above argument suggests, it could be argued, on the contrary, that statistical data can be used to identify and challenge racial discrimination and inequalities. The question behind such an argument thus concerns how much scope there is to take advantage of quantitative research or, at the very least, to limit or resist its worst effects? Rather than assume the political outcome of research from the research method, why not leave open the question of the effects of such research and link such a discussion to an analysis of the use of and struggles over such knowledge by the various interested parties? In other words, in the case of the PSI survey a more strategic evaluation would be rooted in an assessment of the research's uses and effects, rather on the basis of its chosen research method.

This last point also suggests that the same research findings lend themselves to different interpretations. For example, evidence which confirms that disproportionate numbers of African-Caribbean men are forcibly sectioned under the 1983 Mental Health Act can be used to prove the discriminatory role of statutory agencies (police, psychiatrists) in reaching such judgments and moreover that stereotypical assumptions made about young black male behaviour underpin such discriminatory practices (Sashidaran). On the other hand, the same data can, and has been used to suggest that the figures confirm that black people are indeed suffering from mental illness, but this is entirely due to the discriminatory way in which they are treated in the wider society. As Littlewood suggests racism is enough to send anyone mad (cited in Clarke). In the first case, illness is a racist fiction, whilst in the second, racism creates a mad reality. There is a third explanation of the evidence which rests on biological, racist arguments, i.e. that mental illness results from innate racial characteristics. Which interpretation becomes the majority-held view, and the processes by which legitimacy for a particular argument is secured or diminished, is part of the remit of cultural studies, or at least it could be.

Despite the fact that the first two, and the third explanation above sit at different ends of the political spectrum, all three share a tendency common to all quantitative research, that is they turn people into statistical aggregates. We have argued that this is in contrast to a strong cultural studies (and sociological) tradition which has sought to put subjectivity and agency back into the analysis of ethnicity and 'race'.

This latter approach is to be found in an ethnographic research tradition which aims to explore the meanings associated with decision-making processes as well as those attached to cultural differences between different ethnic groups. Sociological methods of symbolic interactionism and ethnomethodological studies of health have been utilised to this end and the overlap in broad terms with cultural studies is marked at these points. Although not in the area of mental health, David Kelleher makes the case for utilising ideas of ethnic difference when it comes to understanding health issues, and in his own work shows how different groups react to and make sense of pain. He acknowledges that there are dangers of reifying such findings and of attributing them to groups in ways which can be interpreted stereotypically. However, according to Kelleher, it *is* possible to argue that ethnicities are not fixed either in terms of characteristics of membership whilst at the same time acknowledging that some differences (e.g. perceptions of pain) are worth taking into account in health research and policy.

The commitment to giving voice to subordinate groups has been an important principle underpinning cultural studies research, albeit with a bias towards young over older people and gender, class and ethnic differences over questions of disability and mental illness. Arguably it has been less common to give voice to the mentally ill, or those defined as such. As we suggested above, access to such groups and the practicalities of conducting such research are factors which help to explain this imbalance. Kelleher's arguments alert us to the dangers of a 'top-down' research approach which may serve only to consolidate existing power/knowledge relations within mental health arenas. Instead his research looks for differences within ethnic groups not from large scale epidemiological surveys but from qualitative interviews with different ethnic groups. This 'bottom-up' research allows research subjects to be just that, i.e. subjects, rather than statistical categories. It provides an opportunity to explore the complexities such as age and gender differences although the size of most qualitative studies make generalisations more difficult. The most important point remains however who is in control of the definitions and labels attached to groups and how are they subsequently used.

Michael Angrosino, an anthropologist who acknowledges the significance of cultural studies in his research, comes close to this 'bottom-up' approach (1998). Instead of seeing the characteristics of the 'mentally ill' as essentially fixed and amenable to objective description (a common anthropological assumption), Angrosino stresses the mediated, dynamic aspects of culture. He also stresses the form of the research over its content which, in his case, meant organising his ideas and data around a short-story, fictional, narrative style. The characters were thus sometimes composites and sometimes exaggerated versions of real-life characters. The events described were often based on events witnessed by the author and sometimes imagined on the basis of what he knew of the people, i.e. evidence he acquired both as a volunteer and later as a participant observer over a period of 10 years.

The overall effect of his research was to 'normalise' a group of men with learning difficulties or 'retards' as they are referred to in US academic literature. In these short dramatic episodes, those usually labelled and represented in statistics or by professionals, played leading roles in dramas in which naivety and ignorance were the prerogative of the narrator. At times their ethnicity was made apparent and at other times it seemed less relevant to other sources of identity, e.g. their gender or just the fact of their being labelled retarded. Asked in interview whether such a fictional form of research could have policy implications, Angrosino replied that sometimes 'fiction' could be more powerful and effective in prompting change than data presented in more abstract, quantitative forms.

A more radical position with regard to racial categorisation linked to subjectivity is to be found in the work of Gilles Deleuze and Felix Guattari (1988). They argue that racism operates by means of a process of identification, in which those who resist such categorisation as racial other, have been subject to exclusion and in some instances genocide (ibid., p. 178). The racist preoccupation with or reification of the body and particularly that of the ('over-coded') face can only be contested by a thorough dismantling of subjectivity. Mental illness is but one possible consequence of the ensuing struggles. Rhizomes, in Deleuze and Guattari's terms, are structures which are both points of racial signification *and* points of escape (ibid., p. 9). Rhizomes thus provide important opportunities for analysis and research which can either consolidate the points of territorialization and segmentation or help to sanction the escape from such categorisation and from subjectivity itself.

Much debate within cultural studies and sociology regarding the appropriateness of one research method, or one term, over another cannot be resolved at an abstract level of discussion. It is not so much about choosing, in principle, between quantitative and qualitative research, or between different categories or concepts e.g. 'black' and ethnic, racism and cultural difference/identity, or passive victim and active subject. Rather, it is to relate the choice of method and terminology to a sense of who the research is for and what are its likely effects. Rather than choosing between quantitative and qualitative research it is arguably more productive to examine the *effects* of different research data. If large-scale surveys confirm the disproportionate numbers of young African Caribbean men being labelled schizophrenic and this makes policy makers including governments etc. sit up and act then this is reason to support such research. On the other hand, if qualitative research ends up hardening popular perceptions of ethnic differences and, possibly unwittingly, helping to create new stereotypes, then from a political standpoint is arguably more problematic than quantitative data which highlights discrimination and/or sanctions positive policy changes.

Cultural studies creates itself as an oppositional form of knowledge, a way of thinking and understanding the world which reveals the powers behind all kinds of normative thinking. The formative work in cultural studies analyses institutional power as the most devious of formations. Most writing around the issue of mental health and race assumes that minority communities are the object of study and debate. A cursory study of the available literature shows the extent of this belief – that ethnicity is a mental health issue only for minority communities and that the mental health experience of minority communities is different in problematic way.

When we look at media accounts of mental health issues, we see that the suggestions of cultural studies writings are often confirmed. Cultural studies has famously championed the importance of popular understandings in any account of social meaning. This has resulted in ways of working which combine methods such as ethnography with more textual analyses of media or popular texts.

Cultural studies has argued that the construction of common sense as a structure of understanding and articulation is central to any hegemonic project – and that the iniquities of our society are shored up by a complex set of popular narratives which shape our understanding and garner our (largely passive) consent for things as they are. Paying close attention to popular representations such as newspapers, television and film has been one strategy for making the construction of this supposed common sense visible and questionable. In particular, extensive work has been carried out in relation to representations of gender and race.

The representation of mental health and illness, on the other hand, has rarely been analysed within the discipline of cultural studies. For this reason, we wish to devote a section of this paper to a discussion of media representations. We hope that these initial suggestions will form a basis for more extensive and sustained work and indicate another method to usefully integrate cultural studies work into an understanding of debates around race and mental health.

On the whole, representations of mental illness and of the mentally ill refrain from the outright hate-mongering of, for example, some infamous cases of racist reporting of 'crime'. While Winston Silcott can be made into the worst of monsters by an openly racist press who decide his guilt and contribute to his wrongful arrest and imprisonment for the killing of PC Blakelock, accounts of those suffering mental illness, even when they are allegedly involved in crime, tend to pretend sympathy for the accused. Rather than depicting an idea of absolute evil and inhumanity, the mentally ill are more often portrayed as victims of unhappy circumstance. This can be seen in recent debates around the rethinking of community care. The New Labour agenda of overhauling the systems and processes of mental health care, including, most significantly, a review of the unhappy state of care in the community, received widespread agreement and applause from the British media. At last, it was implied, here was someone recognising the extreme dangers posed by the mentally ill. The widespread debate around 'The failure of care in the community' which took place across the summer of 1998 took a number of key narrative structures.[1] One was the idea that community-based care laid the general public open to attack by the mentally ill – a media myth which even the media found questionable.

> Contrary to the image projected by the media, mental patients pose a far greater threat to themselves than to the public. About 1,000 commit suicide every year compared to 26 who kill members of the public. Statistically, you are 20 times more likely to be killed by a sane than an insane person.[2]

Closely linked to this was a suggestion that mental health was an issue for the law and order debate and the wider wish to bring calm to dangerous city streets through the use of state-sanctioned force. Although these narratives made no explicit mention of race, the allusion to law and order and agendas could not fail to trigger the usual racialised agendas for a British audience. The construction of urban threat has come to be figured almost exclusively as a racial danger in recent Western cultures. Even when threats are presented as class-based, this has tended to be the racialised account of class as a biologised category.[3] When mental distress is seen as a policy issue because of an alleged threat to public order, popular understandings easily translate this into a racial threat. Thus the announcements that the review of care in the community would include increasing the powers of doctors to force people given a psychiatric diagnosis to take medication, feeds smoothly into the idea that those perceived as dangers to society should be controlled by any means available. In effect, these people are more likely to be from racialised communities, and particularly, to be young black men. The racialised outcomes of regarding mental health issues as part of law and order are seen painfully clearly in the death of Roger Sylvester. Police detained Roger Sylvester, a young black man from Tottenham, under the Mental Health Act on 11 January 1999. In the course of being detained, he suffered respiratory failure and had to be resuscitated in hospital. On 18 January, Roger Sylvester died. His case echoes a long line of deaths in custody in Britain in which young black men have suffered respiratory failure in the course of being restrained. Suggesting that mental health care should become even more closely aligned to the criminal justice and penal systems can only increase this danger.

Community-based Mobilisations: the Case of MIND and ...

In keeping with a strong tradition within cultural studies, we have chosen to conclude this chapter with a view of mental health and ethnicity from the perspective of local community-based organisations in order to examine why and who different forms of ethnic identification have become significant in political campaigns and interventions. The secondary documentation of such groups, in this case MIND in Tower Hamlets and the Franz Fanon Centre in Birmingham can serve to illustrate these processes of self-identification, group mobilisation and political intervention. In the case of MIND, its 'open door' policy has been found to work for some ethnic groups but not for others. As is often the case with a policy which purports to be inclusive, it ended up including the dominant ethnic group to the exclusion of others. The appointment of staff from different ethnic backgrounds, in addition to outreach work in the communities helped to build up its clientele, so that in 1994–95 the Advocacy Project (which involved supporting people often over their right to determine their own treatment), supported 140 people of Bangladeshi origin, 92 white UK, and 47 of African-Caribbean background. The Open House project, which offered a range of activities, including workshops, outings and group work, was used by 89 UK whites, 24 of Bangladeshi and 18 of African Caribbean origin. Other projects include the 'Chance to Work' which provides training in picture framing and the opportunity to develop retailing skills in local shops where the products are sold. Projects have been monitored by ethnicity and where gaps are noted, new initiatives have targeted particular ethnic groups.

Informal patterns of exclusion prompted MIND to run an ethnically specific project – Daryeelka – in response to specific issues relating to the Somali community. The project actually grew out of the Black and Ethnic Communities Project (BECP) for which funding ended in 1994–95. The problems with BECP were a combination of under-resourcing, over-ambition and diffuseness of purpose. Somalis had been long-time settlers in the area due to the proximity of the docks and their role as seamen. In the 1980s a civil war led to a new influx seeking refugee status. Their wartime experiences and their reception in the UK created a need for mental health services which was not then being met by statutory agencies. Three workers were funded in 1994 but this figure was reduced to two in 1996. The range of provision included: an informal drop-in centre which provided advice through an interpreter on housing benefits and form filling, etc.; a women's woodwork group and crèche which was started in 1996, and a lunch club which was started in the spring of 1994.

As a result of the project, people who would otherwise have not known about MIND or sought support began to hear about a project specifically for Somalis. People with different kinds of problems including post-natal depression, post-traumatic stress and substance abuse were identified. Project workers were not only able to establish a relationship with Somalis, but also to debunk the myths surrounding that, eschewing and campaigning for better provision within the statutory sector. As a result, more Somalis became aware of the project and sought help.

We would like to end the piece with another voice. Errol Francis is both a mental health practitioner, programme director of the Franz Fanon Centre in Birmingham, and a researcher in the field of cultural studies. His ideas offer a way forward for thinking through the debates of mental health, culture and cultural studies. Francis explained the role of the centre:

> The background [of the centre] is concerns in the black community in relation to the quality of the mental health services being delivered. The main concerns have been around the over-representation of African-Caribbean people within the mental health system. The main things have been the means by which people go into hospital, i.e. black people tend to go with the involvement of the courts or the police, the type of treatment they get once they are in hospital which tends to be medication-based, using restraints, using restrictions and also the diagnosis of schizophrenia. Against that background there have been growing concerns and these have been voiced for twenty years at least nationally.

Francis highlighted the particular role played by fears of black rage in this institutional context,

What was different here and what made the trust decide to seek special funding to set up this organisation was the incident which occurred in Rackhams, I think about five years ago, where a man called X went into the store and attacked about a dozen white women with a knife and actually slashed their throats. It was thought that he was mentally ill and it actually focused a lot of people's minds in the city around mental health services for black people. It focused the minds of the government, the then Tory government, and they started to set up special funding initiatives for certain inner city areas where they had had similar scandals. In London, too, there were a series of incidents in which young black men went out into the community and attacked white people and where mental illness was given as the reason. There were many of us who felt that it wasn't mental illness that was the motivation in fact for these outrages, but something else going on in the black community around anger and outrage. However, it was seen in a mental health frame so you get in London these special target challenge areas, and also Leeds and here.

The objectives of the project have been set to challenge the pathologisation of black people within the mental health system,

The objectives that we have set are fairly simple. The first one is that we have to improve mental health assessment. Implied in that is to try and get a more natural spread of diagnosis in which schizophrenia is not over-represented. And, where the client's perspective is taken on board, rather than a medicalising of social problems, which is what is actually happening. The second one is that we are aiming to improve access to mental health services and to make it happen earlier and more appropriately, because the evidence shows that it is not happening in the appropriate way. So instead of a police situation – the Mental Health Act – we want to get black people treatment at a primary care level where they can be looked after in their own homes and remain active in the community. The third one is to improve the engagement with the individual client, [to improve] the relationship ... of suspicion between the black client in relation to the white therapist. And to get a better satisfaction level of the individual person and the community, because clearly at the moment people are very dissatisfied.

[The goal] is to try and reduce the level of coercion involved. All these procedures, including the diagnostic procedure, involve violence in relation to the person's needs. That's why we named the centre after Franz Fanon, because we believe that there are various acts of violence being perpetrated against the black person, both in terms of the way in which their psyche is being described and in the way in which they are brought into the system.

Francis described his unorthodox route into mental health work,

> It is a very strange route which started in the early eighties with a group of young
> gay black men in London who were asking questions about why was sexuality
> medicalised, why was it that we were made to feel pathologically abnormal as
> black men. We felt at the time abnormal both in relation to our own culture,
> the black community, in terms of our sexuality and in terms of wider culture
> we felt that our sexuality was made more deviant. We became interested at
> that time in representations of ourselves in culture, and in science as deviant.
> [That was] how we were lead to the question of madness and we discovered
> the work of Michel Foucault and his work answered a lot of questions about
> our sexuality. We came to this point where we asked the question – what was
> more important to our identity, was it our sexuality or our race? Foucault
> helped us to answer this question by saying it was our race, not our sexuality.
> When he says that in the West sexuality is made to be the core of the person,
> we took that as a liberation. A hint that we could discard this sexual label and
> deal with our identity in terms of racialised being. So it freed us to forget about
> our sexual oppression and just look at the ways in which black people were
> oppressed by medicine generally.
>
>   There are a number of things which I bring with me. Firstly, disrespect for
> Western science. I have a sense of hurt and outrage about Western science
> in relation to black people, [about] the way it has inferiorised black people
> through scientific racism and nowhere is this more apparent than in a field like
> psychiatry. So I bring this scepticism. I have not been trained as a psychiatrist,
> so I feel no need to hold professional protocols. I think that has made me
> much more questioning and one of the core things I question is the way in
> which culture is a signifier for vestigial forms of the old racism. Culture here
> is a way of rehearsing genetics through other means. It is a way of rehearsing
> immutable difference through other means and it is a way of rehearsing innate
> pathology. These three levels get disguised through the way that culture is used
> as a fuzzy concept for these traditional ideas of racial difference, so I have
> come to distrust the use of the word.
>
>   It [the concept of culture] gives a lot of short-hand and sloppy thinking to
> mental health work. It encourages people to reinscribe the idea of immutable
> difference in a different way, whereas in the previous language about race
> and biology it was very explicit. I think now with culture it is implicit, so
> we have to be very careful. When you look at the literature in mental health
> work and psychiatry, what you see is a tendency towards a generalisation in
> relation to certain differences inherent in African-Caribbean or Asian people,
> the stereotypes, basically, which notions of culture seem to justify.
>
>   This service was called the African-Caribbean service and I suggested that
> we change the name to the Franz Fanon centre because there was no reliable
> way of describing the client group in terms of genetics or culture and that any

one of these was leading into one of these violences. I think what we need to take on board is have we reached the end of ethnic classification. If we are really going to argue against this background of oppressive science how can we continue the classification ourselves? Does it make any sense?

If nothing else, this is the contribution of cultural studies to argue that culture is not an essential attribute of the individual to be deciphered, but rather that what is at stake is the working of power under the guise of our shared wider culture.

Notes

1   The Failure of Care in the Community', *The Independent*, 30 July 1998 (709).
2   'Real Care', *The Guardian*, 30 July 1998, p. 17.
3   See Campbell, 1993.

References

Angrosino, M. (1998), *Opportunity House: Ethnographic Stories of Mental Retardation*, Sage, London.
Campbell, B. (1993), *Goliath*, Methuen, London.
Cochrane, R. (1983), *The Social Construction of Mental Illness*, Longman, London.
Deleuze, G. and Guattari, F. (1988), *A Thousand Plateaus: Capitalism and Schizophrenia*, The Athlone Press, London.
Fanon, F. (1986), *Black Skin White Masks*, Pluto, London.
Foucault, M. (1965), *Madness and Civilization: A History of Insanity in the Age of Reason*, Tavistock, London.
Greenslade, L. Madden, M. and Pearson, M. (1997), 'From Visible to Invisible: the Problem of the Health of Irish People in Britain', in Marks, L. and Worboys, M. (eds), *Migrants, Minorities and Health: Historical and Contemporary Studies*, Routledge, London, pp. 14–78.
Hillier, S. and Kelleher, D. (eds) (1996), *Researching Culture Differences in Health*, Routledge, London.
hooks, bell (1996), *Killing Rage, Ending Racism*, Penguin, London.
Littlewood, R. and Lipsedge, M. (1989), *Aliens and Alienists: Ethnic Minorities and Psychiatry*, Unwin Hyman, London.
Nazroo, J. et al. (1997), *Mental Health and Ethnicity: Findings from a National Community Survey*, PSI, London.
Rack, P. (1982), *Race, Culture and Mental Disorder*, Tavistock, London.

Chapter 5

Religious Issues in Ethnic Minority Mental Health: Special Reference to Schizophrenia in Afro-Caribbeans in Britain: a Systematic Review

Kate Miriam Loewenthal and Marco Cinnirella

Background

Religion and Mental Health

How does religion affect mental health? About ten years ago, there was some consensus that there was an overall positive association between the two. Underlying this, there are many effects to consider, many aspects of religion, and many aspects of mental health. The last decade has seen a mushroom-like growth of studies and reviews (see Loewenthal, 1995; Bhugra, 1996; Worthington, Kurusu, McCullough and Sandage, 1996). There is scope for methodological improvements, and many interesting questions to be answered. This review is concerned with one set of such questions: religion and mental health among Afro-Caribbeans particularly those living in the UK and the USA, with particular reference to schizophrenia.

Definition of 'Afro-Caribbean' and Scope of Research in this Review

The Hutchinson Encyclopaedia defines an Afro-Caribbean as a 'West Indian person of African descent', and adds that Afro-Caribbeans are descended from West Africans, captured, or bought from African traders by Europeans, who shipped them to European colonies in the West Indies from the sixteenth century onwards, until the abolition of slavery, which occurred in different countries and colonies at different points in the nineteenth century. Since World War II many Afro-Caribbeans have migrated to the UK, the USA and the Netherlands.

There seems to be little or no research material on mental illness on Afro-Caribbeans in the Netherlands, but there is a great deal on African Americans, and on Afro-Caribbeans in the UK, who are mostly descendants of West African slaves shipped to North American colonies, or immigrants from the West Indies.

While it is agreed that Afro-Caribbeans in Britain and African Americans in the USA have many similarities in their history and current circumstances, we have not used the terms interchangeably. We have drawn on research material from both Afro-Caribbeans in Britain and Afro-Americans, as well as on people of African descent in the Caribbean area, in Africa, and occasionally elsewhere.

Schizophrenia among Afro-Caribbeans

This review focuses on one specific set of questions: how might religion affect the reported over-representation of Afro-Caribbean groups among those diagnosed with schizophrenia in the United Kingdom? Possibly related problems are the greater use of compulsory detention under the 1983 Mental Health Act, including police involvement in hospitalization, and the use of restraint and pharmacological agents in control of Afro-Caribbean patients. Such over-representation also exists of Afro-Americans in the USA, and is by comparison both with other ethnic groups in the UK and the USA, and also with Afro-Caribbeans in African and Caribbean countries, where there has perhaps been a less marked degree of recent disadvantage and minority status (Davis, 1975; Ineichen, 1986, 1991; Cope, 1989; Thomas et al., 1993). Sugarman and Craufurd (1994) have concluded that the very high morbidity risk for schizophrenia among British Afro-Caribbeans is entirely due to environmental (not genetic) factors.

An interesting claim has been made by Littlewood and Lipsedge (1978, 1981a, 1981b), and others. Littlewood and Lipsedge based their claim on a series of studies of patients admitted with diagnoses of psychosis to a psychiatric hospital in East London. They suggest that the high rates of psychosis among Afro-Caribbeans are explained by rates of schizophrenia similar to those in other ethnic groups, plus rates based on a large number of acute psychotic reactions with paranoid and religious flavour. These latter disorders are diagnosed as schizophrenia, but resemble acute psychotic disorders described in Africa and the Caribbean, and have a sudden onset with a clear provoking agent. Littlewood and Lipsedge's patients were first-generation immigrants. Littlewood and Lipsedge's suggestions deserve further attention, particularly with regard to forms of psychosis in second-generation Afro-Caribbean immigrants, among whom rates of psychosis are reported to be even higher than in the immigrating generation. There has been no comparable work in the USA.

This review takes up the more general but related issue of the ways in which psychosis in Afro-Caribbeans may be affected by religious factors.

Social History

Afro-Caribbean social history in Britain and USA is dominated by the hideous history of slavery. European slave-traders were buying slaves from the West Coast of Africa in increasing numbers during the seventeenth and eighteenth century, particularly to provide labour for plantation development in the New World (the Caribbean and the Americas), recently colonised by European settlers. The native Indian populations were severely reduced, by desettlement, genocide and European-imported illnesses, and African slaves were a readily-available source of cheap labour for the sugar plantations. Increasing numbers of people from West Africa were kidnapped and sold into slavery, and transported across the Atlantic in horrible conditions of cruelty, filth and disease. Altogether an estimated 10 million Africans were brought to the New World in this way, mostly to the Caribbean area (Curtin, 1969). In the plantations, any family and social networks which had survived kidnapping and transportation were broken up, and the practice of native religion disallowed (Goveia, 1965). This was coupled with cruel retribution for anything other than passive obedience, engendering disorientation, helplessness, and dependence. The abolition of slavery in Europe, the Americas and the Caribbean led to some improvement in social and economic conditions, but these improvements were generally small and the social and psychological legacies of deracination and cruelty remained (Wagley, 1961; Franklin and Moss, 1988). Economic need resulted in steady migration to the Northern United States, and a flood of immigration from the Caribbean to Britain in the 1950s and 1960s. Afro-Caribbeans continue to be beset by racism, exploitation in employment, lack of opportunity, and other forms of social and economic disadvantage in both the UK (Rack, 1988) and the USA, although there have been legislative attempts to remove some of these disadvantages (Franklin and Moss, 1988; Jackson, 1991).

Religion in Afro-Caribbean Life

Afro-Caribbean religion is said to embody responses to oppression and exploitation, enabling the expression of spirituality (Baer, 1984; Griffith and Bility, 1996), the formation of communities (Turner, 1969) and hence social support and identity. The two dominant strands have been native African religions, and European Christianity. The former was suppressed, and the latter imposed upon the plantation slaves and, later, encouraged by missionaries to the freed slaves (Gates, 1980; Brewer, 1988; Chatfield, 1989). The current situation involves a huge range of often syncretistic blends, although the African elements are less overt in British and US black-led Christianity than they are in the Caribbean and its neighbourhood, and in Africa.

New black religious movements include Black Islam (Franklin and Moss, 1988; McCloud, 1995) in the USA, and Rastafarianism (Hickling and Griffith, 1994) in the Caribbean and the UK. However, in the UK and the USA the dominant form of black religion is Christianity with African influences (Jules-Rosette, 1980). Howard (1987) concluded that post-World War II Caribbean Christian immigrants to the UK expected a warm welcome from the existing churches, but found them cold and unfriendly, and so set up their own groups. Most Christian Afro-Caribbeans in the UK are now reported to be affiliated to black-led churches, with predominantly black membership. The most popular forms are Charismatic and Pentecostal Christianity and Seventh Day Adventists. Howard does not offer figures, but of Cochrane and Howell's random community sample (1993) of black men in the UK Midlands, 27 per cent belonged to generally white-led churches (Church of England, Roman Catholic), 52 per cent were Pentecostal (almost or completely black-led), and 4 per cent were Rastafarian (with 18 per cent non-affiliated). Leadership in black-led churches is generally strong and respected, since religious leaders have emerged by force of personality, charisma, popularity and dedication to the needs of their communities. There is emphasis on enthusiastic prayer, which may include the gift of speaking in tongues, dance, and trance-like possession states, and on living a moral, family-centred life, with good physical health practices, and kindness and helpfulness to others (Howard, 1987). Griffith (1980) provides a valuable description of a week-night service in a Pentecostal group in the USA. The service includes extensive and enthusiastic thanks and praise to the Lord for healing and support, as well as the features described above (speaking in tongues, etc.). Healing may be an important religious activity, and services in black-led churches are reported by their participants to be emotionally and spiritually positive experiences

(Griffith and Mathewson, 1981; Griffith, Young and Smith, 1984; Maloney and Lovekin, 1985).

Afro-Caribbean counter-culture is said to emphasise partying, promiscuity, drink and drugs (Howard, 1987), but Cochrane and Howell's figures suggest that members of this counter-culture may be a minority among Afro-Caribbeans.

Religiously, the situations in the USA and the UK are somewhat similar, although the black-led churches in the USA have a longer history than those in Britain, dating from the latter half of the nineteenth century (Franklin and Moss, 1988). Those in Britain date mainly from the post-World War II period.

In contemporary religious life in Africa, the Caribbean, and in black communities in Central and South America, the influence of traditional African religions is more overt, and the social-scientific and medical literature shows many examples of traditional African practices relating to health and mental health, some of which will be described in this review.

Definitions of Religion

There is a variety of definitions and measures of religion (Brown, 1987). Loewenthal (1995) suggests that religion involves belief in spirituality, a divinely-based moral code, and seeing the purpose of life as increasing harmony in the world by doing good and avoiding evil. All religions involve and depend on social organisation for communication of these ideas. Glock and Stark (1965) suggested five possibly orthogonal aspects of religiosity: experiential, ritual, belief, intellectual, and a fifth dimension reflecting the extent to which the first four are actually applied in daily life. In practice, four popular measures of religiosity are: affiliation, self-definition (as religious), practice (attendance, prayer and other activities), and belief.

Search Strategy

The search strategy was based on some of the guidelines indicated by the UK Cochrane Centre National Health Service Research and Development Programme (Chalmers and Haynes, 1994; Eysenck, 1994; Knipschild, 1994; Mulrow, 1994; and particularly Oxman, 1994), and by the York University National Health Service Centre for Reviews and Dissemination (1996). These guidelines suggest selecting clinical trials reaching certain standards of research design. The number of such studies in the field under review was negligible, and meta-analytic work was therefore impossible. However the guidelines were followed insofar as search terms and search strategies were defined. These were as follows:

> Three groups of search terms were used (where acceptable, the suffix * or ? followed a truncated form of words such as religious, religiosity, religion: i.e. relig* or relig? Otherwise the alternatives were spelled out):
>
> *Group 1* (religion) – Relig*, Faith, Belief*, Pentecostal*, Adventist
>
> *Group 2* (ethnicity) – Afr*, Carib*, Black, West (W) Indian, Jamaica, Trinidad, Ethnic*
>
> *Group 3* (mental health, schizophrenia, and religious behaviour which might be seen as symptomatic of disturbance) – Mental*, Schizophren*, Possession, Hallucination, Glossolalia, Trance

For electronic databases of articles, books and thesis abstracts, three groups were first formed by searching for any of the search terms in the group. The final search was for material which included at least one search term from each group.

For databases of book titles and theses (which yielded very little using the above strategy), searches were also made by combining search terms from two groups at a time: e.g. relig* afr*, relig* carib*, relig* black, etc.

Sources Searched

Electronic databases of published articles: Sociofile, Medline, ERIC, Embase, Pascal, PsychLit, BIDS (Social Sciences, Sciences, and Arts and Humanitites) In each case the search was made from the earliest year represented in the database up to the most recent; PsychLit contains articles back to 1972, but the other databases start in or around 1982.

Electronic databases of published books: PsychLit, CUPAC, Libertas, BIDS. As with databases of articles, the search was made from the earliest year represented in the database.

Electronic sources of unpublished material: theses (Dissertation Abstracts

International (1982–96), AsLib (British MPhil and PhD. theses) (1970–92), and worldwide web.

Other sources: information about ongoing work was obtained by personal contact including conference attendance, by correspondence, and via the worldwide web.

The main product of these searches was in the form of titles, author and abstract (or book chapters). This first crop was sifted for relevance, and some items immediately discarded. Others were sorted into two categories:

(a) of some relevance but no further information needed; some items were subsequently discarded as work proceeded.
(b) relevant and original book or article needed. In this latter case the item was either obtained immediately (where available), or via the inter- library loan service. Visual searches were made of the bibliographies of the most fundamental of these books and articles: Griffith (1980); Littlewood and Lipsedge (1981a, 1981b, 1989); Worthington et al. (1996); Bhugra (1996).

Conceptual Approach

The structure of the review that follows two approaches. Firstly we look at pathways into illness (influences on prevalence), using a broad conceptual framework based on Brown and Harris (1978, 1989), and which is generally popular in social psychiatric and related work. The framework involves three wide classes of variables:

STRESS (ADVERSITY) – MEDIATORS (BUFFERS) – DISTRESS (and ILLNESS)

We propose to examine the influences of religion within each of these classes. The second approach is to examine pathways into care. We examine how religion may affect:

REFERRAL – DIAGNOSIS – TREATMENT.

The review focuses on schizophrenia in Afro-Caribbean groups, but some related material has been included, on religion and mental health generally, and particularly in Afro-Caribbeans, and on Afro-Caribbean religion, both in relation to healing, and in relation to behaviours which may be religiously sanctioned and adaptive, but which might give rise to misdiagnosis by psychiatrists and others ignorant of cultural and religious mores.

Religious Influences on Prevalence

Adversity

Here we consider ways in which religion may effect levels and types of adversity (stress), and ways in which religious factors may moderate the effects of adversity. We consider first the beneficial affects of religious factors, and then the possibility of stress-exacerbating effects of religious factors.

First, then, the question whether religious factors may help to minimise adversity. We are not concerned here with general cultural factors – the economic and social difficulties which may be associated with being Afro-Caribbean.

Loewenthal et al. (1996) suggested that patterns of stress – and therefore possibly distress and illness – differed between traditional religious groups and others, among Europeans. Their main conclusion was that severe, disruptive life-events were less likely among traditional religious groups. This in turn had an impact on the prevalence of depression. We could not find comparable data for Afro-Caribbeans in Britain, but a study of black Americans (Gary, 1984) led to roughly comparable conclusions. This study involved 451 non-institutionalized black adults in Virginia, and one conclusion was that less religious respondents experienced more stressful life circumstances. Further work is needed to confirm the suggestion that religious groups and beliefs may serve to regulate social relations, lessening the likelihood of some forms of stress.

Finally, an intriguing case study suggests further positive features of religious beliefs on stress. Heligman, Lee and Kramer (1983) reported on an elderly black lady who was able to tolerate major abdominal surgery without analgesia. There was minimal post-operative discomfort. She attributed this to the presence of protective angels. Psychological testing and interviews showed her to be 'fully in touch with reality'.

The sparse material described so far has thrown up several recurrent and important themes in understanding the roles played by religion in Afro-

Caribbean mental health. First, the probable importance of religion to many Afro-Caribbeans. Second, the importance of religiously-encouraged social support networks. And finally, the occurrence of religiously-based beliefs and ideas which might be taken as evidence of psychological disturbance by professional care workers without sufficient knowledge of cultural-religious norms and values.

Moderating Effects of Religion

Several studies indicate that compared with other groups in Britain and the USA, religion is a more important value for Afro-Caribbeans. Boyd-Franklin (1989) (USA), in a review highlighting five fundamental strengths in black families and implications for treatment, found that one strength is strong religious orientation. Cochrane and Howell (1995) (UK), in a study of a random sample of 200 black and 170 white men, found that similar proportions of blacks (74 per cent) and whites (75 per cent) had religious affiliations but a higher proportion of blacks (29 per cent) than whites (9 per cent) attended regularly. Edwards (1987) (USA), in a study of self-defined religious components of psychological health, with a sample of 25 black adults, eight male and 17 female, found that of the five essential characteristics of a psychologically healthy black American, religion and spirituality were the most important. Ellison (1995) (USA), in a summary of three major surveys, found that average levels of religious engagement are higher among African Americans than among whites. Ferraro and Koch (1994) (USA), using a national sample ('Americans' Changing Lives 1986'), found that the three dimensions of religiosity were strongest among black adults and women. Jones (1990) (USA), in a review of literature on effectiveness of white therapists treating black clients, found that therapists should consider, among other factors, the intense religious orientations of black people. Rosen (1982) (USA), in interviews with 148 senior citizens (aged over 65), found that blacks used religion to a greater degree than did whites, both to cope with adversity and to reduce depression. The above is replete with suggestions and evidence that religion is indeed important to Afro-Caribbeans in the UK and to Afro-Americans, both in absolute terms and relative to other groups.

We now turn to evidence on the question, whether and how religion has a stress-moderating effect among black people. Brown and Gary (1987) (USA), in a study of 177 black males and 274 females found no direct buffering effects of religiosity on mental health, and only among females on physical health. In 1998, in a further study of 245 black females, Brown and Gary found that high religiosity (and perceived social support) was important in reducing distress, especially in the unemployed compared to the employed. Brown and Gary (1994) (USA), in a study of 537 urban black males, found that denominational affiliation was associated with fewer depressive symptoms and that higher frequency of church attendance was associated with less alcohol and cigarette consumption.

Cochrane and Howell (1995) (UK), in a study of a random sample of 200 black men and 170 white men, found that religious observance and belonging to a Pentecostal church were strongly associated with moderation in alcoho,l and a relation between lower alcohol consumption and problems among blacks explained by black religiosity. Ellison (1995) (USA), in a study of a community sample of 1,029 blacks and 1,927 whites, found that denominational affiliation was associated with fewer symptoms among blacks only and that frequency of church attendance was associated with fewer depressive symptoms among whites only; frequency of private devotion was associated with depressive symptoms among both black and whites. Ferraro and Koch (1994) (USA), in their study using the 'Americans' Changing Lives 1986' sample, found that the association between religion and health differs between black and white people. Social support is important for health in both black and whites but the religious consolation hypothesis was supported for blacks only and there was no overall association between religion and health among blacks. Martin (1984) (USA), looked at annual suicide rates and church attendance and found that religiosity (church attendance) was associated with lower suicide among both black and white in both males and females. Millet, Sullivan, Schwebel and Myers (1996) (USA), asked 67 black and 78 white subjects to read vignettes on mental health problems and rate the importance of spiritual and other factors as causes and their effectiveness in treatment. They found that Black American respondents rated spiritual factors as more important in aetiology and treatment than did whites. Platt (1995) (UK), used a sample of 100 church members (Seventh Day Adventists) and 100 non-members and found that religiosity was associated with fewer mental health and health problems. However, the groups were not closely matched for ethnicity, as 79 per cent of the church members were black but only 37 per cent of non-members. Taylor and Jackson (1991) (USA), in a study of 289 urban African-American women found seven variables including religious orientation were significantly related to general mental health symptoms.

The above tells us nothing directly about schizophrenia, and little about the stress-buffering effects of religion, but it does indicate a strong association between religion and various measures of health and mental health: low or absent religiosity is a risk factor for poor (mental) health in black people.

There is evidence on means by which religion may be associated with better mental health among black people. Looking at the area of social support and family, Boyd-Franklin (1989) (USA), in a review highlighting five fundamental strengths in black families and implications for treatment, found that one strength was the bond of the extended family. Brown and Gary (1987) (USA), with a sample of 451 urban black adults, found that the number of near relatives was related to mental health in females and that perceived social support buffered the effect of stress on mental health. Amongst the males, the number of confidants was inversely related to physical health. Caldwell, Greene and Billingsley (1994) (USA), in a review of historical material and their own research programme, found that family support programmes provided by black churches had changed over time. Ferraro and Koch (1994) (USA), mentioned above, found that social support was important for health in both black and whites. Gary (1984) (USA), in a probability sample of 451 black adults, found that low religiosity and aspects of low social support, for example, being divorced or separated or not being an active community participant were associated with more stress. Gary (1995) (USA), using the same sample, found that religion was unrelated to perceived conflict in male/ female relationships. Howard (1987) (UK), in a review of studies on Afro-Caribbean Christianity in Britain, found that church leaders were respected for their personal qualities and turned to for advice and guidance on matters which may enhance family stability, for example, banning extra-marital sex. The importance of church leadership was again highlighted by Stevenson (1990) (USA), with reference to education about teenage pregnancy. Walls and Zarit (1991) (USA), interviewed 98 elderly black people, aged 65 to 104 years, and found that the family network was perceived as more supportive than the church network, but that both contributed to feelings of well-being. However, involvement with organised religious activities and spiritual aspects of religion were found to be unrelated to well-being.

In the area of worship-related activities, Ellison (1995) (USA) found that in a community sample (2,956) of both black and white, the frequency of private devotional activity (e.g. prayer) was associated with depressive symptoms in both blacks and whites. Griffiths (1980) (USA) observed Wednesday night black church services which had an attendance of about 11 per cent of Sunday church services made up mainly of church activists. The service took the form of thanks to God, led by male members, the pastor then led the members in giving testimony and saying how God had helped them cope. Possession and trance states were observed, especially among the women and also glossolalia and members reported feelings of love, warmth and rebirth. Griffiths and

Mathewson (1981) (USA), as described above, found that this religious group compared to the 'healing community', which involves 'communitas' and 'healing charisma'. There was a suggestion that improvements in psychiatric status may be 'more than transient'. Griffiths, Young and Smith (1984) (USA), in interviews with 20 young attenders of these midweek services, aged 18 to 27 years, described feelings and behaviours in relation to four main components of the service; testimony – ineffable, religious; possession – ecstasy, relief; dancing and glossolalia – religious. As a whole, feelings of group closeness, hope, altruism, self-expression and helping others were described. Ness and Weintrob (1981) (USA), describes faith healing in fundamentalist Christian groups and the belief in rootwork among black and white people in the south eastern USA.

A third route by which mental health and religion may be connected is by the socio-cognitive factors of belief and identity. Bartocci (1975) (South Africa), in a study of 33 Bantu and 30 'coloured' patients during their first hospitalisation with psychosis, found that the 'coloured' patients' disorders were more serious (hebephrenic) and that they had no solid cultural background. The Bantus had a structured background with animistic beliefs and a firmer ego/identity. Hickling, Griffith and others (1994) (Jamaica), in a discussion of clinical perspectives on the Rastafari movement, suggested that it may provide an affirmation of black identity and a moral framework. Hill (1987) (USA), observing a Simba Wachanga ceremony and discussing the rearing of the African-American child, found a need for coming of age rituals and other rituals to ensure continuity of culture and cultural identity. Littlewood (1993) (Trinidad), in a medical anthropology study, discusses the relations between pathology and identity. Gessler and Nahim (1984) (Sierra Leone), in a study of 200 in-patients and 207 out-patients at the only western mental hospital, found that the more seriously ill patients were less likely to have social support, were more likely to express western ideas about the causes of mental illness and were more likely to have western treatments than out-patients, suggesting weak identity. Redlener and Scott (1979) (USA), in a case study of a 9-month-old black child admitted to hospital with meningitis and brain damage, with a devout mother and a grandmother who was a minister of the Holiness Church, found a belief in the efficacy of prayer and reform of the sufferer and his/her social network. Snow (1974) (USA), in interviews with members and ministers of the Holiness Church, found beliefs in the efficacy of prayer and repentance.

Religion may lower the prevalence of mental illness among black people by mitigating the effects of stress. First, social support: both church and family support are important to well-being, and family support may be enhanced by church membership. But as with research in other groups, the relations between religion and social support could do with further clarification. Social support is important for recovery and prevention of relapse as well as prevention of initial onset.

Second, worship-related activities have been reported to induce feelings of well-being, comfort and other aspects of positive mood, which are likely to have a beneficial effect on mental health.

Third, religion is associated with social-cognitive factors such as identity, self-esteem and beliefs which can have a positive impact on mood.

In all cases however there is a lack of outcome studies. Additionally we know very little about the relations between the factors described, and schizophrenia, in black people.

We now look at possible adverse effects of religion upon mental health, by belief in sin and suffering and the belief in evil or harmful spirits or witchcraft.

Looking at the belief in sin and suffering, Redlener and Scott (1979) (USA), in the case study previously mentioned, found that the grandmother believed that the child's serious condition was due to the mother failing to pray enough. Snow (1974) (USA), in interviews with members and ministers of the Holiness Church, found a belief that illness can be sent as a punishment for sin or as a reminder to improve. A child's illness could be sent as a result of the parents' sins. Because of this, a doctor might not be able to heal the illness. Littlewood and Lipsedge (1989) (UK), in a case study, observed that the patient was self-harming and self-destructive as she had had a strictly religious and physically abusive upbringing and felt that she was irredeemably bad.

On the subject of belief in evil spirits and witchcraft, Erinosho (1977b) (Nigeria), looking at four case histories of Nigerian patients undergoing psychotherapy, found that all expressed a belief in the evil machinations of others through witchcraft. This belief was not confined to the non-literate. Lefley and Bestman (1977) (USA and Caribbean), in a description and discussion of psychotherapy in Caribbean cultures, covering indigenous healing systems; Voudou (Haiti), Obeah or witchcraft (British West Indies, Virgin Islands, Bahamas), Espiritismo (Puerto Rica), mentions the practice of various forms of hexing. Hillard and Rockwell (1978) (USA), in a case study of an intelligent, well-educated black woman from the rural southern USA suffering from dysesthesia, suggested that the dysesthesia was a conversion reaction, and that it responded to conventional psychotherapy. The patient believed that she was the victim of witchcraft. They suggested that beliefs in witchcraft (rootwork and hexing) should be asked about in patients with unusual symptoms and the appropriate cultural background. Littlewood and Lipsedge (1978, 1981a and 1981b) (UK), in a study of patients admitted with diagnoses of psychosis, found that many Afro-Caribbeans had a paranoid and religious flavour, resembling 'Bouffes delirantes' described in the French West Africa, in which the persecutory content is often linked to witchcraft. Patel (1995) (Africa), reviewing studies of beliefs about the causes of mental illnesses from 11 countries in sub-Saharan Africa, found that causes can include spiritual factors. Stevens (1987) (Africa), reviewing three case histories, suggested that belief in witchcraft and fear of ancestor retribution in Africa and developing countries may play a role in acute psychoses. Ward and Beaubron (1981) (UK), made a study of 20 members of a West Indian Pentecostal group, 16 women and four men, all of whom believed in malevolent spirit possession, and who were tested with the EPI and the neurotic hysteria scale of the MMPI. They found that the 10 subjects who were defined as spirit-possessed scored significantly higher on neuroticism and hysteria than did the control group. They suggested that possession may be a culture-bound disorder.

The important suggestions are that belief in a relation between sin or wrongdoing, and suffering, may actually cause symptoms of distress or illness. However, these beliefs may contain the seeds of cure, insofar as they indicate remedies which may sometimes be effective. A further important effect is that 'Western' health professionals with inadequate knowledge of cultural-religious mores may view such beliefs as signs of mental disorder.

We noted that there was no reported evidence that religion plays a role in creating or exacerbating adversity. However, religiously-associated physical/emotional abuse is a possibility that has been suggested – often controversially – among other groups (Capps, 1992) and could be examined in Afro-Caribbeans.

Overall, the weight of evidence and of suggestions is that religion is important to Afro-Caribbeans, is likely to have beneficial effects (overall) in lowering prevalence of mental illnesses, and that these effects operate via a number of routes. We note however that little of the research relates directly to schizophrenia. Research designs are generally observational or correlational or involve the reporting of clinical case material. Further research could focus on schizophrenia, and involve designs which look at outcome either retrospectively or if possible prospectively.

Religious Influences on Referral

Having looked at religious influences on the prevalence of schizophrenia (pathways into illness) we now look at pathways into care and/or diagnosis. Sometimes there is genuine overlap in research material bearing on the two problems, in which case we have repeated our citations of the studies concerned.

Religious factors may discourage black people from consulting orthodox medical and mental health services, either because it is seen or used as a more effective form of coping or because of religious/social disapproval of the use of orthodox services. Jones (1992) (USA), in a literature review on psychotherapy with African-American women, found that spirituality is an important construct and coping strategy within the African-American culture. Lefley and Bestman (1977) (USA and Caribbean), as mentioned previously, described indigenous healing systems in the Caribbean. Millet, Sullivan, Schwebel and Myers (1996), in their study where 67 black and 78 white patients, read vignettes on mental health problems and rated the importance of spiritual and other factors as causes and their effectiveness in treatment, found that black American respondents rated spiritual factors as more important in aetiology and treatment than did whites. Purdy, Simari and Colon (1983) (USA), gave questionnaires on religion, mental illness and the pastor's role to 32 black and 73 Puerto Rican members of five Pentecostal churches and found that the majority of those surveyed would turn to their pastor rather than to a counsellor or clinician for help with personal or family problems. In the Redlener and Scott (1979) (USA) study of the devoutly religious mother and grandmother and child with meningitis and brain damage, the mother and grandmother said that the baby should be removed from hospital so that proper prayers could be started. The grandmother believed that an illness of the mother had been cured by prayer and the child's condition would not be so serious if the mother had prayed more. Silva de Crane and Spielberger (1981) (USA), looked at the attitudes to mental illness of 309 18–35-year-old Anglo, Spanish American and black undergraduates, and found that blacks and Hispanics had more negative and less benevolent attitudes to mental illness than whites (suggesting possibly a greater degree of stigma).

The material above is rather sparse, but as far as it goes supports the suggestion that religious factors may, for various reasons, discourage black people from seeking help for mental illness from (white) mental health professionals: Afro-Caribbeans may fear that their religious beliefs and values may be misunderstood, they may perceive the mental health professions as ineffective or misguided, they may perceive other (religious) helping agents and activities as more effective, and there may be fear of stigma.

If religious helping agents and activities are seen as effective, what are they? Griffith, Young and Smith (1984) (USA), in interviews with 20 regular attenders of a mid-week black church service, suggested that the service is a mental health resource. The features are testimony, possession, dancing and speaking in tongues and the therapeutic factors include hope, group cohesiveness, altruism and helping. Lefley and Bestman (1977) (USA), when looking at the health needs and provision for Caribbean immigrant groups in Miami, described the belief in hexing and the use of folk healers and the need for a health provision that combines both traditional and scientific approaches to psychotherapy. Mollica, Streets and Boscarino (1986) (USA), in a survey of 116 traditional clergy, including 21 black clergy, found that the black clergy were functioning as a major mental health resource compared with others, some of whose activities were very limited. This was partly due to the emergence of pastoral counsellors who have largely taken over the counselling functions of clergy among non-blacks. Purdy, Simari and Colon (1983), as mentioned above, found that the majority of the sample would turn to their pastor rather than to a counsellor or clinician for help with personal and family problems.

These studies offer a relatively high degree of quantification, and suggest a range of religious resources seen by black people (at least, those who are church members) as efficacious for mental health problems.

Religious Influences on Symptoms/Diagnosis

An important theme which has intruded throughout this review is the regrettable tendency of (usually white) mental health professionals to regard a range of religious behaviours and beliefs by black people as symptomatic of mental illness. Sometimes indeed there may be a genuine mental illness and it is difficult for the professional to tell whether say, a religious ecstasy, is pathological or not (e.g. Littlewood and Lipsedge, 1989; Csordas, 1987). The cases below, however, give some cause for concern regarding the risk of over-diagnosis of mental illness, particularly of schizophrenia, in black people with religious 'symptoms' and suggest that some religiously endorsed or encouraged behaviour may be regarded as psychotic or otherwise disturbed.

Alonso and Jeffrey (1988) (USA), looking at four case studies of Cuban American psychiatric patients, suggested that belief in spirit possession fostered by the syncretic Afro-Christian religion, Santeria, may have complicated diagnosis and treatment. Ananth (1984) (USA) looked at a case study of a 19-year-old black woman who died the day after treatment for a sudden psychosis with hyper-religiosity. The post mortem showed thymoma, showing that in patients with psychosis with hyper-religiosity, an organic cause should be considered. Dobbin (1983) (Montserrat, West Indies). in an anthropological analysis of ethnographic data on the Jombee dance. found that the music and steps were European influenced but that the role of trance-divining, the intervention of ancestor Jombees (spirits who possess the dancers) and the use of Obeah, indicate African roots. Early and Lifeschutz (1974) (USA), a case study of a 10-year-old black girl who experienced religious stigmata, including bleeding, and auditory hallucinations of a religious nature, found that she showed no evidence of psychopathology. Hickling, Griffith and others (1994), as mentioned above, encouraged clinicians to diagnose on phenomenological grounds, rather than social behaviour in the case of Rastafarians whose beliefs and practices include wearing dreadlocks, sacramental use of marijuana and opposition to traditional government. Hall (1994) (USA) is an historical analysis of the religious experiences of blacks in Florida from 1565 to 1906, which traces the development of independent black churches from the period of slavery (when slaves were relegated to separate pews in white dominated churches). The final chapter focuses on the centrality and persistence of possession-like ritual behaviour over the period studied. Hillard and Rockwell (1978) as mentioned earlier, found that the patient believed she was a victim of witchcraft even though the dysesthesia was a conversion reaction which responded to conventional psychotherapy. In Lipsedge's (1996) (UK) medical review of religion and madness, there was little found to support Zilboorg and Henry's 1941 conclusion that madness was widely believed to be caused by possession. A number of cases involving religious phenomenology were examined, holy anorexia, possession, visions, etc., as were the debates regarding whether the sufferer was saintly or mad. Lipsedge points out that religious means were an effective way for women to gain an audience in cultures of female disempowerment. Littlewood and Lipsedge (1989) (UK) described how, in a case study of a female patient in a state of extreme religious enthusiasm ,who was excited and talking or babbling incoherently, the psychiatrist thought this was glossolalia but the members of her Pentecostal church said it was not. Ndetei (1998) (UK) looked at the phenomenology of psychiatric illness in a London hospital and the socio-cultural backgrounds of West Indian, African and Asian immigrants to the UK, using a sample of 593 psychiatric inpatients. The findings were that paranoid and religious phenomenology were associated with African and West Indian groups for cultural reasons rather than their socio-environmental and racial status in Britain. Paranoia was directed to fellow-immigrants rather than to the host population. There was also a suggestion that auditory hallucinations and first rank symptoms of schizophrenia do not have the same diagnostic significance in every culture and that paranoid and religious phenomenology may not have the same clinical significance among Africans and Afro-Caribbeans. Ndetei and Vadher (1984) further found cultural differences in persecutory, grandiose, religious, sexual and fantastic delusions and that all are at relatively higher frequencies in West Indian and African groups. Redlener and Scott (1979) (USA), as previously cited, found that the mother was described by the hospital social worker as relating to the child in a loving but unrealistic manner, saying that the child was special to her and that she fasted and prayed for his recovery and attributed the illness to 'demonic forces' and wanted to take the child home. In court hearings regarding custody, the mother was evaluated as 'paranoid-schizophrenic' and allowed supervised visits only. The child was eventually institutionalised and the suggestion is made that this outcome was the result of incompatibility between medical and religious ideology. Ward (1982) (various) looked at four case histories of 25–38-year-old women from syncretic subcultures in traditional societies and examined spirit possession as a form of personal maladjustment and as a form of social protest. It was suggested that pathological possession states are precipitated by difficulties like those in industrialised societies but are coloured by traditional beliefs. As discussed earlier, Ward and Beaubrun (1981) suggested that possession may be a culture-bound disorder.

The above cases offer a range of descriptive material suggesting that trance/possession, beliefs in evil spirits and witchcraft, and other forms of religious behaviour and beliefs, are particularly likely among people whose background has been influenced by African religion. It is difficult for professionals to distinguish the genuinely pathological from the culturally alien.

An interesting footnote is offered by two studies which suggest the presence and amount of religious symptomatology in schizophrenia is actually unrelated to level of individual religiosity (Littlewood and Lipsedge, 1981b; Arnold, 1993).

Religious and Related Effects in Treatment

Much of the literature of Afro-Caribbean schizophrenia suggests that it is characterized by briefer episodes, faster recovery, and less risk of relapse (Littlewood and Lipsedge, 1981a, 1981b; Stevens, 1987). Here we consider religious influences related to these effects. These religious influences have been discussed elsewhere in this review: religiously-encouraged social support (Jackson and Birchwood, 1996; stronger religiosity, treatment preferences for clergy, religious practices including syncretic rituals, trance, possession, glossolalia and prayer for therapeutic purposes. An important possibility is that religion influences the form and possibly the occurrence of a 'culture-specific' brief psychosis in Afro-Caribbeans, which may not even be a true psychosis in some cases. Even where it is, the prognosis is said to be very good compared to 'Western' schizophrenia.

The main thrust of the available evidence is that these religious influences contribute to the better prognosis of Afro-Caribbean schizophrenia. The chief possible adverse effects of religion lie in the risk of misdiagnosis of religious behaviour and beliefs as schizophrenia.

We look finally at some more remote religious influences on Afro-Caribbean mental illness, its cures and the use of religious therapeutic practices among black people outside the UK and USA. Csordas (1987) (Brazil) looked at case vignettes from interviews with a Brazilian psychiatrist who was an elder of the Candomble cult and found that the patient's recovery was assisted by referral, where wished to a Candomble practitioner and by cooperation between the psychiatrist and religious specialists. Erinosho (1977a) (Nigeria), in a retrospective study of 208 treated schizophrenics and their next of kin, found that a substantial number of patients from all educational levels had previously sought help from native healers or syncretic churches. Griffith (1983) (Jamaica) interviewed 39 patients, 15 staff, the pastor and clinic director of a church-based healing ministry, where the clinic offered health care, integrating religious and medical/psychological beliefs. The patients were led in prayer before referral for medical treatment or psychological counselling. Idowu (1992) (Nigeria) described the Oshun festival – traditional healing of the mind and soul – involving bathing in the Oshun river, and which fosters self-esteem and group ties. Lefever (1996) (Cuba) analysed socio-anthropologically the Santeria religion which is a syncretism of African religions, Roman Catholicism and French Spiritism. It was felt not merely to be an attempt to conceal the worship of African gods but as a way of harnessing and appropriating the power of the masters. Peltzer and Ebigbo (1989) (Africa) looking at an edited collection of descriptions of a wide range of traditional forms of healing considered psychosocial and psychotherapeutic aspects of traditional forms of healing used in hospitals and among some Christian groups. Roach (1992) (Trinidad) studied the use of Obeah in the treatment of mental illnesses believed to be caused by evil spirits. Umoren (1990) (Nigeria) looked at explanations and treatment of mental illness among the Annang and found that explanations are based on a strongly religious world view. Possession and non-possession mental disorders are identified. The case did not involve possession and treatment included relaxation, suggestion, manipulation, chains and tranquillising medicine.

The above show a range of overtly African-influenced religious practices and beliefs related to mental illness. Although it has been stressed that this kind of information needs to be taken on board by mental health professionals working with black people, there have been no outcome studies in this area.

The use of culture-sensitive, collaborative, multicultural approaches have been advocated in various ways. Views that black people need to be weaned away from 'unscientific' beliefs in religious factors now seem outmoded in the face of a two-pronged attack – in one direction from those favouring multicultural approaches in medicine and psychiatry, and in the other direction from an increasing body of scientific evidence that religious factors may play important preventive and therapeutic roles in mental illness. Several postures on multiculturalism have been outlined (MacLachlan, in press); most authors report that Western-trained professionals are pragmatically taking into account other ('non-Western') beliefs, and where indicated, are referring for treatment which is consistent with those beliefs (Burlew, 1992; Brent and Callwood, 1993; Jackson; 1986; Jones, 1990; Lefley, 1981; Lefley and Bestman, 1977; Richardson, 1991; Sandoval, 1979; Stevenson, 1990).

For example, Csordas (1987) describes several case vignettes from a Brazilian psychiatrist who is an initiated elder of the Afro-Brazilian Candomble cult. The cases involved cross-referral from the psychiatrist to religious practitioners, and sometimes back again. Of particular interest in Csordas' account is the psychiatrist's observation that some of the religious practitioners are able to distinguish between a genuine religious trance (called orixa), a simulated one, and a hysterical crisis, a feat which the psychiatrist says is beyond the psychiatrist. In the latter case they will tell the client to see a doctor.

Some mental health practitioners have tried to incorporate aspects of traditional healing into their practice – kind of psychiatric syncretism. However some authors (Oyarebu, 1982) incline to the view that it is wiser for Western and religious forms of healing to coexist (and cross-refer where necessary).

A careful set of suggestions is made by Maclachlan (in press), who recommends that the clinician should draw up a 'problem portrait'. This is a description of all the things that are 'wrong' with the patient (according to the patient), what s/he thinks caused them, and what s/he thinks other members of their social group/s think cause problems like this. This will enable the clinician to draw up treatment goals in collaboration with the patient, and to draw on healing resources that are seen as appropriate, often using several different kinds of healing resource and cross-referring where necessary.

Summary and Conclusions

What then are the religious influences on schizophrenia among Afro-Caribbeans?

Religion is important to Afro-Caribbeans in the UK and to Afro-Americans, both in absolute terms and relative to other groups. Via a number of routes, religious factors may lower prevalence and improve prognosis. This is a bit speculative because most of the evidence relating religion to mental health among Afro-Caribbeans deals with forms of mental illness other than schizophrenia. Clearly there is space for research on the ways religious factors – social support, worship-related activities and social-cognitive factors – relate to prevalence, referral and recovery in schizophrenia. It is suggested that the direction of these effects is likely to be to lower prevalence and referral, and improve recovery. If so, these effects cannot explain any higher rates of schizophrenia referral among Afro-Caribbeans.

However there is also the suggestion that religious factors may influence symptoms, sometimes causing a risk of over-diagnosis of schizophrenia.

It is unlikely, however, that the high risk of schizophrenia among Afro-Caribbeans can be explained solely in terms of the added likelihood of 'culture-specific' psychosis influenced by cultural-religious factors. If this were so, it would be hard to explain the reported rise in risk of schizophrenia among second-generation immigrants to the UK. Moreover, 'culture-specific' psychosis is reported in African countries and elsewhere, where rates of schizophrenia are said to be as low as in indigenous European and other groups. These phenomena might be better understood with better information on religiosity in relation to schizophrenia.

The only way in which religious factors are likely to contribute to raised rates of schizophrenia is however in over-diagnosis of schizophrenia among disturbed Afro-Caribbeans presenting with a 'religious flavour' to their disturbance. But this is speculative and deserves closer study.

Religious methods of healing are to an increasing extent being taken into account by mental health professionals, including those working among Afro-Caribbean groups. It is likely that this trend will continue. It is to be hoped that outcome studies will appear in this field.

Acknowledgements

We would like to thank Emma Lowers for her help in the early stages of the literature search, and the library staff of the Bedford Library (Royal Holloway, University of London) and of Senate House (University of London) for advice and assistance in the main phases of the literature search, particularly Adrian Machiraju and Anne Sergeant of the Bedford Library for their advice in formulating a search strategy and in implementing it.

We would also like to thank the Department of Health for financial assistance with the literature search.

References

Alonso, L. and Jeffrey, W.D. (1988), 'Mental Illness Complicated by the Santeria Belief in Spirit Possession', *Hospital and Community Psychiatry*, 39, pp. 1188–91.

American Psychiatric Association (1987), *Diagnostic and Statistical Manual of Mental Disorders*, 3rd edn, revised, APA, Washington DC.

American Psychiatric Association (1994), *Diagnostic and Statistical Manual of Mental Disorders*, 4th edn, revised, APA, Washington DC.

Ananth, J., Davies, R. and Kerner B. (1984), 'Psychosis Associated with Thymoma', *Journal of Nervous and Mental Disorder*, 172, pp. 556–8.

Arnold, C.C. (1993), 'Religiosity and Delusional Content among Individuals with Schizophrenia', MSW thesis, California State University, Long Beach, California.

Baer, H.A. (1984), *The Black Spiritual Movement: a Religious Response to Racism*, University of Tennessee Press, Knoxville.

Bartocci, G. (1975), 'Transcultural Psychiatry: an Investigation of Symptoms in Two Racial Groups', *Lavoro Neuropsichiatrico*, 56, pp. 17–38.

Bhugra, D. (ed.) (1996), *Psychiatry and Religion: Context, Consensus and Controversies*, Routledge, London.

Boyd-Franklin, N. (1989), 'Five Key Factors in the Treatment of Black Families', *Journal of Psychotherapy and the Family*, 6, pp. 53–69.

Brent, J.E. and Callwood, G.B. (1993), 'Culturally Relevant Psychiatric Care: The West Indian as a Client', *Journal of Black Psychology*, 19, pp. 290–302.

Brewer, P.D. (1988), 'The Baptist Churches of South Trinidad and their Missionaries', MTh thesis, Glasgow University.

Brown, D.R. and Gary, G.E. (1987), 'Stressful Life Events, Social Support Networks, and the Physical and Mental Health of Urban Black Adults', *Journal of Human Stress*, 13, pp. 165–73.

Brown, D.R. and Gary, G.E. (1988), 'Unemployment and Psychological Distress among Black American Women', *Sociological Focus*, 21, pp. 209–21.

Brown, D.R. and Gary, L.E. (1994), 'Religious Involvement and Health Status among African-American Males', *Journal of the National Medical Association*, 86, pp. 825–31.

Brown, G.W. and Harris, T.O. (1978), *The Social Origins of Depression*, Tavistock Press, London.

Brown, G.W. and Harris, T.O. (eds) (1989), *Life Events and Illness*, Unwin Hyman, London.

Brown, L.B. (1987), *The Psychology of Religious Belief*, Academic Press, London.

Burlew, A.K.H. (ed.) (1992), *African American Psychology: Theory, Research and Practice*, Sage, Thousand Oaks, CA.

Caldwell, C.H., Greene, A.D. and Billingsley, A. (1994), 'Family Support Programmes in Black Churches: a New Look at Old Functions', in Kagan, S.L. and Weissbourd, B. (eds), *Putting Families First: America's Family Support Movement and the Challenge of Change*, Jossey-Bas, San Francisco.

Capps, D. (1992), '"Religion and Child Abuse: Perfect Together", Presidential Address of the Society for the Scientific Study of Religion 1991, Pittsburgh, Pennsylvania', *Journal for the Scientific Study of Religion*, 31, pp. 1–14.

Chalmers, I. and Haynes, B. (1994), 'Reporting, Updating and Correcting Systematic Reviews of the Effects of Health Care', *British Medical Journal*, 309, pp. 862–5.

Chatfield, A.F. (1989), 'A Sociology of Trinidad Religion, with Special Reference to Christianity', MTh thesis, Leeds University.

Cochrane, R. and Howell, M. (1995), 'Drinking Patterns of Black and White Men in the West Midlands', *Social Psychiatry and Psychiatric Epidemiology*, 30, pp. 139–46.

Cope, R. (1989), 'The Compulsory Detention of Afro-Caribbeans under the Mental Health Act', *New Community*, 15, pp. 343–56.

Csordas, T.J. (1987), 'Health and the Holy in African and Afro-American Spirit Possession', *Social Science and Medicine*, 24, pp. 1–11.

Curtin, P.D. (1969), *The Atlantic Slave Trade: a Census*, University of Wisconsin Press, Madison.

Davis, L.G. (1975), *The Mental Health of the Black Community: an Exploratory Bibliography*, Council of Planning Librarians, Monticello, IL.

Dobbin, J.D. (1982), 'Doo'en Dee Dance: Description and Analysis of the Jombee Dance of Montserrat (West Indies)', PhD thesis, Ohio State University.

Early, L.F. and Lifschutz, J.E. (1974), 'A Case of Stigmata', *Archives of General Psychiatry*, 30, pp. 197–200.

Edwards, K.L. (1987), 'Exploratory Study of Black Psychological Health', *Journal of Religion and Health*, 26, pp. 73–80.

Ellison, C.G. (1995), 'Race, Religious Involvement and Depressive Symptomatology in a Southeastern U.S. Community', *Social Science and Medicine*, 40, pp. 1561–72.

Erinosho, O.A. (1977a), 'Social Background and Pre-admission Sources of Care among Yoruba Psychiatric Patients', *Social Psychiatry*, 12, pp. 71–4.

Erinosho, O.A. (1977b), 'Cultural Factors in Mental Illness among the Yoruba', *International Journal of Group Psychotherapy*, 27, pp. 511–15.

Eysenck, H.J. (1994), 'Meta-analysis and its Problems', *British Medical Journal*, 309, pp. 789–92.

Ferraro, K.F. and Koch, J.R. (1994), 'Religion and Health among Black and White Adults: Examining Social Support and Consolidation', *Journal for the Scientific Study of Religion*, 33, pp. 362–75.

Franklin, J.H. and Moss, A.A., Jr (1988), *From Slavery to Freedom: A History of Negro Americans*, 6th edn, Alfred Knopf, New York.

Gary, L.E. (1984), *Pathways: a Study of Black Informal Support Networks*, Mental Health Research and Development Centre, Institute for Urban Affairs and Research Howard University, Washington.

Gary, L.E. (1985), *Black Male-Female Relationships: an Empirical Assessment*, Institute of Urban Affairs Howard University, Society for the Study of Social Problems Association Paper, Washington.

Gates, B.E. (ed.) (1980), *Afro-Caribbean Religions*, Ward Lock, London.

Gesler, W.M. and Nahim, E.A. (1984), 'Client Characteristics at Kissy Mental Hospital, Freetown, Sierra Leone', *Social Science and Medicine*, 18, pp. 819–25.

Goviea, E.V. (1965), *Slave Society in the British Leeward Islands at the End of the Eighteenth Century*, Yale University Press, New Haven.

Griffith, E.E. (1980), 'Possession, Prayer and Testimony: Therapeutic Sspects of the Wednesday Night Meeting in a Black Church', *Psychiatry*, 43, pp. 120–28.

Griffith, E.E. (1983), 'The Impact of Sociocultural Factors on a Church-based Healing Model', *American Journal of Orthopsychiatry*, 53, pp. 291–302.

Griffith, E.E. and Bility, K.M. (1996), 'Psychosocial Factors and the Genesis of New Afro-American Religious Groups', in Bhugra, D. (ed.), *Psychiatry and Religion*, Routledge, London.

Griffith, E.E. and Mathewson, M.A. (1981), 'Communitas and Charisma in a Black Church Service', *Journal of the National Medical Association*, 73, p.. 1023–7.

Griffith, E.E., Young, J.L. and Smith. D.L. (1984), 'An Analysis of the Therapeutic Elements in a Black Church Service', *Hospital and Community Psychiatry*, 35, pp. 464–9.

Hall, R.L.B. (1984), 'Do, Lord, Remember Me : Religion and Cultural Change among Blacks in Florida, 1565–1906', PhD thesis, Florida State University.

Heligman, R.M., Lee, L.R. and Krager, D. (1983), 'Pain Relief Associated with a Religious Visitation: a Case Report', *Journal of Family Practice*, 16, pp. 299–302.

Hickling, F.W. and Griffith, E.E. (1994), 'Clinical Perspectives on the Rastafari Movement', *Hospital and Community Psychiatry*, 45, pp. 49–53.

Hill, P., Jr (1987), 'Passage to Manhood: Rearing the Male African-American Child', paper presented at the Annual Conference of the National Black Child Development Institute, Detroit.

Hillard, J.R. and Rockwell, W.J.K. (1978), 'Dysesthesia, Witchcraft and Conversion Reaction: a Case Successfully Treated with Psychotherapy', *Journal of the American Medical Association*, 240, pp. 1742–4.

Howard, V. (1987), *A Report on Afro-Caribbean Christianity in Britain*, University of Leeds Department of Theology and Religious Studies Community Religions Project Research Papers, Leeds.

Idowu, A.I. (1992), 'The Oshun Festival: an African Traditional Religious Healing Process', *Counselling and Values*, 36, pp. 192–200.

Ineichen, B. (1986), 'Compulsory Admission to Psychiatric Hospital under the 1959 Mental Health Act: the Experience of Ethnic Minorities', *New Community*, 13, pp. 86–93.

Ineichen, B. (1991), 'Schizophrenia in British Afro-Caribbeans: Two Debates Confused?', *International Journal of Social Psychiatry*, 37, pp. 227–32.

Jackson, C. and Birchwood, M. (1996), 'Early Intervention in Psychosis', *British Journal of Clinical Psychology*, 35, pp. 487–502.

Jackson, G.G. (1986), 'Conceptualizing Afrocentric and Eurocentric Mental Health Training', in Lefley, H.P. and Pedersen, P.B. (eds), *Cross-cultural Training for Mental Health Professionals*, Charles C. Thomas, Springfield, IL.

Jackson, J.J. (ed.) (1991), *Life in Black America*, Sage, Newbury Park, CA.

Jones, N.S.C. (1990), 'Black/White Issues in Psychotherapy: a Framework for Clinical Practice', *Journal of Social Behaviour and Personality*, 5, pp. 305–22.

Jones, P. (1992), 'African-American Women: the Psychotherapeutic Process as a Coping Style', paper presented at the American Psychological Association, Washington, DC.

Jules-Rosette, B. (1980), 'Creative Spirituality from Africa to America: Cross-cultural Influences in Contemporary Religious Forms', *Western Journal of Black Studies*, 4, pp. 273–85.

Knipschild, P. (1994), 'Systematic Reviews: Some Examples', *British Medical Journal*, 309, pp. 719–21.

Lefever, H.G. (1996), 'When the Saints go Riding in: Santeria in Cuba and the United States', *Journal for the Scientific Study of Religion*, 35, pp. 318–30.

Lefley, H.P. (1981), 'Psychotherapy and Cultural Adaptation in the Caribbean', *International Journal of Group Tensions*, 11, pp. 3–16.

Lefley, H.P. and Bestman, E.W. (1977), 'Psychotherapy in Caribbean Cultures', paper presented at the American Psychological Association, San Francisco.

Lipsedge, M. (1996), 'Religion and Madness in History', in Bhugra, D. (ed.), *Psychiatry and Religion: Context, Consensus and Controversies*, Routledge, London.

Littlewood, R. (1993), *Pathology and Identity: The Work of Mother Earth in Trinidad*, Cambridge University Press, Cambridge.

Littlewood, R. and Lipsedge, M. (1978), 'Migration, Ethnicity and Diagnosis', *Psychiatrica Clinica*, 11, pp. 15–22.

Littlewood, R. and Lipsedge, M. (1981), 'Some Social and Phenomenological Characteristics of Psychotic Immigrants', *Psychological Medicine*, 11, pp. 289–302.

Littlewood, R. and Lipsedge, M. (1981), 'Acute Psychotic Reactions in Caribbean-born Patients', *Psychological Medicine*, 11, pp. 303–18.

Littlewood, R. and Lipsedge, M. (1989), *Aliens and Alienists: Ethnic Minorities and Psychiatry*, 2nd edn, Unwin Hyman, London.

Loewenthal, K.M. (1995), *Religion and Mental Health*, Chapman and Hall, London.

Loewenthal, K.M., Goldblatt, V., Gorton, T., Lubitsch, G., Bicknell, H., Fellowes, D. and Sowden, A. (1996), 'The Costs and Benefits of Boundary Maintenance: Stress, Religion and Culture among Jews in Britain', *Social Psychiatry and Psychiatric Epidemiology*.

MacLachlan, M. (in press), *Culture and Health*, Wiley, Chichester.

Maloney, H.N. and Lovekin, A.A. (1985), *Glossolalia: Behavioural Science Perspectives on Speaking in Tongues*, Oxford University Press, New York.

Martin, W.I. (1984), 'Religiosity and United States Suicide Rates, 1972–1978', *Journal of Clinical Psychology*, 40, pp. 1166–9.

McCloud, A.B. (1995), *African American Islam*, Routledge, New York.

Millet, P.E., Sullivan, B.F., Schwebel, A.I. and Myers, L.J. (1996), 'Black Americans' and White Americans' Views of the Etiology and Treatment of Mental Health Problems', *Community Mental Health Journal*, 32, pp. 235–42.

Mollica, R.F., Streets, F.J., Boscarino, J. and Redlich, F.C. (1986), 'A Community Study of Formal Pastoral Counselling Activities of the Clergy', *American Journal of Psychiatry*, 143, pp. 323–8.

Mulrow, C.D. (1994), 'Rationale for Systematic Reviews', *British Medical Journal*, 309, pp. 597–9.

Ndetei, D.M. (1988), 'Psychiatric Phenomenology across Countries: Constitutional, Cultural or Environmental?', *Acta Psychiatrica Scandinavica*, 78/supplement, 344, pp. 33–44.

Ndetei, D.M. and Vadher, A. (1984), 'Frequency and Clinical Significance of Delusions across Cultures', *Acta Psychiatrica Scandinavica*, 70, pp. 73–6.

Ness, R.C. and Wintrob, R.M. (1981), 'Folk Healing: a Description and Synthesis', *American Journal of Psychiatry*, 138, pp. 1477–81.

Oxman, A.D. (1994), 'Checklists for Review Articles', *British Medical Journal*, 309, pp. 648–51.

Oyarebu, K.A. (1982), 'An Assessment of the Current Status of Mental Illness in Bendel State of Nigeria: Implications for Public Mental Health Policy and Education', DRPH thesis, University of Texas at Houston School of Public Health.

Patel, V. (1995), 'Explanatory Models of Illness in Sub-Saharan Africa', *Social Science and Medicine*, 40, pp. 1291–8.

Peltzer, K. and Ebigbo, P.O. (eds) (1989), *Clinical Psychology in Africa, the Caribbean and Afro-Latin America: a Textbook for Universities and Paramedical Schools*, Social Psychiatry Research Institute, New York.

Platt, S.L. (1995), 'The Comparative Study of Health Lifestyle and Beliefs in a Religious and Non-religious Group', MSc dissertation: St George's Hospital Medical School, University of London.

Purdy, B.A., Simari, C.G. and Colon, G. (1983), 'Religiosity, Ethnicity and Mental Health: Interface the '80s', *Counselling and Values*, 27, pp. 112–21.

Rack, P.H. (1988), 'Psychiatric and Social Problems among Immigrants', *Acta Psychiatrica Scandinavica*, 78/supplement, 344, pp. 167–74.

Redlener, I.E. and Scott, C.S. (1979), 'Incompatibilities of Professional and Religious Ideology: Problems of Medical Management and Outcome in a Case of Paediatric Meningitis', *Social Science and Medicine*, 138, pp. 89–93.

Richardson, B.L. (ed.) (1991), *Multicultural Issues in Counselling: New Approaches to Diversity*, American Association for Counselling and Development, Alexandra, VA.

Roach, R. (1992), 'Obeah in the Treatment of Psychiatric Disorders in Trinidad: an Empirical Study of an Indigenous Healing System', MSc thesis, McGill University.

Rosen, C.E. (1982), 'Ethnic Differences among Impoverished Rural Elderly in Use of Religion as a Coping Mechanism', *Journal of Rural Community Psychology*, 3, pp. 27–34.

Sandoval, M.C. (1979), 'Santeria as a Mental Health Care System: an Historical Overview', *Social Science and Medicine*, 138, pp. 137–51.

Silva de Crane, R. and Spielberger, C. (1981), 'Attitudes of Hispanic, Black and Caucasian University Students toward Mental Illness', *Hispanic Journal of Behavioural Sciences*, 3, pp. 241–55.

Snow, L. (1974), 'Folk Medical Beliefs and their Implications for Care of Patients', *Annals of Internal Medicine*, 81, p. 83.

Stevens, J.R. (1987), 'Brief Psychoses: Do they Contribute to the Good Prognosis and Equal Prevalence of Schizophrenia in Developing Countries?', *British Journal of Psychiatry*, 151, pp. 393–6.

Stevenson, H.C. (1990), 'The Role of the African-American Church in Education about Teenage Pregnancy', *Counselling and Values*, 34, pp. 130–33.

Sugarman, P.A. and Craufurd, D. (1994), 'Schizophrenia in the Afro-Caribbean Community', *British Journal of Psychiatry*, 164, pp. 474–80.

Taylor, J. and Jackson, B.B. (1991), 'Evaluation of a Holistic Model of Mental Health Symptoms in African American Women', *Journal of Black Psychology*, 18, pp. 19–45.

The Hutchinson Encyclopaedia (1964), Helicon Publishing, Middlesex.

The University of York NHS Centre for Reviews and Dissemination: Information Sheets 1–7 (1996), University of York NHS CRD Centre, York.

Thomas, C.S., Stone, K., Osborn, M., Thomas, P.F. (1993), 'Psychiatric Morbidity and Compulsory Admission among UK-born Europeans, Afro-Caribbeans and Asians in central Manchester', *British Journal of Psychiatry*, 163, pp. 91–9.

Turner, V. (1969), *The Ritual Process: Structure and Anti-Structure*, Routledge and Kegan Paul, London.

Umoren, U.E. (1990), 'Religion and Traditional Medicine: an Anthropological Case Study of a Nigerian Treatment of Mental Illness', *Medical Anthropology*, 12, pp. 389–400.

Wagley, C. (1961), 'Recent Studies in Caribbean Local Societies', in Wilgus, C. (ed.), *The Caribbean*, Gainesville, FLA.

Walls, C.T. and Zarit, S.H. (1991), 'Informal Support from Black Churches and the Well-being of Elderly Blacks', *Gerontologist*, 31, pp. 490–95.

Ward, C. (1982), 'A Transcultural Perspective on Women and Madness: the Case of the Mystical Affliction', *Womens Studies International Forum*, 5, pp. 411–18.

Ward, C. and Beabrun, M.H. (1981), 'Spirit Possession and Neuroticism in a West Indian Pentecostal Community', *British Journal of Clinical Psychology*, 1981, 20, pp. 295–6.

Worthington, E.L., Kurusu, T.A., McCullough, M.E. and Sandage, S.J. (1996), 'Empirical Research on Religion and Psychotherapeutic Processes and Outcomes: a 10-year Review and Research Prospectus', *Psychological Review*, 119, pp. 448–7.

Zilborg, G. and Henry, G.W. (1951), *A History of Medical Psychology*, Allen and Unwin, London.

Chapter 6

Law and Mental Health: Some Implications for Ethnic Minorities in England

Prakash Shah and Dion Hanna

Introduction

The main aim of this chapter is to analyse the level and type of coverage given to mental health issues concerning ethnic minorities in the literature within the legal field. A general survey of some key legal areas is made, including the fields of anti-discrimination law, immigration law, and the criminal law system. Then the literature about the psychiatric detention system under the mental health legislation is examined. Account is taken of existing work in other disciplines to evaluate the progress that has been made towards a more informed understanding of ethnic minority experiences. Despite its reliance on norms of formal equality it can be seen that in the mental health field, English law reserves special treatment for people on the basis of their race or ethnicity. On the other hand, we found that the legal literature largely fails to give this impression.

This review commences with a general discussion of the situation of ethnic minorities within the English legal system which, underpinned by assimilationist assumptions, can be seen to have either ignored or bypassed their customary or religious laws. Then some specific areas of English law are considered. These include issues such as the impact of immigration laws, the protection offered by British anti-discrimination legislation and the criminalisation of some ethnic minorities. In this part we have not relied on a systematic review to search for the relevant literature. Rather, we have relied on information generally available to us as researchers and teachers in the field of ethnic minorities and the law in Britain.[1] We acknowledge that a fuller review would necessitate the examination of literature in several other legal areas covered by English law, in particular, the laws relating to families and children.

The second part of this review focuses on the more specific issue of the British mental health legislation and its impact on ethnic minorities. For this section a systematic review was carried out within the limited resources available. This involved a search of legal databases and indexes to reported cases, as well as library catalogues at the Institute of Advanced Legal Studies, School of Hygiene and Tropical Medicine, the School of Oriental and African Studies and the King's Fund Institute.

We were struck by the dearth of literature in the law-based resources, a fact which we believe is not unrelated to awareness generally about issues important for ethnic minorities. One of the implications is that lawyers, judges, magistrates, the police and others wishing to know more about this field will have to look outside the narrow legal discipline. In recent years the literature by, for or about the 'caring professionals' has mushroomed and, despite some advances in practice, it seems that patterns of institutional racism continue to bedevil the experiences of ethnic minorities. We point to some accounts of individuals experiences of the impact of the state upon their lives. Thus, just as the legal fiction of equality masks grave distances in the legal position of various ethnic groups within Britain, 'scientism' and its dogma of universal applicability masks the stealthy ethnocentric distinctions that officials or mental health practitioners make.

English Law and Ethnic Minorities

In the period after the Second World War, immigration from non-European territories and the development of a sizeable non-white ethnic minority population in Britain have called into question the legal framework of liberal quasi-secularism that reluctantly admits of plurality. Thus one author points to the official assimilationist legal expectation that the new minorities should 'do as the Romans do' (Poulter, 1986, p. v). But if one's perspective shifts from the official English law, one can see that ethnic minorities continue to independently weave the demands of the official legal system into their traditional laws, thus creating, for example, distinct British South Asian laws, thus defying simplistic official expectations of assimilation (Menski, 1993, for South Asians). One consequence of official incapability to recognise such legal facts in the UK is that ethnic minorities bypass the English legal requirements altogether, a factor that may contribute further to official ignorance of ethnic minority legal concerns. The capacity of ethnic minorities to mobilise independently in the legal field is shown, for example, in the work of the Sharia Council which takes on the role of dealing with legal problems of Muslims in Britain in situations where English law offers little recourse (Badawi, 1995).

Officials and lawyers may remain in ignorance of legal practices of the many ethnic minorities and are easily led to relying upon stereotypes in their official dealings with them. Recently, training programmes in 'racial sensitivity' for police (Oakley, 1989) and judicial officers (see Judicial Studies Board, 1996) have been instituted and their outcomes will be of interest. Importantly, one study has found that lawyers are identified with state authorities among ethnic minority communities and also that lawyers themselves do not wish to specialise in areas of demand among ethnic minorities.[2] The problem goes beyond simply securing the proportionate entry of ethnic minorities into the legal professions and judicial benches. One could here also usefully re-evaluate the assimilationist bases of legal education offered to law students, both from 'white' and minority backgrounds (Menski, 1997b). We notice that similar issues are cropping up in medical fields where there are indications that Asian doctors cannot identify the needs of ethnic minorities.

The above-mentioned training initiatives do suggest that official bodies cannot be immune from taking into account the specificity of ethnic minority needs. To some extent the official law has recognised a role for itself through the Race Relations Act 1976, under which private actions for damages may be brought for acts of discrimination or under which organisations may come under the microscope of the Commission for Racial Equality (CRE). However, critical studies in this area have revealed that judges have applied this law in a way that has generally discounted the concerns of ethnic minorities in employment and effectively given endorsement for the continuation of discriminatory practices (Gregory, 1987). Employers such as local authorities have also effectively learnt how to stave off discrimination-based legal challenges against their practices (Joy, 1995).

The 1976 Act has also been criticised for omitting to mention 'religion', thus depriving Muslims, Hindus and Rastafarians of protection. On the other hand, protection for 'ethnic groups' has been judicially interpreted to apply to some and not others. Thus the English, Welsh, Irish, Jews and Sikhs may be considered as ethnic groups, but such recognition has not been held out by the Court of Appeal for Rastafarians.[3] Such second-rate treatment of some ethnic minorities is also evident in other areas of law, and is particularly worrying in the field of criminalisation and the use of the Mental Health Act powers, where Black ethnic minorities in general, and Rastafarians in particular, seem to be targeted. Racial harassment in both public and private places is a daily reality for many ethnic minorities. The scale and nature of such harassment is only recently becoming clearer in recent studies which have pointed to a large proportion of incidents involving ethnic minorities as victims being racially motivated (Virdee, 1995; FitzGerald and Hale, 1996). In the criminal law field there already exists the power for judges to take into account racial motivation in sentencing.[4] However, reporting of incidents among ethnic minority groups varies (in particular, 'Pakistanis' and 'Afro-Caribbeans' report incidents much less) and there is a general lack of satisfaction when incidents are reported as involving a racial factor (FitzGerald and Hale 1996). Indeed, Virdee's (1995) study indicates that where incidents were reported to the police no further action was taken, while police officers themselves took to harassing the complainants.[5] Virdee also argues that there is little that official legal mechanisms can achieve, especially for the prevalent 'low-level' forms of racial harassment such as verbal abuse and bullying.

Negative experiences of police attitudes are amplified when consideration is given to the criminalisation of some ethnic minorities in Britain. It is known that some groups consistently report negative experiences with police and Black youth, in particular, have higher rates of being stopped, questioned, arrested and cautioned or charged (Ellis and McLaughlin, 1991; Brown, 1997, pp. 19–27). Much research has been directed to establishing which links in the chain of criminalisation account for the over-representation of African-Caribbean (or Black) people within the criminal law system (for a discussion of the emerging issues see Cook and Hudson, 1993). Continuing deaths of African-Caribbean and African people who are detained under either immigration or police powers are a cause of further concern. The hard fact that the criminal court system could discriminate against Black people was recently shown by Hood's (1992) study, which has been the subject of discussion in judicial training seminars. However, the gap between academic knowledge and legal practice is vast. A case reported in 1994 brought fourth the following comment from the trial judge:

> You are four coloured men. I do not want you to think for one moment that if you were four white men standing here you would be getting a moment less by way of sentence than you will in fact get. You are being sentenced for robbery, not for the colour of your skin.

On appeal the sentence was reduced, the Court of Appeal stating that the colour, race or religion of defendants was irrelevant because *all were equal in the eyes of the law*. The Court felt that the trial judge's comments would leave a lingering feeling that colour affected the length of the sentence.[6] Any conclusion about the enlightening power of training seminars for judicial officers must surely be reserved in the light of such persistent 'colour blindness', although a less generous view may dismiss such comments as mere judicial politicking.

A huge literature has grown on the subject of the extent to which mental illness can be linked to the migration process itself and the culture conflicts that this may involve (Furnham and Bochner 1986). While these debates are certain to go on it is known that migration divides many families and the strain on individuals is exacerbated by the restrictions imposed by the immigration laws specifically designed to limit the entry of family members of ethnic minorities already settled in Britain.

Official views about the strength of family support among ethnic minorities, which may indeed be borne out by the feeling of obligation on the part of family members (Fenton, 1987; Atkin and Rollings, 1993, p. 14), need to take into account this oppressive dimension of state law. The notorious 'primary purpose rule' was targeted at South Asian couples, whereby the state attempted to carry out an agenda of limitation of numbers and constructive repatriation (Sachdeva, 1993) in the process affecting the health of many Asian women (Menski, 1998). The formal abolition of that rule in 1997 may be no more than a political response, as anecdotal evidence still indicates that spouses from the Indian subcontinent continue to be refused family reunion on other criteria. Mothers, especially from the West Indies, and later from the Philippines, also suffered long periods of separation from their children who had remained behind in countries of origin. In turn, they were targeted by the immigration laws, which imposed the need to show that parents had 'sole responsibility' for their children (Cheney, 1993; Bhabha and Shutter, 1994, pp. 129–61). In recent years asylum has become a major legal issue, and asylum seekers have been placed under all sorts of restrictions, including routine detention and denial of social benefits and housing. These will no doubt also have their impact for the mental health of ethnic minorities as recent studies are beginning to show (Medical Foundation, 1994).

The general survey of English law and its response to ethnic minorities made above gives cause for concern in several ways. The legal system has generally failed to incorporate a recognition that ethnic minorities have pursued their own forms of legal organisation. At the outset, therefore, the system has been more preoccupied to uphold the view that by consistently treating everyone in the same way it achieves certain just ends, regardless of their culture or ethnicity. From the perspective of ethnic minorities therefore the underpinnings of the legal system appear assimilationist as conformity is a precondition for legal benefits. In specific fields, such as the enforcement of the Race Relations Act or protection from racial harassment, the official legal agencies have generally failed to respond to ethnic minority demands. The response of key agencies like the police has been to retain control rather than to extend protection evenly, and is manifested in disproportionate criminalisation, particularly of Black people. Immigration laws have primarily been concerned to limit non-white immigration and continue to impact upon ethnic minorities in so many ways. The law and the legal system are therefore sites of culture conflict and oppression. The type and level of impact on the mental health of ethnic minorities remains an unexplored field, although much could no doubt be said about the psychological implications of this kind of culture conflict. Further, given the negative experiences of ethnic minorities with the legal system it can be doubted whether legal mechanisms specifically in the mental health field can offer adequate protection against the use of coercive powers that are themselves legitimated by the official law.

Ethnic Minorities and the British Mental Health System

For this part of the review, a more systematic, though not exhaustive, survey of existing resources was carried out. The *Index to Legal Periodicals and Books* (which only documents English language sources) and the Index to Foreign Legal Periodicals were examined on CD ROM (only the entries in English in the latter were noted).[7] The index Canadian Legal Literature for the years 1995–97 was also examined.[8] We immediately realised that it is in the non-legal sources that one finds the greatest level of existing research about ethnic minorities in the British mental health system. Two important bibliographies were found – Karmi and McKeigue (1993) and SHARE (1997).[9] Library catalogues at the King's Fund Institute (which proved the most valuable), the School of Hygiene and Tropical Medicine, the School of Oriental and African Studies and the Institute of Advanced Legal Studies were also used.[10] We also took into account information collected over the years by Werner Menski, Director of the Group for Ethnic Minority Studies (GEMS) at SOAS.

Mental Health Law in England and Wales

The main legislation empowering different agencies to exercise coercive powers against persons on the basis of a diagnosis of their mental condition is the Mental Health Act 1983. There are several detailed studies on the provisions of and the practical operation of the Mental Health Act (Jones, 1997; Hoggett, 1996; Cavadino, 1989). These studies are reviewed further below in relation to their treatment of ethnic minorities. The important powers under the 1983 Act are those of forcible psychiatric admission. These are split into Part II and Part III of the Act respectively. What follows is only a summary of the main powers.

Part II admissions come under Sections 2, 3 or 4 of the Act and are considered as the civil sections. Section 2 allows admission on the basis of an application by a nearest relative, or court, or a social worker and two registered medical practitioners, one of whom must be a qualified psychiatrist. It allows detention for up to 28 days. The application must be made in the interest of a person's own health and safety or with a view to the protection of other persons. Section 3 allows detention for up to six months (renewable for yearly periods thereafter) and can be achieved in a similar manner although, if a nearest relative objects, court authority is needed. Section 4 allows compulsory detention for assessment for up to 72 hours and it can be effected on the authority of only one doctor. This type of admission can be extended by complying with Section 2 powers. The majority of compulsory patients are committed to psychiatric hospitals in the interest of themselves or other people under these sections as a result of an application made by a social worker or the nearest relative and supported by one or two doctors (Cope 1989). That gives sufficient authority to detain and sometimes to treat a patient against his or her will. Section 136 allows a police officer to remove a person who appears to be in need of care and control to a place of safety, which includes a police station. The object of the section is to secure a speedy assessment by a doctor and social worker. Special provisions apply to persons detained in police stations, and who are deemed to be mentally disordered or handicapped. There is a possibility to appeal to a Mental Health Review Tribunal if detention is under any Mental Health Act powers.

The 'forensic' sections are the powers available to the courts or a direction of the Home Secretary to order a person into detention, after he or she has been accused of having committed a criminal offence. Detention in psychiatric care may thus be ordered at any time up to and including the sentencing stage and also after a person has been sentenced. Powers of the courts are not restricted to the Mental Health Act, but also appear in other legislation.[11]

In both types of 'sectioning' power, doctors and psychiatrists enjoy a good deal of discretion to bring their diagnostic powers to result in a person's detention. Social workers, the police, courts, probation officers, nursing staff also all have a role to play in the institutional mental health system.

Existing Review Literature

Atkin and Rollings (1993, pp. 29–40) review of statutory community health provision, as part of a wider review of community care, offers a general view about the attitudes of practitioners within the health and social services, as well as the experience of South Asian and West Indian minorities (often classed together as 'Black') in contact with them. A definite indication is given of the over-representation of Black people in aspects of social services activity (for example, Black children in care and numbers of Black youths in detention centres) which involve overt social control and institutionalisation, and of their over-representation in psychiatric institutions. Black clients' experiences are generally not satisfactory, leaving them angry and estranged. Social policy tends to function on the paradigm of 'colour-blindness', corresponding to the dominant official legal attitudes, social workers often overemphasising cultural difference or being totally ignorant of its relevance. Similarly, a particular study summarised by Atkin and Rollings (1993, p. 36) suggests that 'health services do not seem to consider difference and diversity, and assume their policies, procedures and practices are appropriate for everyone. This results in unfavourable treatment and unequal access for black and ethnic minority people'. The literature on 'mental health', 'general practice' and 'community nursing' reveals a more detailed picture along similar lines. Even younger Asian doctors, it seems, are failing to take into account complaints from older Asian patients. Echoing Atkin and Rollings general findings is Watters' (1996) critique of institutional approaches to the mental health needs of ethnic minorities using examples from South Asians and Afro-Caribbeans experiences.

He notes that a number of initiatives have been undertaken to provide special services to ethnic minorities but that they are often short-term in nature and have acted as a buffer to fend off demands for change in the mainstream of health services. More specifically, Watters (1996, p. 116) notes that under the Community Care Act 1990 less emphasis will be placed upon targeting people who are perceived as under-utilising services to increasing surveillance and control of those perceived to be 'dangerous'.

Browne (1993), in his review of the existing literature on race and psychiatry, states that there is a great deal of research on psychiatry and Black people's experience showing that there is Black over-representation among patients in psychiatric hospitals (or coming to psychiatry), and that most of these hospital admissions are accompanied by diagnoses of serious mental illness or schizophrenia. For Browne the term 'Black' indicates a person of African origin whether born in Africa, the Caribbean or in Britain although, to be sure, there are more studies related to African-Caribbeans, whether migrants themselves or British-born. He notes that an early response of researchers was to assume that the high rate of mental illness was to do with the migration process itself. That assumption was abandoned when high rates of admission continued among second-generation Blacks. Other studies were conducted to investigate this but they were based on the basic premise that Black people were themselves somehow deviant.[12]

The literature which emerged in the late 1980s and the early 1990s was, according to Browne (1993), more far reaching, especially in the area of compulsory admission to psychiatric units under the Mental Health legislation, and that is confirmed by other studies not reviewed by Browne. They show that throughout the process of compulsory admissions there has been a disproportionate exercise of powers against Black people:

1 Significantly more 'migrants' from West Africa and the Caribbean had been shown *not* to have been referred to hospitals by their GPs (Rwegellera, 1980). That was echoed more recently for African-Caribbeans (Moodley and Perkins, 1991). The admission of Black patients is more likely to be the result of police and social service referrals (Mama, 1992, p. 9).

2 Black people are more likely to be perceived as threatening, incoherent and disturbed (Pipe et al., 1991).

3 Black men are more likely to receive diagnoses of psychotic illnesses and, in particular, schizophrenia or drug-induced psychosis (Dunn and Fahy, 1990; Moodley and Perkins, 1991; Crowley and Simmonds, 1992; Mama, 1992, p. 9).[13] The schizophrenia diagnosis is even higher in British-born African-Caribbeans (Harrison et al., 1988). Illicit drugs were identified in discharge summaries as a contributing factor in the 'formal' admission of African-Caribbeans at nearly 10 times the 'White' rate, also possibly suggesting that routine testing for drugs is carried out on at least some ethnic groups (Crowley and Simmonds, 1992).

4 Black people are more likely than Whites to be given neuroleptic drugs (Dunn and Fahy, 1990). Black people, particularly African-Caribbeans, receive more physical treatment, such as electroconvulsive therapy (ECT), oral and injected drugs in higher dosages, and they are less likely to

receive non-physical forms of treatment such as counselling (Littlewood and Lipsedge, 1982; Mama, 1992, p. 94).

5 Black people are more likely to be put on compulsory admission (Dunn and Fahy, 1990; McGovern and Cope, 1991) and one-third were likely to have been treated in forensic units at some time (McGovern and Cope, 1991). The compulsory detention rate for African-Caribbean youth has been found to be 25 times higher than for white youth (Cope, 1989).

6 Black men and women are more likely to be sectioned under Section 136 of the Mental Health Act 1983 by the police (Dunn and Fahy, 1990; Pipe et al., 1991; Moodley and Perkins, 1991). A study of schizophrenia admissions in the London Borough of Harrow showed a significantly higher level of police involvement in African-Caribbean cases (Perera et al., 1991).

7 Young African-Caribbean men were more likely to be placed under 'forensic' psychiatric detention (that is, through the criminal justice system) (Cope, 1989; McGovern and Cope, 1991). African-Caribbeans are more likely to be referred from the prison system while on remand and more likely in these circumstances for urgent psychiatric treatment (Cope and Ndegwa, 1990, study of a Regional Secure Unit). Magistrates are more likely to opt for hospital orders or psychiatric probation orders for African-Caribbean defendants, who were also more likely to be diagnosed as suffering from mental illness and likely to spend longer remanded in prison custody (Browne, 1991).

8 Higher proportions of African-Caribbeans who were compulsorily detained believed there to have been nothing wrong with them (Moodley and Perkins, 1991).

9 It has been pointed out that British literature omits any real consideration of Black women, while studies which include gender analyses have tended to be colour blind (Mama, 1992, p. 93). However, Chigwada (1991) found that Black women tend to be treated under the mental health legislation in a discriminatory manner in several of the respects identified above: they are more likely to be dealt with under Section 136; to be given psychotropic medication; and to be detained beyond the relevant legal limits.

10 Up to 40 per cent of African Caribbean people in National Health Service beds are there as psychiatric patients (Black Patients and Health Workers Group, 1983; Mama, 1992, p. 91).

We were unable to locate any analyses of the coroners' inquests into the deaths of Michael Martin (1984), Joseph Watts (1988) and Orville Blackwood

(1991), in which juries had all returned verdicts of 'accidental death'. However, the inquiries by the Special Hospitals Service Authority (1989 and 1993) are informative. The 'Report of the Committee of Inquiry into the Death in Broadmoor Hospital of Orville Blackwood and a Review of the Deaths of two other Afro-Caribbean Patients: "Big, Black and Dangerous"', in particular, makes very interesting reading. In that report many of the findings about discrimination in the mental health system cited above are referred to, some discussion is made about the attitudes of staff in Broadmoor, and proposals are made with a view to increasing staff awareness of ethnic minority issues.

A number of other recent studies have taken a more interrogative approach to the views and decision making of professionals and officials. Bowl and Barnes (1990) found that the main sources of referral to approved social workers (ASWs) were ones which had been identified in an earlier study as not likely to pass on cases resulting in compulsory detention. Yet there was found to be a significant over-representation of African-Caribbeans in compulsory detentions under Sections 2 and 4 of the Mental Health Act. 'The assessment by an ASW appears therefore to amplify the discriminatory effects of referral patterns, reinforcing the tendency of Afro-Caribbeans to be subject to compulsory detention' (Bowl and Barnes, 1990, p. 14). A main conclusion of their research was that local authorities generally tended to adopt a 'colour-blind' approach and not to provide for ethnic minority needs. Browne (1995) reports that perceptions of Black people were consistently reported to be negative among general practitioners, police officers and ASWs.

At the 'forensic' stages Browne (1995, pp. 70–71) concluded from a series of interviews with magistrates, probation officers, solicitors, court clerks and psychiatrists that:

> Decision-makers appeared more likely to err on the side of caution with black mentally vulnerable defendants and to be affected by a heightened perception of dangerousness with regard to this group, thus mirroring the actions of their civil section counterparts.

In this respect it is useful to refer to some of the evidence in the events leading up to the death of Joseph Watts at Broadmoor in August 1988. He had not been allowed to have a picture of Haile Selassie on the walls of his ward. Many members of his patient care team had no knowledge of religious beliefs, and Watts himself had stated that mention of his Rastafarian beliefs would lead to punitive action by way of increased medication (he had even been told by a staff member to 'shut up about religion' or his medication would be increased). Staff had referred to Watts as a 'gorilla' and a 'monkey' (Special Hospitals Service Authority, 1988). The more recent report from Broadmoor is even clearer with respect to the attitudes of staff who did not seem to be aware of racism or the special needs of ethnic minority inmates.

Even the cultural and religious significance of food was not recognised (Special Hospitals Service Authority, 1993, pp. 52–5).

The View from the 'Other' Side

> In a sense what appears to be the most telling account of the ways in which race influences the decisions of professionals comes out not from their own reports, but from the account of the (black) people about whom these decisions are made, for it is here and only here that we will begin to understand the nature of racist practice – in the very violent effect it has on ordinary people's lives (Browne, 1993, p. 75).

The often violent treatment meted out to African and African-Caribbean people within the mental health system is not without literary support. Bryan, Dadzie and Scafe's contribution (1985), supported by accounts of cases which the authors have dealt with, remains a very powerful account of the treatment of Black women at the hands of the state as employer and policeman. Among the areas of concern highlighted is a dissatisfaction with the health and welfare system where professionals' treatment of Black women seems to be organised around premises that do not respect a woman's right to control her own fertility or her right to look after her family. Horrific treatment in prison, including the denial of food according to religious demands, forcible injection with tranquillisers and solitary confinement appear to be a common occurrence. The Black Health Workers and Patients Group (1983) also tell of ethnic minorities barbaric treatment by the legal and health systems, including case studies about the uses of psychiatric diagnoses, treatment by the police and the court and prison system. Similarly, Browne's (1995) recent account also contains two case studies which reveal, along similar lines, how the criminalization and sectioning systems work hand-in-hand to institutionalise African-Caribbeans. With such treatment being experienced daily by some ethnic minorities it is small wonder that detainees feared that the authorities in Broadmoor were 'killing them off' (Special Hospitals Service Authority, 1993, p. 52).[14]

Studies on Mental Health Law

We have recounted above some of the existing literature which shows that where Black people (Africans and African-Caribbeans) are concerned, professionals use the mental health system at all levels to the former's detriment. To what extent do the existing studies and guide-books on the operation of the mental health legislation evince an acknowledgement that there are problems in this area of the law? To what extent do the books continue to deal with the issues in a 'colour-blind' manner?

Clive Unsworth's (1987) study of the history and politics behind the mental health legislation does not attempt to take a perspective incorporating ethnic or cultural factors. Campbell and Heginbotham (1991) analyse the types of discrimination faced by the mentally ill, and refer to the models of the race and sex discrimination laws, but they do not recognise the 'double discrimination' faced by those from ethnic minorities classified as mentally ill. Peay's (1989) study of decision making by the Mental Health Review Tribunal in cases of patients at a Special Hospital is generally very sensitive. Despite the fact that one of its research objectives was to examine the way in which tribunals reached their decisions, no specific indication is given about the detainees ethnicity as a factor integral to the Tribunal's decisions. A more recent work which is supposed to act as a users guide to the Tribunal's operation and the legal questions that may arise under the 1983 legislation appears to be totally ignorant of ethnicity issues (Eldergill, 1998). Although there is a large section on assessing the presence of mental disorders no indication is given that such medical information may contain cultural biases. *Jones' Mental Health Act Manual* (1994), a section-by-section guide to the relevant statutory materials, is similarly unconscious of ethnic minority issues, except when it points out that a social worker's duty is to interview clients in a 'suitable manner'. That phrase was inserted into Section 13 of the 1983 Act due to concern expressed in Parliament over language difficulties faced by ethnic minorities (Jones, 1994, p. 52).

A review of studies on the exercise of police powers to detain after the Police and Criminal Evidence Act 1984 contains a small section on 'mentally disordered or mentally handicapped people' which makes no reference to ethnicity (Bucke and Brown, 1997, pp. 7–9). Prins's (1986) study of the 'forensic' sections of the Mental Health Act and other powers that the courts enjoy does not refer to ethnicity, race or culture. Dell and Robertson (1988) concentrate on male prisoners at Broadmoor Hospital and their diagnosis (either psychotic or psychopathic), admission, treatment and discharge. Although the reports by the committees of inquiry into the deaths of Joseph Watts and Orville Blackwood are very aware of the fact that African-Caribbean prisoners are over-represented in Broadmoor (Special Hospitals Service Authority, 1989 and 1993), Dell and Robertson make no attempt to analyse the implications of their ethnicity for the detainees concerned.

The studies cited so far seem to have made virtually no attempt to assess the impact of the mental health laws as they operate in a multi-ethnic context. Especially given the interest about over-diagnosis of certain mental illnesses and the involvement of the police in initiating committals, this lack of awareness shows an unwillingness to question the assumptions of formal legal equality. Further, there may be nervousness among critical legal scholars to question the culture-neutral fictions predominant in Western psychiatry which other professional orthodoxies simply tend to defer to.

Two writers who do make some reference to the type of difficulties to be faced by African-Caribbean people are Michael Cavadino (1989) and Brenda Hoggett (1996). Cavadino shows an awareness of several studies already reviewed about Black people's treatment in the mental health system. Hoggett mentions an early case concerning a woman from Jamaica as an example of the black experience of the mental health laws. She was arrested under Section 136 of the Mental Health Act by police who had come on the scene to inquire about a neighbour dispute, was taken to a police station, and thereafter committed to hospital from where she was released within a few hours. Her bid to sue for false imprisonment in the courts failed.[15] Here there is a definite awareness that *something* is wrong with the system. Unfortunately, two or three-page analyses do not suffice. While writers like Hoggett and Cavadino, unlike the former group, instinctively feel that there is a problem here with respect to how the law treats (some) ethnic minorities, their (limited) analyses do carry a danger that there is a continual reproduction of stereotypes of mental health, as with the 'criminogenic' pathologies which legitimise criminalisation of the same groups.

Conclusions

In the first part of this review we attempted to reflect on some emergent literature in selected legal fields to indicate where there may be intersections between mental health issues for ethnic minorities and the official English legal system. They are presented as doorways through which further exploration of the complex issues arising could take place. Then we have tried to examine how the Mental Health Act powers have affected ethnic minorities. Since most of this study has concentrated on issues concerning African-Caribbeans in Britain, it is pertinent to point out that when discussion about the position of ethnic minorities takes place, there are dangers, pointed to by Menski (1997, p. 72) in the context of law teaching in fields of concern to ethnic minorities:

> ... the repercussions of linking Africans and Afro-Caribbeans with topics like race and crime are alarming. The uncritical reproduction of official stereotypes is certainly problematic; it seems essential to discuss why the law has specific problems with certain groups ... inadvertent racism remains a professional hazard constantly shared by all participants.

Another caution which has exercised our minds is the danger of conflating a multiplicity of experiences under general terms such as Black, African-Caribbean, African, West Indian, Asian and so forth, which all empirical studies rely upon to base their findings. In commenting on these we have not intended any implication of essentialization of identities. However, whatever the problematic associated in the use of general terms, we have found some of this material valuable in guiding us through the mazes of law and medicine, in which certain reproductive cycles based on broad ethnic categories recur. We remain conscious of the fact that further work remains to be done in the same field for South Asian and other ethnic minorities (and majorities) and the trajectories of their relationships with the official system.

Thus we have pointed to some research literature in other fields which takes into account the different levels of decision making to analyse the points at which discriminatory practices in the compulsory admission system could be identified. We also point to some accounts of individuals' experiences in the (mental) health system. Our main observation is that legal research directed to studying the mental health system is woefully inadequate and, largely, does not even bother to take literature from other fields into account. Even where this is done, to what extent can one be confident of relying on research studies elsewhere which may contain certain slants? For example, Littlewood (1992, p. 145) in his review of research on differing patterns of psychiatric diagnosis for ethnic minorities bemoans the fact that most explanations assume that 'the conventional biomedical definition of schizophrenia reflects something "real": objectively justifiable ... and potentially independent of the perception of ethnicity by the psychiatrist'. But these are precisely the studies which progressive legal writers seem to rely on. Thus, while endless pages can be written about whether discrimination within the legal system exists, as has already been done in the criminological field, the idea persists that, fundamentally, the law is and should continue to be the same for everybody.

It seems that legal writers need to do much catching up here and we would not dismiss the rich potential in interdisciplinary communication, but would only point out that a broader view needs to be taken of precisely what the character of these contacts is going to be. To what extent does the law in alliance with professional groups delegitimise non-Western cosmologies of mental well-being? Stone and Matthews' recent work on *Complementary Medicine and the Law* is aware that 'certain systems of traditional medicine remain popular and well-supported by ethnic communities [*sic*] within Britain' (1994, p. 61) although they acknowledge that the official legal system has largely kept its distance. What space is there for the retention of, and support for, these therapies, increasingly popular with many groups of people in Britain today? What is the role of religion and faith here? For future work we look forward to investigations about how pluralist approaches could be built into legal studies of mental health. In this regard the path paved by the critical work of Fernando (1991) is worthy of note. First making an exposé of the historical and present day ethnocentrisms in Western psychiatry, and then attempting to summarise a great deal of learning about non-Western cosmologies of mental health, he goes on to formulate a proposal for pluralist mental health provision, with a cohabitation of Western and non-Western medical knowledge, but with freedom from the dominance and coercion exercised by Western notions and practices of psychiatry. Confronting these issues will imply a radical critique of the kind of state-sanctioned terror which has been unleashed upon some minority groups but also inevitably lead us to re-examining what pluralist mental health laws will look like.

Notes

1   The reviewers in particular would like to acknowledge the invaluable support given to this research by Werner Menski, Senior Lecturer in South Asian Laws at the School of Oriental and African Studies.

2   For a report of the study conducted by Bristol University for the Law Society's race relations committee, see the *Law Society Gazette*, 6 October 1993 or *New Law Journal*, 1 October 1993. The study speculates that perceptions may change if there were more solicitors from ethnic minorities.

3   *Crown Suppliers (PSA) v Dawkins* [1993] Industrial Court Reports 517. Even here there are ambiguous signals. In *Samuels v Capitol Security Services Ltd* (*EOR Discrimination Case Law Digest*, No. 31, Spring 1997, p. 3) a Stratford industrial tribunal allowed a case of a British Afro-Caribbean man wearing locks. The Tribunal reasoned that the discrimination

had been on the basis that 'It is a style of hair which, by its nature, is peculiar to black people'. In this way the 'ethnic group' test was bypassed.

4   *R v Ribbans, Duggan and Ridley, The Times*, 25 November 1994, CA.

5   For a recent case where a young Somali woman who complained of a racial assault was herself arrested by the police see *Farah v Commissioner of Police of the Metropolis* [1997] 1 All ER 289, CA. The Court of Appeal held that while officers could individually be liable under the Race Relations Act 1976, the Commissioner of the Met. could not be liable vicariously for their acts.

6   *R v George, McKay, Hayes and Hinds, The Times*, 9 November 1994.

7   There is much material on law and mental health in other languages although, from what the present writers could make out, not specifically or obviously related to cross-cultural situation. The search terms 'mental health', 'psychiatry', 'psychiatric hospitals', 'ethnic minorities' and 'race' were used (where two or more words are used entries in which either appears would be apprehended).

8   Under the terms 'mental health', 'psychiatric hospitals', 'racism', 'ethnicity', 'ethnic relations'.

9   Both contain notes on the sources. The former includes commentaries about the major issues emerging from the existing research. The latter was compiled from the King's Fund Library and as well as other data sources, including DHSS data.

10   The search terms 'Black', 'ethnic minority', 'mental health' and 'race' were used.

11   For example the Criminal Justice Act 1991, Section 4, carries a reminder to judges that they should consider psychiatric detention as an option.

12   Many empirical studies have focused on Afro-Caribbeans and, to a lesser degree, West Africans' vulnerability to psychotic illnesses, in particular schizophrenia. Most are of an epidemiological nature, attempting to find the reasons for high rates of such diagnoses (see studies cited in Karmi and McKeigue, 1993, pp. 74–81).

13   The analysis of social factors in the construction of 'cannabis psychosis' by Ranger (1989) shows that race and culture are strong determinants of that diagnosis.

14   Sayce (1995) provides some insights about fears of deaths in custody and discusses the Clunis and Blackwood cases, although she is rather silent on ethnicity and race issues.

15   *Carter v Metropolitan Police Commissioner* [1975] 1 Weekly Law Reports 507, CA.

References

Atkin, K. and Rollings, J. (1993), *Community Care in a Multi-racial Britain: a Critical Review of the Literature*, HMSO, London.

Black Health Workers and Patients Group (1983), 'Psychiatry and the Corporate State', *Race and Class*, XXV, pp. 49–64.

Bowl, R. and Barnes, M. (1990), Race, Racism and Mental Health Social Work: Implications for Local Authority Policy and Training', *Research, Policy and Planning*, 8(2), pp. 12–18.

Browne, D. (1991), *Black People, Mental Health and the Courts*, NACRO, London.

Browne, D. (1993), 'Race Issues in Research on Psychiatry and Criminology', in Cook, D. and Hudson, B. (eds) (1993), *Racism and Criminology*, Sage, London, pp. 64–76.

Browne, D. (1995), 'Sectioning: the Black Experience', in Fernando, S. (ed), *Mental Health in a Multi-ethnic society: a Multi-disciplinary Handbook*, Routledge, London, pp. 11–35.

Bryan, B., Dadzie, S. and Scafe, S. (1985), *The Heart of the Race. Black Women's Lives in Britain*, Virago, London.

Bucke, T. and Brown, D. (1997), 'PACE Ten Years On: a Review of the Research', Home Office Research Study No. 155, Home Office Research and Statistics Directorate, London.

Campbell, T. and Heginbotham, C. (1991), *Mental Illness: Prejudice, Discrimination and the Law*, Dartmouth, Aldershot.

Cashmore, E. and McLaughlin, E. (eds) (1991), *Out of Order? Policing Black People*, Routledge, London and New York.

Cavadino, M. (1989), *Mental Health Law in Context. Doctor's Orders?*, Dartmouth, Aldershot.

Cheney, D. (1993), Valued Judgements?: a Reading of Immigration Cases', *Journal of Law and Society*, pp. 23–38.

Chigwada, R. (1991), 'The Policing of Black women', in Cashmore, E. and McLaughlin, E. (eds), *Out of Order? Policing Black People*, Routledge, London and New York, pp. 134–50.

Cook, D. and Hudson, B. (eds) (1993), *Racism and Criminology*, Sage, London.

Cope, R. (1989), 'The Compulsory Detention of Afro-Caribbeans under the Mental Health Act', *New Community*, 15(3), pp. 343–56.

Cope, R. and Ndegwa, D. (1990), 'Ethnic Differences in Admission to a Regional Secure Unit', *Journal of Forensic Psychiatry*, 1, pp. 365–78.

Crowley, J.J. and Simmons, S. (1992), 'Mental Health, Race and Ethnicity: a Retrospective Study of the Care of Ethnic Minorities and Whites in a Psychiatric Unit', *Journal of Advanced Nursing*, 17, pp. 1078–87.

Dell, S. and Robertson, G. (1988), *Sentenced to Hospital. Offenders in Broadmoor*, Oxford University Press, Oxford.

Dunn, J. and Fahy, J.A. (1990), 'Police Admissions to a Psychiatric Hospital: Demographic and Clinical Differences between Ethnic Groups', *British Journal of Psychiatry*, pp. 373–8.

Eldergill, A. (1998), *Mental Health Review Tribunals. Law and Practice*, Sweet and Maxwell, London.

Fenton, S. (1987), *Ageing Minorities: Black People as they Grow Old in Britain*, Commission for Racial Equality, London.

FitzGerald, M. (1993), 'Ethnic Minorities and the Criminal Justice System', Royal Commission on Criminal Justice, Research Study No. 20, HMSO, London.

FitzGerald, M. and Hale, C. (1996), 'Ethnic Minorities, Victimisation and Racial Harassment', Home Office Study No. 154, HMSO, London.

Furhman, A. and Bochner, S. (1986), *Culture Shock*, Methuen, London and New York.

Glover, G.R. (1989), 'Differences in Psychiatric Admission Patterns between Caribbeans from Different Islands', *Social Psychiatry*, 24, pp. 209–11.

Gregory, J. (1987), *Sex, Race and the Law. Legislating for Equality*, Sage, London.

Harrison, G., Ineichen, B. and Smith, J. (1984), 'Psychiatric Admissions in Bristol. (1) Geographical and Ethnic Factors. (2) Social and Clinical Aspects of Compulsory Admissions', *British Journal of Psychiatry*, 145, pp. 600–11.

Harrison, G., Owens, D., Holton, A., Neilson, D., and Boot, D. (1988), 'A Prospective Study of severe Mental Disorder in Afro-Caribbean patients', *Psychological Medicine*, 18, pp. 643–57.

Hood, R. (1992), *Race and Sentencing*, Clarendon, Oxford.

Hoggett, B. (1996), *Mental Health Law*, Sweet and Maxwell, London.

Jones, R. (1994), *Mental Health Act Manual*, Sweet and Maxwell, London.

Joy, F. (1995), 'Cast Aside', *Community Care*, No. 1088, 28 September, pp. 16–17.

Judicial Studies Board (1996), Fourth Annual Report of the Ethnic Minorities Advisory Committee, London.

Karmi, G. and McKeigue, P. (1993), *The Ethnic Health Bibliography*, North East and North West. Thames Regional Health Authority.

Littlewood, R. (1992), 'Psychiatric Diagnosis and Racial Bias: Empirical Interpretive Approaches', *Social Science and Medicine*, 34(2) pp. 141–9.

Mama, A. (1992), 'Black Women and the English State: Race, Class and Gender Analysis for the 1990s', in Braham, P., Rattansi, A. and Skellington, R. (eds), *Racism and Anti-racism: Inequalities, Opportunities and Policies*, Sage and Open University Press, London.

McGovern, D. and Cope, R. (1987), First Psychiatric Admissions Rates of First and Second Generation Afro-Caribbeans', *Social Psychiatry*, 22, pp. 139–49.

McGovern, D. and Cope, R. (1991), 'Second Generation Afro-Caribbeans and Young Whites with a First Admission Diagnosis of Schizophrenia', *Social Psychiatry*, 26, pp. 95–9.

Medical Foundation for the Care of Victims of Torture (1994), *A Betrayal of Hope and Trust: Detention in the UK of Survivors of Torture*, Medical Foundation, London.

Menski, Werner (1993), 'Asians in Britain and the Question of Adaptation to a New Legal Order: Asian Laws in Britain?', in Israel, M. and Wagle, N.K. (eds), *Ethnicity, Identity, Migration: The South Asian Context*, Centre for South Asian Studies, University of Toronto [South Asian Studies Papers, No. 6], pp. 238–68.

Menski, W. (1997), 'Race and Law', Ireland, P. and Laleng, P. (eds), *The Critical Lawyers Handbook 2*, Pluto, London and Chicago, pp. 61–75.

Menski, W. (1998), 'South Asian Women in Britain, Family Integrity and the Primary Purpose Rule', in Bradley, H., Fenton, S. and Barot, R. (eds), *Ethnicity, Gender and Social Change*, Macmillan, London.

Moodley, P. and Perkins, R. (1991), 'Routes to Psychiatric In-patient Care in an Inner London Borough', *Social Psychiatry and Psychiatric Epidemiology*, 26, pp. 47–51.

Nazroo, J. (1997), *The Mental Health of Ethnic Minorities*, Policy Studies Institute, London.

Oakley, R. (1989), Community and Race Relations Training for the Police: a Review of Developments', *New Community*, 16(1), pp. 61–79.

Oakley, R. (1995), 'Police Training on Community and Race Relations: the Role of the Specialist Support Unit', *The Police Journal*, January, pp. 32–8.

Perera et al. (1991), *Ethnic Aspects: a Comparison of Three Matched Groups*.

Peay, J. (1989), *Tribunals on Trial. A Study of Decision-making under the Mental Health Act 1983*, Clarendon Press, Oxford.

Pipe, R., Bhat, A., Matthews, B. and Hampstead., J. (1991), 'Section 136 and African/Afro-Caribbean Minorities', *International Journal of Social Psychiatry*, 37, pp. 14–23.

Poulter, S. (1986), *English Law and Ethnic Minority Customs*, Butterworths, London.

Prins, H. (1986), *Dangerous Behaviour, the Law and Mental Disorder*, Tavistock Publica tions, London and New York.

Ranger, Chris (1989), 'Race, Culture and "Cannabis Psychosis": the Role of Social Factors in the Construction of Disease Categories', *New Community*, 15(3), pp. 357–69.

Robilliard, St John A. (1984), *Religion and the Law. Religious Liberty in Modern English Law*, Manchester University Press, Manchester.

Rwegellera, G.G.C. (1980), 'Differential Use of Psychiatric Services by West Indians, West Africans and English in London', *British Journal of Psychiatry*, 137, pp. 428–32.

Sayce, E. (1995), 'Response to Violence: a Framework for Fair Treatment', in Crichton, J. (ed.), *Psychiatric Patient Violence*, Duckworth, London, pp. 127–50.

SHARE (1997), *Mental Health (a Bibliography)*, King's Fund Institute, London.

Special Hospitals Service Authority (1989), 'Report of the Inquiry into the Circumstances leading to the Death in Broadmoor Hospital of Mr Joseph Watts on 23 August 1988', SHSA, London.

Special Hospitals Service Authority (1993), 'Report of the Committee of Inquiry into the Death in Broadmoor Hospital of Orville Blackwood and a Review of the Deaths of two other Afro-Caribbean Patients: "Big, Black and Dangerous"', SHSA, London.

Stone, J. and Matthews, J. (1994), *Complementary Medicine and the Law*, Oxford University Press, Oxford.

Unsworth, C. (1987), *The Politics of Mental Health Legislation*, Clarendon, Oxford.

Virdee, S. (1995), *Racial Violence and Harassment*, Policy Studies Institute, London.

Watters, C. (1996), 'Representations and Realities: Black People, Community Care and Mental Illness', in Ahmad, W.I. and Atkin, K. (eds), *Race and Community Care*, Open University Press, Buckingham and Philadelphia, pp. 105–23.

Chapter 7

Black Families

William Obomanu

In recent years there has been an overlap in the interest shown by a variety of disciplines in the concept of the family. The concept of family values has been taken up by politicians in relation to the effect on society of the perceived demise of the traditional family. In the academic and health fields, anthropologists, family therapists, sociologists and psychiatrists have been concerned to widen the concept of 'the patient' to include the family and, where relevant the wider community. There has been much adverse comment on the contribution made by therapeutic services in dealing with the distress experienced by members of Britain's ethnic minorities as they cope with the stresses of adapting to life in Britain, a contribution which has often been found to be wanting due to a lack of understanding on the part of the professionals about the issues involved. This chapter aims to review recent papers presenting a number of perspectives on the family in order to discuss the issues involved in delivery of culturally relevant therapy on the family model. In terms of formal family therapy there is little systematic research in this area in this country and as a result the paper will draw on relevant experience and research from the US.

People of non-European origin have been in the British Isles since the sixteenth century, and there were some Africans in the retinue of King James IV of Scotland during the fifteenth century, but there is little systematic data available today about early Black populations in Britain. Historical sources suggest that African communities developed in London, Bristol and Liverpool, and were estimated to number as many as 14,000–15,000 (2 per cent of the contemporary population of London) by the end of the eighteenth century (Shyllon, 1974). The majority of these were brought from the West Indies to work as personal slaves. This population, largely of African origin, was supplemented by free seamen from Nelson's navy and the merchant marine. The Black population then seems to have disappeared from public view, perhaps because many Black men living in Britain died without issue and there were few Black women. Inter-racial cohabitation or marriages were known and commented upon (Walvin, 1973). Until the early twentieth century small populations of Blacks (a few thousand) could be found in London, Bristol, Cardiff, Liverpool and other ports. These were mainly men of West African origin, rather than the descendants of the earlier population, and the numbers of Blacks did not increase again until recruitment drives in the West Indies during the First World War. Asians, present since the nineteenth century, attracted less attention. Most were free servants rather than slaves, or were grandees and their children (Visram, 1986), and by the end of the nineteenth century small numbers of Chinese had begun to settle, again largely in port towns. At the 1931 census, 86,963 persons born in India were said to be living in England and Wales, 5,232 born in the African colonies, and 10,468 born in the West Indies and South Americas. However, a large proportion of these would have been White people of British origin. By 1954 it was estimated that the 'Negro minority' in England had risen to 43,000, including the indigenous black population (Banton, 1955). Since the Second World War large-scale immigration to the UK from the New Commonwealth has produced increasing cultural and racial diversity. The 1991 census estimates that, before adjustments for under-reporting, approximately 3 million of the UK population is from an ethnic minority group (5.5 per cent of the total population).

The last few decades have witnessed increasing amounts of research into the circumstances of ethnic minority populations in Great Britain. The Policy Studies Institute and its predecessor, Political and Economic Planning (PEP) have conducted four major programmes of epidemiological research into the social and economic condition of Britain's racial minorities, in 1966–67, 1974–75, 1982 and 1992 (Jones, 1993). These studies made detailed comparisons with the white majority population, and concluded that racial minorities as a whole had substantially lower living standards than white people did. Previous research suggested that, in terms of employment, people of Afro-Caribbean and South Asian origin have historically been over-represented in poorly paid jobs, even when qualification levels were taken into account. In housing, people from the ethnic minorities tended to be in lower-quality housing. Research in the 1960s showed that much racial disadvantage stems from discrimination in the labour and housing markets (Daniel, 1968). Research in the early 1980s showed that despite some changes since the 1970s, the overall position of racial minorities remained one of substantial disadvantage compared to the white population (Brown, 1984). Thus, three decades after the first major waves of immigration from the Caribbean and Indian subcontinents, research on ethnic minorities in Britain showed remarkable consistency with earlier patterns. Clearly, regardless of race, any immigrants who have to adapt to life in a new country would expect to face some disadvantage and difficulties for a time. However factors limiting opportunities for newly arrived immigrants, such as overt discrimination, poor job opportunities and limited access to good quality housing may have set a pattern that continued after the constraints themselves had ceased. Against this, there is also evidence of a strong dynamic among ethnic minority communities, which drives them to develop beyond the social and economic niches that they fill for the first 20 years. Since the 1970s an expanding literature has focused on the functioning of ethnic minority families. The bulk of this work, mostly American, has emphasised the harmful effects of racism, poverty and political powerlessness so that positive aspects of ethnicity such as traditions, coping skills and belief systems are neglected. Since many of the political realities of life in Britain are similar to those of African-Americans many parallels can be drawn between the two. However, it is important not to gloss over the fact that there are important differences between them too, and that the passage of time has changed certain characteristics within each population.

Ethnic values and identities are retained for many generations after immigration. Fourth generation Americans have been demonstrated to differ from the dominant culture in terms of lifestyles, behaviour and values, suggesting that even in the 'melting pot' of the United States ethnicity remains an important determinant of family patterns, belief systems and cultural identity (Greeley, 1969). Similarly, distinctive patterns of family and household sizes and structures for different groups can endure across many generations, and data from the 1910 US Census showed the existence of substantial racial differences in family and household structure. Compared with Whites, African-American households were less likely to consist of a single nuclear family and more likely to be headed by women. This appears to still be the case in the USA today. Continuities such as these in living arrangements within ethnic groups suggest that the influence of economic, cultural and demographic factors also remain important (Morgan, 1993). Although there is now a substantial American literature in this field there is little comparable available for Britain, partly due to the fact that there were no large ethnic minority groups in Britain until recent times. Data on ethnic minority groups has only become widely available since the 1970s through large-scale official surveys such as the Labour Force Survey (LFS) and National Dwelling and Housing Survey NDHS and a number of other specialised surveys (see Brown, 1984). These surveys have provided insights into living arrangements of ethnic groups (Haskey, 1989, Berrington, 1994; Commission for Racial Equality, 1988; Department of the Environment, 1993). Their findings demonstrating the concentration of disadvantage in many ethnic minority populations have stimulated a number of policy responses relating to the issues of equal opportunities, race relations and the provision of special support for disadvantaged communities. Since the 1991 British Census included for the first time a question on ethnicity, Britain has become the only Western European country to have explicit questions on ethnicity in its census (apart from the Channel Islands). The official explanation for the introduction of these questions, were set out in the Census White Paper of 1991, justifying their inclusion on the grounds of general public welfare and race relations. The main thrust of the argument is that, in order that resources can be allocated in line with the special needs of particular communities, more detailed data was required on the living arrangements, employment and age-structure of different groups. The 1991 census data now allows these areas to be examined in more detail (Murphy, 1996).

The Family as the Basic Social Group

A general problem in analysing data on families is the sheer diversity of people's living arrangements. When we speak of a 'household' or 'the family' the implication is of a unit of social organisation which is in some way distinctive. However, definitions of the family overlap, frequently contradict each other, and can change over time, demonstrating a mutability which has led to the family being referred to as a 'zombie' category; that is, a social category which is 'dead and yet alive' (Beck, 1999). Most definitions of the terms are imprecise, allowing several alternative definitions so that the family can be defined as a geographical unit, as an economic unit in which individuals are dependent upon one another, or as a social unit of individuals who live together. There are differences in the size of households and families; the roles played within them by men and women; and the extent to which households comprise one person or family, or are constituted by more complex units. The composition of the family group varies greatly between cultures, as does the role it plays in the lives of individual family members. In urban industrialised societies the nuclear family is now the norm, contrasted with the extended multigenerational pattern seen more commonly worldwide. Often, in poorer areas of the world, the larger family unit acts as a self-contained community or self-help group while still linked to the wider society. In all settings, within the family resources are shared as are everyday tasks and responsibilities. Regardless of the cultural context the family usually includes members who are not biologically related to the family, and therefore forms a social as well as a biological entity and usually such 'fictive kin' may include close friends, neighbours or health professionals. It can be useful to view the family as a small-scale society with its own distinctive organisation and culture since, although 'family cultures' are usually notably similar to the wider societal culture, they are rarely identical to it. Like larger societal institutions and other groups families have their own world views, gender roles, history, and develop particular patterns of communication which may heavily influence individual members ways of communicating distress to one another or outside bodies such as healthcare professionals and therapists.

Underpinning modern critical notions of the family is a view that, as a result of trends towards individualisation, social institutions of industrial society such as class, family and gender have become 'disembedded' so that people are increasingly freed from historically inscribed roles. The individualisation created by this unmooring of institutions creates new forms of social commitment but may at the same time render other roles obsolete. While undermining the support and security formerly found through institutions such as religious faith, individualisation liberates people from traditional roles and constraints in a variety of ways. As social classes are 'detraditionalised' in terms of family structures, housing conditions, leisure activities, voting patterns and so on individuals are released from traditional roles as they utilise the new mobility between different status-based classes that has become available to them. For example, women are said to have become released from a 'status-fate' of compulsory housework and husband support, creating a new negotiated family composed of multiple relationships. As a consequence of the decline of traditional class and status groups individuals become the agents of their own identity and livelihood and are more able to replace the family unit with other friendships and alliances.

An example of the size of the social changes associated with these changes is the dramatic increase in single person households over the last 20 years such that in most large cities they now comprise over 50 per cent of all households. These and similar 'post-modern' arguments stress the breakdown of traditional categories and constraints and in doing so often highlight the opposing effects of a new standardisation based on the employment market. In other words the individual is removed from traditional commitments and support relationships but exchanges them for the constraints of existence within the labour market. A corollary of such arguments is that associated with this burgeoning dependence on the labour market is an increasing reliance on extra-familial structures such as state education, welfare state regulations and on fashions in medical, psychological and pedagogical care.

The boundary between the family and public spheres is marked out by various oppositions; between public and private, category and person, market and household, and interest and emotion. Unlike the market values that characterise public life, within the family members are reluctant to put monetary values or time limits on obligations or sentiments to other family members. A historical perspective shows a change in the typical family structures seen in the pre-industrial era and those seen in modern industrial times. Within North Europe and other Western countries the nuclear family has largely replaced the extended family, usually defined as a residential unit composed of the nuclear family living together with married offspring and their children. Opposition of the family and market domains in this way has contributed to a view of the nuclear family as a kind of 'super-personality' (Gubrium and Holstein, 1990). Others have argued that such views are reductionist and that their use of oppositions tends to obscure the subtler inter-penetration of kinship and economics in modern societies, and the permeable nature of the boundary between household and market. As Medick and Sabean (1988) argue 'emotional needs imply social structures and can only be fulfilled within relationships whose structure is shaped by complex material forces'.

Notwithstanding the diversity of family forms and the statistical abnormality of the 'normal' two-parent family unit the normative stereotype persists and the notion of the nuclear family household remains a central theme in academic and popular thinking, at least in relation to industrialised Western societies. Often it is characterised as a sacred private sphere, free from coercive state intervention or a 'haven in a heartless world' (Lasch, 1977). According to this view within the family can be found an affective antidote to the impersonal world of short-term market relationships that exist between people outside the family. Any account of the functions of the modern family must accommodate, to some degree at least, the many forms of family that exist in today's society and the necessarily varied and complex ways these forms relate to other institutions in society. Most views delineate a control function, with families represented as part of a system in which they interact with formal institutions to form a web of socialisation and control. The American sociologist, Talcott Parsons (1949), regarded the modern family as a response to the societal differentiation brought by the Industrial Revolution. He distinguished two irreducible functions as being the primary socialisation of children and the stabilisation of adult personalities within the society. Parsons viewed the nuclear family as the agency best adapted to creating a personality type suited to the demands encountered within a highly rational industrial society and considered the psychological experience children receive within the family patterns their later participation in the occupational milieu and in the wider society. He based his argument on a presumption that the nuclear family has a role as the centre of emotional support and affective expression which is situated in a society where all other spheres are given over to detachment and calculation and also remains a place to which individuals return to refuel their emotional lives. This championing of the harmony between the nuclear family and industrial society has been criticised as an apology for capitalist values. Another more critical view of the relationship between modern society and the nuclear family is articulated by Richard Sennett (1978), who considered the advent of the nuclear family as a manifestation of people's progressive retreat from an increasingly hostile society. Sennett observed that since the thirteenth century the family has moved from a large corporate form strongly enmeshed in society at all levels to the nuclear form we are more familiar with today. He saw this as problematic since such a growth of privacy results in the formation of intensive family structures that deny children the chance to build a fund of experience with a wide range of people from an early age. This may then lead to ineptitude when they are faced with unfamiliar challenges outside the family as young adults. Unlike Parsons, Sennett challenged the view that the conjugal nuclear family is the form best suited for industrial society and suggested that the more communal extended family form might suit the needs of modern society better. Despite their different conclusions, both Sennett and Parsons construct arguments that tend to reflect the sociological concern with processes within society as a whole rather than focusing on the individuals within the family.

Black Families and Households

Attempting to systematically study and describe the 'Black family' presents additional difficulties to those outlined above. There are the problems discussed above related to the different definitions of 'Black' that have been used in different studies. In addition, defining an 'ethnic minority household' is problematic if the household includes members of more than one ethnic minority. The best source of information about contemporary family living arrangements, the 1991 Census, also highlighted special difficulties in the interpretation of results for ethnic families, such as that caused by their relatively young age structure compared to indigenous White families. Another such methodological hurdle in making comparisons between different ethnic groups is that, since average household and family size and structure vary during the family cycle, observed overall differences among and between ethnic groups may reflect demographic factors rather than being the consequence of either choices or external constraints. Despite these factors, broad comparisons can still be made between different groups. It seems likely that following the census in 2001 fresh data will allow more detailed comparison of both differences and trends. In the following passage some findings of the 1991 census about differences between the living arrangements of ethnic minority households in the UK are outlined, followed by a brief discussion of their implications. In the following discussion, the terms used will be the main classificatory terms employed by the 1991 census; i.e. 'Black' will be taken broadly as 'non-white', i.e. including Black-Caribbean, Black-African, Indian, Pakistani, and Chinese.

Patterns of Family Structure

Households are made of family units. As defined in the 1991 census nuclear families consist of a couple (married or cohabiting) with or without never-married children, or a lone parent with never-married children. Grandparents with never-married children constitute a nuclear family even if there is a 'missing middle generation'. In the case of a three-generation group consisting of the grandparents, never-married child and grandchildren the last two are said to form the family unit. Thus the primary classification of family types is by whether or not a household contains a couple and whether or not children are present. The most noteworthy finding of the census was the high prevalence of lone parenthood among the Black women. South Asians were found to be much more likely to be living as part of a couple with children, and much less likely to be living outside a family unit than all other groups. The lifetime experienced varied markedly between groups. An illustrative example is that while a third of White men experience the 'empty nest syndrome' around the age of 50, for Pakistani/Bangladeshi men this stage in the family cycle is reached at that rate only by the age of 70, by which time about two-thirds of Whites are in this situation. By contrast, there is no stage where more than one third of Black women are in the empty nest phase.

Analysis of living arrangement is commonly done using the headship rates, i.e. the proportion of those in a particular age, sex or other group who are designated as 'head of household'. Among teenagers the lowest rates are found among the Indian group (0.4 per cent) and the highest among Black women. For adult men the patterns are broadly similar at younger ages but in the middle working years, Black and (to a lesser extent) White men have lower rates than all the Asian ethnic groups. This has been linked to marriage differences in that a much higher proportion of Asian men tend to be married at these ages. However the situation is reversed at older ages so that at age 75, about 90 per cent of Black and White men, but only about 50 per cent of South Asian ethnic group men are household heads. In contrast the rates start to decline among South Asian men before the age of 50. For women, patterns of headship rates are broadly similar for the three Asian groups on the one hand and for Black and White women on the other. Among White and Black women there is a tendency for the rates to decline until about age 50 and then increase. Among the Asian groups the rates are generally lower and show a steady rise with age. These trends reflect the different marriage patterns of the various groups; differences in the propensity of non-married women to head their own household; and differences in the likelihood of non-married women being designated 'head of household.' About half of Black women in their thirties are heads of household compared with about one in 10 South Asian women, and headship rates for married women are highest for Black women (apart from elderly women). White men have the highest headship rates overall. It may be an indicator of the role and status of women that one in five married Black women are the head of their household compared with one in 20 South Asian women, with White women in an intermediate position.

According to the 1991 Census the average household size, however defined, was largest among the South Asian (Indian sub-continent) groups, especially the Pakistani/Bangladeshi group (about two and a half times larger on average than among Whites (the smallest group). These large average household sizes are due both to larger numbers of adults and of children, but principally to more children. Only 0.4 per cent of people overall live in the largest household sizes (9–11); this figure rises to 13 per cent among Pakistani/Bangladeshi households.

Complex Households

The prevalence of extended family living (more than one family in a household) is relatively low overall. However, the census results indicate that all the ethnic minority groups are more likely than the White group to be living as part of an extended family, especially the South Asian group. Overall a third of the South Asians are living in a nuclear family with other permanent residents as well, and they are at least three times more likely than other groups to be living in a household containing at least two family units (about 15 per cent). The low over-all prevalence of extended family living should be viewed against the fact that prevalence is a cross-sectional measure and refers to the living arrangements on one particular day (in April 1991). Much higher proportions of the population is likely to have lived in such conditions at some point in their life. This was demonstrated in a 15-year longitudinal study of middle-aged women in the US, between a quarter and a third of White women, and two-thirds of Black women had lived in an extended family setting at some stage (Beck and Beck, 1989).

The proportion of complex households has been declining over time in Britain (Wall, 1983), with an apparently accelerating decline in the 1980s (Murphy and Berrington, 1993). This is despite the fact that the northern European pattern has been relatively simple for some centuries (Hajnal, 1982). In general, living in complex households is more common at certain stages of the life cycle: as young children, young adults and among older people, but the levels differ between groups. For South Asian groups, between 10 and 20 per cent of all age groups are likely to be living in complex households, whereas for the non-Asian groups the figure is at no stage more than 5 per cent. Given the relative scarcity of elderly South Asian people to form such households, such a high prevalence begs the question of how much this is a preferred living arrangement as opposed to a constraint imposed by inadequate housing. Comparisons of the 1991 Pakistani/Bangladeshi pattern with that of England and Wales in 1851 shows marked similarities, as do the respective average household sizes. These finding emphasise the similarities between South Asian household structures and those formerly seen in Britain, although it should be borne in mind that this does not imply the mechanism which lead to these similarities or allow one to adduce a trend in household structure. In households with more than one family, ethnic minority groups are more likely to share with relatives. This may be because they are more likely to be recent migrants and may be a transient effect (Haskey, 1989). Against this interpretation is the observation that the long-established Indian group tends to exhibit the greatest complexity. About one in six of the Indian group live in three-generation households, typically comprising a couple with children living with an elderly parent or parents. Blacks have the highest proportion of households containing a grandparent and grandchild with the intervening generation not in the household, and the typical three generation household is a young lone mother living with her parents. Multi-family households are not necessarily three-generation households but it seems that ethnic minority groups are more likely to have more distant relations living in their households than the White group. While vertically extended families are most common among the Indian group, the Pakistani/Bangladeshi and the Other-Asian groups are more likely to be horizontally extended, with more brothers and sisters living with the household head. 1991 census results suggest that among non-Asian groups, household extension is frequently a forced, or non-preferred arrangement. The situation is not quite so clear among the South Asian groups. In every group those higher up the social scale are more likely to be in a single-family home, with little difference in the pattern between the different groups. There is no evidence that higher social status groups are likely to seek extension (Murphy, 1996).

Strengths and Weaknesses of Black Families

Regardless of socioeconomic circumstances, Black children are aware from an early age of the negative value placed on their racial group by the dominant culture (Williams and Morland, 1976). Pinderhughes (1979) highlighted the influence on Black culture of the 'victim system', a circular feedback process which threatens self-esteem and reinforces problematic responses in communities, families and individuals. However not all Black children have poor self-esteem as a result of internalising these values, and Rosenberg (1979) found the self-esteem of Black school children no different from that of white school children. This finding highlights the existence of significant discrepancies between wider societal attitudes and those of particular ethnic minorities. According to Pinderhughes the victim system produces values that are the result of oppression and which emphasise cooperation to combat political impotence. These values include strict obedience to authority in response to perceived oppression, strength, toughness of character, present-time orientation (since the past is painful and there is no future), suppression and channelling of feelings into music, art and other creative activities, and belief in luck, magic and spirituality. Those most severely victimised hold values of autonomy and isolation as a defence against the stresses that engulf them, derived from a sense of abandonment rather than from a conscious effort towards growth or self-actualisation. Combinations of African, mainstream and victim values were found, such that Billingsley (1968) subsequently identified 12 different types of family structure but concluded that most black families do not correspond to any single category.

Hill (1972) reviewed the strengths of Black families, identifying a number of cultural themes seen in their adaptation to all contexts. These included: strong kinship bonds, a high degree of flexibility in family roles and high religious commitment. In his analysis he concluded that the themes he identified underline the diversity within black families and communities which confer coherence. Black families are often reluctant to seek mental health services. They distrust mainstream institutions generally and rely on 'mutual aid systems' (Martin and Martin, 1978) such as extended family ties and church organisations. This finding seems to hold true across class boundaries (McAdoo, 1977). According to data from the 1910 US census, the black kinship system is demonstrably larger than that among the white population; for example larger proportions of Black families take relatives into their home and the kinship system offers help with financial aid, childcare and other forms of mutual support. This situation is not necessarily beneficial to all the family members since, although strong kinship bonds provide valuable sustenance in times of trouble, extended family problems can also become integral to the family (Stack, 1974).

Billingsley (1968) highlighted high flexibility in gender roles within the black family, a view that has been supported by research that suggests that an egalitarian pattern of gender roles typifies black families (Scansoni 1975). This fluidity of roles is usually presumed to be result from socioeconomic imperatives and put down to the fact that historically Black women have had greater access to occupational opportunities than Black men. The consequence is that many black fathers perform domestic and emotional functions while the mother performs the instrumental or economic functions within the household. This situation does not in itself necessarily mean that the family is matriarchal, since it is a response to contextual economic factors rather than a manifestation of an innate cultural preference or difference. However many Black women consider motherhood a more important role than that of a wife, suggesting that their relationship with their partner can become a subsidiary one.

The role of religion in Black family and community life remains more prominent than in the increasingly secular modern White culture. Black churches have a major role in the provision of concrete social services such as senior citizens; activities, childcare and parenting groups, as well as latent functions such as release of emotions and leadership development. Although the role of the organised Christian churches dates back to the era of slavery, a belief in the supernatural remains common. In general, church culture heavily influences the individual's belief system and is often determinant of attitudes to healthcare systems and treatment modalities. Many Black people would rather leave problem-solving to God than take a chance with often unbelieving therapists. Religious beliefs can also be intimately related to political considerations and exert a subtle influence on beliefs, attitudes to healthcare agencies and to health seeking behaviour. For example, denominations such as the Rastafarian faith are rooted in resistance to slavery and its members may view Western treatments as potential contaminants, preferring alternative treatments such as herbalism, homeopathy or acupuncture.

Therapy and Black Families

Contemporary family therapy arose out of psychoanalytically informed thinking. The early practitioners were either psychoanalysts themselves or closely involved with the early psychoanalytic movement. Many of the early pioneers repudiated the psychoanalytic tradition, particularly in the United States. In the United Kingdom, however, psychoanalytic theoretical developments increasingly focused on the role of the emotional environment and the importance of the mother-infant relationship on individual emotional development. Work by Bettelheim and Erikson emphasised the influential role of the family and social environment but their work never became part of mainstream American theory. By contrast object relations theory was developed further in the United Kingdom and applied in the fields of marital therapy, general practice and hospital practice. Group analysis also developed from psychoanalytic ideas, and object relations theory was increasingly applied to group treatments by Ezriel, Bion and Turquet. Increasingly groups were seen to comprise individuals who took up roles that were similar to members of a family. This perspective developed such that therapeutic groups were conceptualised as taking up various family roles that were similar to those adopted in the group member's original family. Skynner worked with the family as a special form of group, as distinct from a 'stranger' group but soon came to view the family as a unique institution and as the main target of therapeutic endeavour instead of the individual within the family.

The 'Milan Team' (Palazzoli et al., 1971) split from the psychoanalytic model in order to explore a more interactional model, initiating a research project with a range of families who presented with a variety of problems. The team was influenced by Watzlawick (1967) in developing a framework that distinguished between the 'process' and 'content' of interpersonal communications. Under this model of family therapy symptoms were viewed as content and the interaction around the symptom as the process. This led to a focus on the systemic meaning and history of a symptom as well as a consideration of the current interactions between family members.

The group drew extensively on the anthropologist Gregory Bateson's ideas about 'multiple levels of context' in interpersonal systems and his dictum that 'without context there is no meaning'.

In systemic family therapy the family is often seen as a system in which patterns of interrelationships can influence both health and disease. Systems or cybernetic theory suggests that family dynamics are often aimed at maintaining a state of equilibrium between family members, by employing mechanisms such as 'scapegoating' or 'anointing' particular family members. Minuchin (1981) showed how certain family structures are more likely to produce disorders, for example, eating disorders in some of its members. Family cohesion and continuity are maintained by producing and maintaining the disorder in the 'identified patient' whose recovery may result in the break up or dysfunction of the 'pathological' family. Focusing on the individual alone will tend to frustrate a full understanding of the problem and identification of therapeutic interventions which might alter the equilibrium to a position where the family and identified patient can identify actions which will enable them to become healthy. Other theorists have conceptualised a 'family script', which is transmitted between generations. These scripts are ways of viewing the world and include emotional responses, which are often outside conscious awareness. They provide a sense of stability and continuity as well as avoiding potentially dangerous conflicts within the family. The role may even determine how and when people become ill or die and depends on the transmission of values so that different generations of the family are aware of their roles within the family script. The scripts can be maintained by the families' own private myths and folklore which may have originated centuries ago and which may exert an ongoing negative or beneficial effect on the health of family members.

More recent theoretical developments have resulted in greater rapprochement between psychoanalytic thinking and family therapists. Psychoanalytic research has tended to promote 'health' through a self-conscious examination of the therapist-patient relationship while in family therapy a number of pictures can be seen. One approach is to involve all family members in individual psychotherapy or psychoanalysis. This is in distinction to seeing the whole family together and giving interpretations to it as an entity with prominence being given to transference and counter-transference experience and fantasies. In this last approach the issues to be tackled and flow of material in sessions are left to the family, reminiscent of the paradigmatic psychoanalytic method of free association. Many family therapists can no longer be described as psychoanalytic since they pick out for special attention particular areas of family functioning such as intergenerational issues and individuation (Bowen, 1976), family loyalties Boszormenyi-Nagy and Spark (1973). Developments such as brief focal therapy (Malan, 1963, 1976) showed a tendency to challenge dogmas such as the belief that change could only occur as the result of long-term work, and to the abandonment of adherence to consensus about proper methods of therapeutic intervention. Early family therapists noted that a wide variety of methods appeared to be effective when applied to families, leading to comments that the theories advanced to legitimise such methods seemed to be little more than rationalisations for the interventions (Ferber, Mendelsohn and Napier, 1973). A product of this phenomena was that the needs of the family were defined by the theories (or formulations) developed for each family. The psychoanalytically oriented view assumed that a suitable formulation of family life would point the way to appropriate therapeutic action, and the formulation had primacy since it was possible to make a formulation which defined intervention as unlikely to have therapeutic efficacy.

Most family therapies available within the National Health system derive from psychodynamic psychotherapies, developed in European, and embedded in a particular socio-cultural and historical context. The model makes assumptions about norms for day-to-day life, notions of the family and individual roles in child-rearing. In addition the model implicitly assumes various culturally mediated issues such as concepts of personhood, obligations to family and community, independence, and other moral social values. Even assuming that the therapy achieves legitimacy by being founded on a universal psychology shared understanding of these aspects of life are likely to be fundamental to the success of any therapy. In individual therapies, since therapist and client are distinct unique beings, there is always an interpersonal and intercultural dimension to any cross-cultural therapy. Relating to a family with totally different life experiences in order to form a therapeutic alliance requires the therapist to make a bridge across which they can comprehend the difficulties of the family under treatment and this is only possible if the therapist gathers sufficient information about the family to allow awareness of cultural difference. Additionally, in order for the therapy to be effective it is necessary for the therapist to set family problems in their historical context. Both of these endeavours may be compromised when working with families of a different cultural background since the therapist may, through no particular fault of their own, have a sketchy knowledge of the culture concerned. The lack of such specific knowledge will result in either therapeutic nihilism or a reliance on vague or erroneous stereotypes that may not actually apply to the family under treatment.

The Relationship between Culture and Family Dynamics

McGoldrick et al. (1982) examined a selection of mini-ethnographies of the families of different American ethnic groups and the problems faced by therapists in dealing with them. In England, Lau (1984) has pointed out how West European or North American therapists may misdiagnose family patterns from other cultures as deviant or even pathological while Maranhao has argued that 'family oriented ethnic groups' are often described as if their differences from the 'Anglo-Saxon' family type were pathological by definition. DiNicola described the relationship between a family's mental health and the culture of origin in terms of 'cultural costume', defined as, 'the particular set of recipes the individuals or families of a community have to give meaning and shape to their experiences and to communicate these experiences through shared ceremonies, rituals and symbols'. Each family culture is a particular and sometimes unique expression of the broad repertoire of cultural beliefs and behaviours of the family. The cultural costume may become a 'cultural camouflage' when it is invoked as an explanatory smokescreen which obscures the elucidation by professionals of individual states of mind or patterns of interactions within the family. For instance, if an individual's mental health is compromised by such behaviour this cultural camouflage may frustrate professional efforts aimed at improving the individual's mental health since the individual will 'camouflage' the issues by employing arguments which counter the advice or interventions of the professionals. This is especially likely where family structures are unfamiliar to the professional involved such as one parent (e.g. West Indian families) or multigenerational extended families living in the same household (e.g. Asian, Chinese or Greek Cypriot families). Lau points out that 'breaks are not expected between the generations and continuity in the group depends on the presence of three generations' in many cultures outside the post-industrial West. This results in different meanings being attached to notions of family, individual personhood and autonomy. Barot has suggested that, when dealing with ethnic minorities, a focus on the culture of the family is insufficient unless account is also explicitly taken of wider analyses of institutional and structural factors, such as unemployment, poor housing, racial discrimination and the effects of migration. These external factors may, in addition to adversely affecting family members, also act to weaken the traditional culture and cohesion of these families so that 'culture' alone is no longer a viable explanation for many of the pathological breakdowns in normal family functioning.

Conclusion

The 1991 UK Census included, for the first time, a question on ethnicity in order to address perceived disadvantage faced by ethnic minority groups in Britain. This review has described aspects of ethnic minority families in Britain using the findings of the 1991 Census, which shows that substantial differences continue to exist between household and family patterns of different minority groups, and that these are more marked than those found between other socioeconomic groups within the population. Although, as a cross-sectional survey, the census is unable to identify trends taken with previous research from a variety of disciplines, its findings support the proposition that the conditions of ethnic minorities in the UK are changing, and that this process is likely to continue. Given that it is a snapshot survey, the 1991 Census cannot show the evolution of trends over time, and in particular the extent to which British-born ethnic minorities are moving towards patterns which are more typical of the population as a whole. As a result of this, the question remains as to how far the distinctive living arrangements identified are due to factors such as recent arrival, socioeconomic disadvantage, racial discrimination and harassment, the political context or cultural preferences. What the findings do clearly demonstrate, however, is the futility of treating the different ethnic groups as a single entity. Despite similar experiences of discrimination, the varying responses of the different groups are often opposed, rather than showing similar patterns. For these reasons it is difficult to predict the future of each group's living arrangements, apart from the vague postulation that as the proportion of British-born ethnic minorities increases, some convergence might be expected. Some emerging trends may impact more on certain ethnic groups, as seen in the US where birthplace effects are largely irrelevant but where shifts away from 'traditional' family arrangements have been greater for Blacks than for Whites (Bianchi and Farley, 1979). This phenomenon would tend to increase rather than reduce differences. There is some evidence that British-born blacks are more dissimilar to the overall pattern than those born overseas (Heath and Dale, 1994). In recent years there has been a debate about non-traditional family living arrangements, such as co-habitation and lone parenthood from some politicians, academics and other commentators. In Britain, unlike the US, there has been little specific connections made with the specific patterns of particular ethnic groups. The discourse in the US has centred around notions of 'choice' and negative images have been associated with particular groups, especially the Black and Hispanic groups. Although living arrangements can be assumed to be within the bounds of individual choice, the same is not true for skin colour, (which is the basis of the classification of ethnicity in the 1991 Census). Given the dramatically different patterns of living arrangements seen between ethnic groups in Britain, notions of 'choice' are likely to be of little help in understanding the cultural influences behind the 1991 Census results. Preferences are likely to be formed in different ways so that, for example, in groups where extra-marital childbearing is common, and where potential husbands have poor socioeconomic expectations, the conventional Western European nuclear family model may not be an option. The central role of the family and household environment for the socialisation of children means that attachment of negative images to particular living arrangements may have significant effects in terms of setting up self-fulfilling prophesies of low self-esteem and social disadvantage.

References

Banton, N. (1955), *The Coloured Quarter*, Jonathan Cape, London.

Beck, U. (1999), *New Times (3)*, pp. 18–21.

Beck, W. and Beck, S.H. (1989), 'The Incidence of Extended Households among Middle-aged Black and White Women: Estimates from a 15 Year Panel Study', *Journal of Family Issues*, 10(2), pp. 147–68.

Berrington, A. (1994), 'Marriage and Family Formation among the White and Ethnic Minority Populations in Britain', *Ethnic and Racial Studies*, 17(3), pp. 517–46.

Bettelheim, B. (1950), *Love is not Enough; the Treatment of Emotionally Disturbed Children*, Free Press, New York.

Bianchi, S.M. and Farley, R. (1979), 'Racial Differences in Family Living Arrangements and Economic Well-being: an Analysis of Recent Trends', *Journal of Marriage and the Family*, 41(3), pp. 537–51.

Billingsley, A. (1968), *Black Families in White America*, Prentice Hall, Englewood Cliffs, NJ.

Bion, W. (1961), *Experiences in Groups*, Tavistock, London.

Boszormenyi-Nagy, I. and Spark, G.M. (1973), *Invisible Royalties*, Harper and Row, New York.

Bowen, M. (1976), 'Theory in the Practice of Psychotherapy', in Guerin, P.J. (ed.), *Family Therapy*, Gardner Press, New York.

Brown, C. (1984), *Black and White Britain*, Policy Studies Institute, London.

Commission for Racial Equality (1988), *Housing and Ethnic Minorities: Statistical Information*, Commission for Racial Equality, London.

Dale, A. and Marsh, C. (eds) (1993), *The 1991 Census Users' Guide*, HMSO, London.

Daniel, W.W. (1968), *Racial Disadvantage in Britain*, Penguin Books, Harmondsworth.

Department of the Environment (1993), *Housing in England: Housing Trailers to the 1988 and 1991 Labour Force Surveys*, HMSO, London.

Erikson, E.H. (1963), *Childhood and Society*, Norton, New York.

Ezriel, H. (1956), 'Experimentation with the Psychoanalytic Session', *British Journal of Philosophy of Science*, 7, pp. 25–41.

Ferber, A., Mendelsohn, M., and Napier, A. (1973), *The Book of Family Therapy*, Houghton Mifflin, Boston.

Greeley, A.M. (1969), *Why Can't they be Like us?*, Institute of Human Relations Press, New York.

Gubrium, J.F. and Holstein, J.A. (1990), *What is Family?*, Mayfield, California.

Hajnal, J. (1982), 'Two Kinds of Pre-industrial Family Household Formation Systems', *Population and Development Review*, 8, pp. 449–94.

Haley, J. (1977), *Problem-solving Therapy*, Jossey-Bass, San Francisco.

Haskey, J. (1989), 'Families and Households of the Ethnic Minority and White Populations of Great Britain', *Population Trends*, 57, pp. 8–19.

Heath, S. and Dale, A. (1994), 'Household and Family Formation in Great Britain: the Ethnic Dimension', *Population Trends*, 77, pp. 5–13.

Hill, R. (1972), *The Strengths of Black Families*, Emerson Hall, New York.

HM Government (1988), 1991 Census of Population (Census White Paper), Cm430, HMSO, London.

Jones, T. (1993), *Britain's Ethnic Minorities*, Policy Studies Institute, London.

Lasch, C. (1977), *Haven in a Heartless World: the Family Besieged*, Basic Books, New York.

Lau, A. (1984), 'Transcultural Issues in Family Therapy', *Journal of Family Therapy*, 6, pp. 91–112.

Malan, D.H. (1963), *A Study of Brief Psychotherapy*, Plenium, New York.

McAdoo, H.P. (ed.) (1977), *Black Families*, Sage, Beverley Hills, CA.

McGoldrick, M., Pearce, J. and Giordano, J. (eds) (1982), *Ethnicity and Family Therapy*, Guildford, New York.

Medick, H. and Sabean, D.W. (1988), *Interest and Emotion: Esssays on the Study of Family and Kinship*, Cambridge University Press, Cambridge.

Minuchin, S. and Fishman, C. (1981), *Family Therapy Techniques*, Harvard University Press, Cambridge, MA.

Morgan, S.P., McDaniel, A., Miller, A.T. and Preston, S.H. (1993), 'Racial Differences in Household and Family Structure at the Turn of the Century', *American Journal of Sociology*, 98(4), pp. 799–828.

Murphy, M. (1996), 'Household and Family Structure among Ethnic Minority Groups', in *Ethnicity in the 1991 Census (Volume 1)*, HMSO, London.

Murphy, M. and Berrington, A. (1993), 'Household Change in the 1980s: a Review', *Population Trends*, 73, pp. 18–26.

Parsons, T. (1949), *The Structure of Social Action*, Free Press, New York.

Pinderhughes, E. (1982), 'Afro-Americans and the Victim System', in McGoldrick, M., Pearce, J. and Giordano, J. (eds), *Ethnicity and Family Therapy*, New York, Guildford

Scansoni, J. (1971), *The Black Family in Modern Society*, Allyn and Bacon, Boston.

Selvini Palazzoli, M., Boscolo, L., Cecchin, G.F. and Prata, G. (1978), *Paradox and Counterparadox*, Aronson, New York.

Shyllon, F.O. (1974), *Black Slaves in Britain*, Oxford University Press for the Institute of Race Relations, Oxford.

Skynner, A.C.R. (1976), *One Flesh: Separate Persons: Principles of Family and Marital Therapy*, Constable, London.

Stack, C. (1974), *All our Kin: Strategies for Survival in a Black Community*, Harper and Row, New York.

Turquet, P. (1975), 'Large Group Processes', in Kreeger, L.C. (ed.), *The Large Group Process: Dynamics and Therapy*, Constable, London.

Visram, R. (1986), *Ayahs, Lascars and Princes: the Story of Indians in Britain 1700–1947*, Pluto Press, London.

Wall, R. (1983), 'The Household: Demographic and Economic Change in England 1650–1970', in Wall, R., Robin, J. and Laslett, P. (eds), *Family Forms in Historic Europe*, Cambridge University Press, Cambridge.

Walvin, J. (1973), *Black and White: the Negro in English Society 1555–1945*, Allen Lane, New York.

Watzlawick, P., Jackson, D.D. and Beavin, J. (1967), *Pragmatics of Human Communication: a Study of Interactional Patterns, Pathologies and Paradoxes*, Norton, New York.

Chapter 8

The Mental Health of British Afro-Caribbean Children and Adolescents

Tami Kramer and Matthew Hodes

Introduction

This chapter will consider social adjustment and psychiatric disorders amongst Afro-Caribbean children and adolescents in the UK. Research in this area has been gradually accumulating over the last few decades but findings have not previously been drawn together and discussed as a whole. The findings regarding Afro-Caribbean youngsters will be compared with the findings of their peers from the White majority and other ethnic minorities. Their utilisation of child and adolescent mental health services will also be considered. It is hoped that this focus on the mental health of the youth from one community will make the review more coherent. The scope of the review has necessarily been limited by the availability of research findings.

Mental health is closely linked to people's sociocultural background. This chapter begins with a brief discussion of the pattern of Afro-Caribbean migration to the United Kingdom, associated socioeconomic adversity and family life. The relevance of such risk and protective factors for the development of psychopathology is explained. Given the importance of school and education, and their relevance for understanding antisocial behaviour, these topics are considered before the sections on conduct disorder and delinquency. The other main psychiatric disorders that occur in children and adolescents and patterns of service use are described. The final section outlines some of the limitations of the existing research and proposes some future research directions.

We have used the term Afro-Caribbean wherever sources are clearly describing people originating from the Caribbean. Many sources use the term Black, which refers to both Africans and Afro-Caribbeans, who make up the great majority of this group. We use the term Black when referring to the combined group. Studies that are clearly about Africans in Britain have been excluded.

Historical Background and Context

The British Isles have received waves of immigrants, including non-White immigrants for hundreds of years. By the latter part of the eighteenth century there were 30,000 Black people in Britain (Benson, 1981). However the Second World War created a demand for men for the British armed forces and war industries. From 1948 larger scale migration from the Caribbean began. Work opportunities in the free market and what were then public services (e.g. British Rail, London Transport and the National Health Service) offered employment to many immigrants especially people from the Caribbean region (Peach, 1996). Migration peaked in the early 1960s and started to diminish by the mid-1970s, and by then the population had reached about 550,000 (Peach, 1996). The size of the Afro-Caribbean community was similar in 1991, although the proportion born in the UK had increased (53 per cent of those who classified themselves as Black-Caribbean were born in the UK; this excludes additional people of Afro-Caribbean descent who consider themselves to be Black British, classified in the census as Black-Other; Peach 1996). Few of those under 20 years were born in the Caribbean (Peach, 1996).

The people of the Caribbean are heterogeneous, as they have come from different islands with varied cultures, languages and colonial histories. However, Jamaicans formed the largest single group (over half) of the community in the UK with much smaller numbers from other islands (Peach 1996). On arrival in the UK the frequent experience of racism and discrimination (particularly with regard to housing and employment opportunities) served to diminish inter-island rivalries and differences, and led to the development of strong community links. Early links were evident with the formation of community organisations (e.g. West Indian Unity Association 1956, West Midlands Caribbean Association in 1959 etc.) and shared experiences such as the 1958 race riots in Nottingham and Notting Hill. Currently community links are reflected in residence patterns. Afro-Caribbeans live predominantly in South East England, 58 per cent in Greater London, with another 16 per cent in the West Midlands (Haskey, 1997). Community links are also reflected in religious links and choice of partner (60 per cent Afro-Caribbeans who are living with a partner are living with an Afro-Caribbean, Peach 1998).

Family Life

Many aspects of family organisation in the Caribbean have been outlined elsewhere. Changes in family life are likely to take place due to migration. During the early years families will have experienced the stress of separation if parents came to the UK ahead of their children. Children themselves may have experienced migration. Nevertheless, Afro-Caribbean family organisation within the UK shows both similarities and differences with that of White British families.

An early study examined the home circumstances and family patterns of Afro-Caribbean families with 10 year old children living in an inner London borough and compared them with non-immigrant White families (Rutter et al., 1975). By this time only 4 per cent of Afro-Caribbean families had children still living in the Caribbean. Rates of one and two parent families were similar in Afro-Caribbean and White communities. However, Afro-Caribbeans had significantly larger families.

Current data reveals that Afro-Caribbean households have higher than average cohabiting couple families with dependent children, and lone parent families, with mainly female headed households (Whitmarsh and Harris, 1996) (rates of cohabiting parents with dependent children: Afro-Caribbeans – 35/1000, all groups – 17/1000; rates of lone parents: Afro-Caribbeans – 202/1000, all groups – 52/1000 (Haskey, 1996)). This is relevant, because in general, children growing up with single parents are at increased risk of adjustment difficulties. In addition, Afro-Caribbean families are no longer large and extended families (which may offer increased support with childcare) (Peach, 1996). Regarding the quality of relationships, marital and parent-child relationships were similar (Rutter et al., 1975). There was considerable overlap in the patterns of discipline. Afro-Caribbean children were considered more 'self-reliant' (i.e. more cleaned their own shoes, tidied their own things, made their own beds, travelled by bus alone and used the cooker without supervision) although the Afro-Caribbean parents exercised more control on how their children spent their free time.

The relationship between family experience and the quality of care of the children is complex (Dunn, 1994). Adverse social factors (such as poverty, homelessness), family factors (such as conflict, neglect, abuse, parental ill-health) and child factors may interact to result in family breakdown and reception of children into local authority care.

For some time evidence has accumulated that Afro-Caribbean children are over-represented within the care system (Barn, 1990). Bebbington and Miles

(1989) investigated the family backgrounds of 2,500 children admitted to care in England. Children of two Afro-Caribbean parents were not over-represented in the care system although children from mixed unions were. Living with one adult only was the single greatest risk factor for admission into care. Since more Afro-Caribbean children are known to be living with one parent only, they are likely to be at increased risk for going into care. Another study of a poor borough in London found that Black children were disproportionately represented in the care system (Barn, 1993). They entered care for reasons of socio-economic difficulties, family relationships and mother's mental health, while most White children entered for parental neglect/inadequacy, failure to thrive, child abuse, delinquency, school non-attendance and the child's behaviour. The police referred more Black children for delinquency and the health service more Black mothers for reasons of mental health. Black children had a better chance of being placed in a foster family and had more regular parental contact.

Social Adversity

The Afro-Caribbean community in the UK has faced economic hardship, adversity and racial discrimination, apparent in patterns of employment and housing (Commission for Racial Equality, 1990; Daniel, 1968). Rutter et al. (1975) demonstrated that very few Afro-Caribbean parents held non-manual jobs and the proportion in menial and unskilled occupations was double that in non immigrant families. This was despite similar levels of training and education in fathers and better educated mothers. This skew towards manual categories remains true for Afro-Caribbean men (with two-thirds in manual occupations compared with half of the White male working population) while for females, rates are currently more similar to White females (Peach, 1996).

However, as far as unemployment is concerned, rates in Afro-Caribbean males and females (23.8 per cent and 13.5 per cent respectively) are far higher than in White males and females (10.7 per cent and 6.3 per cent respectively), with rates for young males aged 18–19 particularly high (43.5 per cent). The history of discrimination and difficulties may be associated with ambivalent or negative attitudes to employment by some Afro-Caribbean youngsters, although this may occur more amongst males (Alexander, 1996). Recent data suggests that young Black females have been able to acquire qualifications, and achieve significant advances and higher incomes in the employment market, compared with White females (Whitmarsh and Harris, 1996).

As far as housing is concerned, the picture is more complicated and has changed over time. Rutter et al. (1975) described how, on arrival, Afro-Caribbeans had difficulty securing accommodation and many were forced to live in over-priced accommodation of a poor standard. Overcrowding was more than twice as frequent in Afro-Caribbean homes. Significantly more bought properties because of lack of other opportunities and significantly fewer were able to get council properties. Between 1961–91 the proportion of the White population in council housing has remained similar (24 per cent), while the proportion of Afro-Caribbeans has increased (from 2 per cent in 1961 to 45 per cent in 1991). In both White and Afro-Caribbean populations the proportion in owner occupied accommodation has increased (42 per cent–67 per cent; 27 per cent–48 per cent respectively) and for both groups private rentals have decreased (Peach, 1998). However, there is evidence that a far larger proportion of Black families live in flats as opposed to houses, live in overcrowded accommodation and spend nearly twice as much on repairs, an indicator of dwelling age (Whitmarsh and Harris, 1996).

The Afro-Caribbean community in the UK has been exposed to persistent racial discrimination apparent in interpersonal encounters. This may take many forms such as name-calling, bullying and violent attacks. The murder of Stephen Lawrence demonstrates the most extreme form of such abuse. The Inquiry (Macpherson, 1999) into Stephen Lawrence's tragic death highlighted how police incompetence and the appallingly high level of discrimination towards Black British people were related to institutional racism. The experience of racism is of crucial relevance to the identity and adjustment of young Afro-Caribbeans (Fernando, 1995). There is apparently no research that specifically and directly investigates adaptation to change (which takes place within the individual, the family and the social world). Change such as migration may be a stressor for children's psychological development. Originally, separations occurred within families. Fathers often came to the UK first, followed by wives or partners, while their children who were often cared for by grandmothers came later. Even now, decades after many Afro-Caribbeans originally came to the UK for work, family separation continues as the older generation may return to the Caribbean for retirement. This may reduce the availability of much valued family support from the grand-parental generation.

Childhood disturbance and maladjustment is determined by the interaction of individual vulnerability in association with family and social adversity. These risks often co-occur and may be cumulative. For example, loss of parents who migrated may be followed by later separation from grandmothers to whom the children became attached. On arrival in the UK there may be exposure to poor housing, and financial difficulties. Research has shown that disruption of relationships and stressful life events are associated with increased psychiatric morbidity in children (Goodyer, 1990; Bailey and Garralda, 1987; Belsky and Cassidy, 1994). Despite exposure to similar risks, individuals vary with regard to their coping, the development of disturbance and outcome (Rutter, 1987). Factors that protect against adversity include individual attributes which may be partly inherent characteristics, such as high intellectual ability, or temperamental characteristics such as flexible, easy temperament and positive self concept, or characteristics that are acquired through learning and experience. Other protective factors include family strengths (including warm and effective parenting) and social supports outside the family (including friends or relatives, school, church etc.) (Werner, 1992). These principles for investigating adjustment and psychiatric disorders underpin research with many social and cultural groups including young Afro-Caribbeans in the UK (Quinton, 1994).

The Afro-Caribbean families who have migrated to the UK will have experienced exposure to different cultures, adversity as well as new opportunities. A central theme in this review is the extent to which adversity or protective factors influence any discernible variation in adjustment and psychiatric disorder between the Afro-Caribbean youngsters in the UK and their peers in the Caribbean, and peers from other communities in the UK.

School and Educational Achievement

Adaptation to the demands of school represents a major developmental challenge for all children. In addition to achieving educational objectives children are required to conform to behavioural expectations and develop skills for successful peer interaction. School failure may lead to a lack of qualifications and skills, and poorer opportunities in the labour market. By contrast successful progress through school enables the transition to higher education or training and employment. School and educational success may be a key turning point in an individual's life (Rutter, 1994). The opportunities that education provides are especially important for the Afro-Caribbean community, who like many immigrant groups, have traditionally had high expectations.

For three decades there has been concern about the academic achievement and progress of Afro-Caribbean children within the UK. Concern arose initially out of studies of reading performance (Bagley, 1971; Yule et al., 1975), IQ testing (Yule et al., 1975) and exam attainment (Tomlinson, 1983; Swann Report, 1985). Yule et al. (1975) carried out the first population based study of 10-year old children in Inner London. Although Afro-Caribbean children scored well below non-immigrant children on reading and intelligence, to those of English, Scottish, Irish and Welsh children, the authors identified a number of factors which may have contributed to the findings: the skewed social class distribution and increased adverse social circumstances of the immigrant families, the possible limitations of intelligence tests for children from different cultures, and school variables (with immigrant children more likely to attend less favourable schools). In addition to the differences in reading attainment Mortimer et al. (1988) detected poorer performance among primary school children in mathematics. Despite these differences, these children had more favourable views of reading (in 3rd year) and maths (in 1st year). Amongst these children, attainments in writing and oral skills were similar to those of English, Scottish, Irish and Welsh children.

There has been controversy about how Afro-Caribbean children's attainment changes over time. Specifically, the question asked is whether Afro-Caribbean children with lower early attainment progress similarly, better or worse than other children with lower early attainment. Mabey (1981), Scarr et al. (1983) and Mortimer et al. (1988) report progressive Afro-Caribbean children with lower early attainment progress similarly, better or worse than other children with lower early attainment. Mabey (1981), Scarr et al. (1983) and Mortimer et al. (1988) report progressive decline in performance over time relative to White English children. Mackintosh and Mascie-Taylor (1985) fail to show any widening of the gap between Black and White children's reading scores. By contrast, Maughan et al. (1985) report progress of Black girls to be similar to Whites, with only a trend towards a slight decline in the performance of Black boys. Maughan and Rutter (1986) studied the relationship over time between ratings of verbal reasoning, reading, non-verbal IQ tests and public examination results (at age 11 years, 14 years, 16 years and at school leaving if later). They revealed that Afro-Caribbean pupils performed similarly to White pupils with a comparable level of earlier attainment i.e. performance did not improve or decline. However, Afro-Caribbean pupils, especially Afro-Caribbean girls, had actually improved their relative position to a considerable extent by the time they left school. Although they were under-represented in the highest exam pass grades, they were more likely than Whites to have achieved at least some graded results and fewer left school without formal qualifications. In line with these findings population data reveals that Black students are more likely than White students to be in full-time education between 16–18 years (Whitmarsh and Harris, 1996). The proportion doing academic courses, as opposed to vocational courses, are similar to Whites, but lower than in other ethnic minorities. Again there are gender differences, with more Afro-Caribbean girls taking academic courses than Afro-Caribbean males (Whitmarsh and Harris, 1996).

Attendance and behaviour at school are also important aspects of progress in school. Regarding primary schools, attendance was better for Afro-Caribbean pupils (Mortimer et al., 1988). However, high rates of permanent exclusion of Afro-Caribbean children are a cause for concern. While the rate overall for the country in 1996/1997 was 0.19 per cent, the rate for Afro-Caribbean children was 0.76 per cent (DFEE, 1998). Research specifically investigating this is lacking, but a higher level of reported disruptive behaviour in schools is likely to be relevant.

Mortimer et al. (1988) studied further the contribution of school variables to primary school children's progress. In terms of behaviour, teachers made more individual contacts with Afro-Caribbean children and heard them read more often, suggesting they may be trying to meet the individual needs of these pupils. Teachers ratings of ability were related to children's attainments and not ethnicity, when other background factors were accounted for. Therefore, overt teacher behaviour and attitudes are individual needs of these pupils. Teachers ratings of ability were related to children's attainments and not ethnicity, when other background factors were accounted for. Therefore, overt teacher behaviour and attitudes are unlikely to be the cause of lower attainments in these children although transmission of expectations can be more subtle. No systematic bias was found in the way schools affected children of different ethnic backgrounds. Schools effective in promoting progress in one group were good for children from other backgrounds. However, Afro-Caribbean children were over-represented in schools that were ineffective in promoting progress of all pupils, irrespective of ethnic background.

Conduct Disorder

Most children exhibit anti-social behaviour at some time. Conduct disorders however are characterised by severe and persistent anti-social behaviour such as physical aggression, vandalism, stealing, truancy, fire-setting, running away, lying etc. These disorders are associated with high levels of impairment (school failure and exclusion, peer problems, family disruption) and comorbidity (substance misuse, mood disorders, self-harm and suicide).

Past research indicates that rates of disturbance as a whole, in Afro-Caribbean children, are similar to rates in indigenous children. These include studies of the community (Earls and Richman, 1980; Nicol, 1971) and school (Cochrane, 1979) across a broad age range (3–14 years). However a number of differences have emerged. Rates of conduct disorder were increased in Afro-Caribbean girls (Rutter, 1974; Cochrane, 1979). School-based conduct disorder (i.e. based on teacher reports) was increased in Afro-Caribbean children while rates at home (i.e. based on parental reports) were similar to indigenous children (Rutter et al., 1974). The increased rates may be linked to poorer reading and apparent lower intellectual ability as measured by IQ tests (Yule et al., 1975). Reading delay and learning difficulties are known to be linked to conduct disorder. Greater difficulty at school may lead to behaviour disturbance at school which does not generalise to home. Alternatively Afro-Caribbean parents may have different expectations from White English parents and be more tolerant of their children's behaviour.

In a more recent study, Afro-Caribbean pupils were rated as having more school based behaviour problems which were 'learning behaviour problems', rather than aggression or anxiety. In this study the increase was linked to poor reading attainment and not ethnicity (Mortimer et al., 1988).

The social and familial correlates for disorder were largely similar in Afro-Caribbean and White English children (Earls and Richman, 1980; Rutter et al., 1974). However disorder in Afro-Caribbean children was not associated with parental psychiatric disorder, parental criminality and marital discord (Rutter et al., 1974).

It is known that physical illness may contribute to child behavioural difficulties. Of relevance here is that in children with sickle cell disease, which occurs largely in Afro-Caribbean children, teachers describe more behaviour problems, although the parents of these children do not perceive an increase in either behavioural or emotional difficulties. These behaviour problems were more likely to occur in children of single mothers with poor mental health (Midence et al., 1996).

Substance use and abuse, which frequently occurs in association with conduct disorder (Berman and Noble, 1993; Robins and McEvoy, 1990), has been increasing over the last decade (Robins and McEvoy, 1990). There is little research looking at rates of substance use and abuse in Afro-Caribbean children. One study found rates of alcohol use in Afro-Caribbean children (aged 9–15 years) to be similar to White children (Health Education Authority, 1992). Another large study found lower reported rates of drug use in Black youth (14–25 years) than White youth (24 per cent vs 37 per cent respectively had ever used drugs) (Graham and Bowling, 1995).

Crime and Delinquency

Delinquency is a legal category referring to offending in young people. Persistent offending may be preceded and accompanied by abnormalities of conduct (such as truancy, aggressiveness etc.), but it is not the same as conduct disorder. Many risk factors for conduct disorder such as reading delay, family disturbance and offending, unemployment and poverty, are also risk factors for delinquency (Farrington, 1995). Offending behaviour increases during adolescence, with a peak between ages 15–17 years. Most crime is committed by male teenagers and young adults, and rates overall have increased steadily since the Second World War. Up until the 1970s, crime rates in Afro-Caribbeans were thought to be low to average, but since then there is evidence of increased rates of arrest and imprisonment (Smith, 1995).

Rates of crime are measured in three main ways: (i) victim surveys; (ii) self-reports of offending; and (iii) crime statistics.

Victim surveys of over-16-year olds (Whitmarsh and Harris, 1996) reveal that Black people are more likely to have been victims of personal and household crimes, and experience more fear of crime. Black victims are less likely than South Asians to perceive the crime they have experienced as racially motivated. Also, Afro-Caribbeans are over represented as offenders in reports where the victim claims to have seen the offender (Smith, 1994), although this may be the result of selective perceptions by White victims.

Self-reports of offending in 14–25-year olds revealed that overall Black and White young people committed similar rates of offences while South Asians had lower rates (Graham and Bowling, 1995). Violent offences were most common among the Black group (one quarter of the Black group vs less than one fifth White group) (Graham and Bowling, 1995). This increase in aggression may reflect a response to more frequently being victims, or experiencing increased environmental adversity. Vandalism was less common than in either White youth or Pakistani youth. Black young women were more likely to have committed any offence than other young women (Graham and Bowling, 1995).

Crime statistics show that Afro-Caribbeans are more likely than Whites or South Asians to be stopped and searched by police and rates of arrest per population are increased. Adult Afro-Caribbeans are over-represented in the prison population (Home Office, 1991). Higher proportions of Afro-Caribbean than White juveniles are prosecuted following arrest (Smith, 1994) and more Afro-Caribbeans under 17 are detained under Section 53(2) of the Children and Young Persons Act, in a young offenders institution for serious offenders (Puri, Lambert and Cordess, 1995). These findings have led to concern that the criminal justice system discriminates against those from Black communities along each stage, from arrest to imprisonment. However, Smith (1994) has argued that racial discrimination alone does not account for the higher levels of Afro-Caribbeans in the criminal justice system. Amongst the reasons are the findings that South Asians are also subject to discriminatory treatment by many institutions, but have low levels of involvement with the criminal justice system compared with White British and Afro-Caribbeans.

Suicide and Deliberate Self-harm

Rates of *suicide* increase over the adolescent years. Suicide in those under 15 years is rare (rate in UK: 0.8/100 000) and increases between 15–19 years (rate in UK: 7.6/100 000) (Shaffer and Piacenti, 1994). Neither death certificates nor coroners reports include information on ethnicity. Place of birth is used as a proxy. Within the UK, levels of suicide do vary according to place of birth (with higher rates in Indians, Irish and non-Commonwealth Africans, lower rates in Pakistanis and Bangladeshis; Balarajan, 1995). Rates overall in Afro-Caribbeans have been found to be similar to those from England and Wales (Balarajan, 1995), or lower (Soni Raleigh, 1992). However, place of birth is less useful in this age group when the majority of this group would have been born in this country. Findings from Soni Raleigh's study (1996), suggest that rates of suicide in the UK reflect rates in the country of origin and not a shift towards rates in the UK. For those who actually migrated, this study does not demonstrate a clear change in rates. Whether this is maintained through successive generations remains unclear. It is also unclear whether suicide is increasing for young Afro-Caribbean males as it is for others (Shaffer and Piacenti, 1994).

Rates of deliberate *self-harm* (including self-poisoning and self-injury) increase markedly during the adolescent years and vary over time (Hawton and Fagg, 1992). Rates in this study from Oxford, UK (10–14-year olds: 104/100,000; 15–19-year olds: 446/100 000) are higher than those found in adolescents in Port-of-Spain, Trinidad (10–18-year olds: 94/100 000) (Neehal and Beharry, 1994). In the US, studies of high school children show a link between ethnicity and self-harm (Centres for Disease Control, 1991; Blum et al., 1992) with similar rates in Whites and Blacks, but higher rates in Hispanics and Native Americans. Burke (1976) found no Afro-Caribbeans under 15 years old admitted for self-poisoning in Birmingham between 1969–1972. He also found lower rates of self-poisoning in Afro-Caribbean immigrants of all other ages in Birmingham (especially in males). Merril and Owens' (1987) study of hospital admissions, following deliberate self-harm, found lower rates in Afro-Caribbeans aged over 25 years, but similar rates in 16-24-year olds. Both studies revealed rates in the Afro-Caribbeans in Birmingham which were higher than rates in the Caribbean (Burke, 1974), suggesting that they increased with migration.

From these studies it appears that rates of DSH may be lower in Afro-Caribbeans, especially in the late teens and early adulthood, suggesting the presence of culturally determined protective factors. These may include:

i)   culturally shaped sense of autonomy and self-efficacy, related to gender role, such as centrality in family life (Littlewood, 1995). This may also be reinforced by relative success in school and employment;
ii) family factors, including less conflict with parents regarding adolescent role transition (as compared to South Asian families (Goldberg and Hodes, 1992)); and
iii) community factors, such as religious beliefs, more expressive communication of distress, less opportunity for spread of the behaviour by contagion.

Despite the presence of protective factors, risk appears to increase with migration. Possible explanations for the increase with migration include (i) the stress of migration; (ii) exposure to new stresses in the UK which may be particular to the Afro-Caribbean community, e.g. racism, discrimination etc.; (iii) once people have been here for some time, they may become more vulnerable to risks in a similar way to the rest of the population. This last factor may explain why Merril and Owen (1987) found no difference in rates in those under 25 years, a group who would have spent a larger proportion of their lives in the UK.

Suicide and deliberate self-harm are associated with psychiatric disorder, most commonly depressive disorder, anxiety disorder, alcohol and substance abuse disorder (Gould et al., 1998; Shaffer et al., 1996). However, it is unclear if these findings are relevant to Afro-Caribbean children and adolescents in the UK. There is no research regarding the presence of depression and anxiety amongst Afro-Caribbean children in the UK.

Eating Disorders

Eating disorders refer to anorexia nervosa, bulimia nervosa and partial syndromes. Anorexia nervosa is characterised by fear and dislike of fatness associated with vigorous attempts to reduce weight by food avoidance, vomiting or other techniques, resulting in such weight loss that menstruation ceases. Bulimia nervosa is characterised by binge eating with behaviours that counteract the fattening effects of eating such as food avoidance or vomiting, associated with fear and dislike of fatness. Bulimia nervosa may be associated with normal weight or obesity. Both disorders have in common fear or dislike of fatness, and sufferers, usually female adolescents or young women, may experience one and then the other disorder.

In recent years the links between culture and eating disorders has attracted much attention (Dolan, 1991; Nasser, 1997; Vandereycken and Hoek, 1992). Earlier views that these disorders occur exclusively in young White women from affluent Western societies have been challenged by their identification in many sociocultural groups, including Black American (Robinson and Anderson, 1985) and Black British women (Dolan et al., 1990; Holden and Robinson, 1988; Lacey and Dolan, 1988). No epidemiological studies that investigate eating disorders amongst adolescent Afro-Caribbeans in the UK have been carried out. The existing literature consists of case reports and some community studies investigating eating attitudes (Reiss, 1996) and bulimia nervosa amongst adult Afro-Caribbean British (Lacey and Dolan, 1988).

The small number of reports of anorexia nervosa in Afro-Caribbean adolescents suggest it is very rare (Holden and Robinson, 1988). It is striking that most reports of anorexia nervosa amongst ethnic minority adolescents in UK concern South Asian youngsters (Bendal et al., 1991; Bryant-Waugh and Lask, 1991; Markantonakis, 1990). Bulimia nervosa also appears to be very rare amongst adolescent Afro-Caribbean adolescent females. This may be because the disorder typically starts in late adolescence or early adulthood, and perhaps because it occurs less in this community (Lacey and Dolan, 1988).

It is important to consider why Afro-Caribbean female adolescents may be protected against developing eating disorders compared with their peers. Two factors appear relevant. Firstly, an important issue is attitude to body shape and dieting. This is relevant because dislike of fatness and associated dieting are important in leading to the onset of eating disorders (Patton et al., 1990). There is consistent evidence that Afro-Caribbean female adolescents are more positive towards their body shape than their peers. A study of adolescents, aged 11–18 years in London secondary schools, has shown that the Afro-

Caribbean girls were more positive towards their body shape, showing less dissatisfaction and less dieting compared with White and South Asian peers (Wardle and Marsland, 1990). This occurred although they had a higher body mass index i.e. were heavier in relation to their height. Another large study of adolescents found that Afro-Caribbeans were less likely to have significantly abnormal eating attitudes in association with low self-esteem (Thomas and James, personal communication). These questionnaire studies are entirely consistent with anthropological accounts that indicate that a fuller body shape has positive associations with fecundity and maturity (MacCormack and Draper, 1987). Adolescents' attitudes to body shape are influenced by their mothers attitudes in diverse cultures (Hill et al., 1990; Mukai et al., 1994). It has been found that Afro-Caribbean mothers in London regarded plumper girl body shapes as attractive compared with White British mothers who found slimmer shapes attractive (Hodes et al., 1996).

The second reason why Afro-Caribbean female adolescents may be protected against eating disorders concerns their strong sense of identity, self-worth and ability to influence their position in the world (Littlewood, 1995). Evidence for this comes from studies indicating the important position of women in Afro-Caribbean family structures (Smith, 1988). They also have achieved important positions in school (Blatchford, 1997), training (Whitmarsh and Harris, 1996) and employment domains. Feminist perspectives on eating disorders have argued that women's lack of real autonomy, effectiveness and ability to assert themselves is related to the propensity to develop eating disorders (Striegel-Moore, 1993).

Schizophrenia

Schizophrenia is rare before adolescence and increases in incidence in late adolescence and early adulthood (Zigler and Levine, 1981). Despite this, a large body of research has been carried out with adult White and adult Afro-Caribbeans, although the data regarding schizophrenia in the younger population in the UK is very limited. Issues of adult incidence and prevalence are discussed elsewhere in Volume II.

Since schizophrenia increases markedly during late adolescence and early adulthood it seems likely that the risk factors are operating in childhood and adolescence. Also, the risk for the development of the disorder is probably higher in families of those with early onset-illness (Werry, 1992). Despite this, and in light of the adult literature, there is little research in the UK on the relative rates of disorder, the contribution of biological versus psychosocial risks, management or outcome of schizophrenia in young Afro-Caribbeans. Goodman and Richards' (1995) study of child and adolescent clinic attenders from one area of London, found that psychotic disorders were over-represented in second generation Afro-Caribbeans. If this finding reflects genuine differences in rates in the community, it would be in line with some adult studies. Although the authors explain why referral bias alone is unlikely to account for this finding, a study of prevalence in the community (with accurate data on the size of the local Afro-Caribbean community) is required to confirm this.

Developmental Disorders

Autism is a rare disorder (incidence 4/10,000) which is more common in males (males: females 3:1). It is characterised by social abnormalities, language abnormalities and stereotyped repetitive patterns of behaviour that become apparent before a child's third birthday. It is generally accepted that autism is a biologically determined neurodevelopmental disorder with a predominant genetic contribution to aetiology (Bailey, Phillips and Rutter, 1996). Physical environmental factors (obstetric and perinatal complications, congenital infections) may contribute in a small proportion of cases.

Only two relevant studies have been identified. In Camberwell, London, increased rates of autism in Afro-Caribbean children were found (3.4 per cent of referred Afro-Caribbean children had autism and related disorders vs 0.8 per cent other children) (Wing, 1979). From the same area of London, a more recent study found Afro-Caribbean clinic attenders included an increased proportion of females with autism and a high rate of more severe mental retardation (Goodman and Richards, 1995). These findings may reflect a higher proportion of autism secondary to severe environmental insults and a lower proportion due to genetic loading. Family studies are needed to clarify this. Afro-Caribbean families in this study had evidence of increased socioeconomic adversity, with significantly fewer heads of household in non-manual occupations, significantly more large families and a trend for more unemployment. The link with socio-economic status and poverty (which may be linked to increased risk of environmental insults) needs further clarification.

There is little research on mental retardation in Afro-Caribbeans in the UK. Akinsola (1986) found that children from ethnic minorities with severe mental retardation had more severe disabilities (including sensory impairments, neurological functioning, and social behaviour). The sample size was not large enough to consider Afro-Caribbean children separately or clarify the reasons for this finding, which may relate to bias in assessment of the children or differences in aetiology of retardation (e.g. communicable diseases, perinatal damage).

Service Utilisation

Ethnicity of children and adolescents in the UK has been shown to be strongly associated with their pattern of service use. Indian children and adolescents are more likely to consult their GP for all problems than other groups, including Afro-Caribbeans (whose rates are similar) (Cooper, Smaje and Arber, 1998). In one of the few studies looking at service utilisation for a specific disorder, enuresis (bedwetting at night), it has been shown that even though Afro-Caribbean children have this problem more commonly than their peers, they attend for help less frequently (Rona et al., 1997). Afro-Caribbean, Indian, Pakistani and Bangladeshi children and adolescents are less likely to use all hospital outpatient and inpatient services than their White counterparts (Cooper, Smaje and Arber, 1998). These differences persist after controlling for socioeconomic and health status (Cooper, Smaje and Arber, 1998). These findings suggest that minority children have less access to secondary health care and it is possible that they are receiving poorer health care because of this.

Studies of referrals to two different child and adolescent mental health services revealed contradictory referral patterns according to ethnic group. One study found that GPs referred more White children, while specialist doctors and education referred more Black children (Daryanani et al., 1998). A study of a service in central London which served a highly multicultural population (183 attenders originated from 43 countries) found that White UK children were less frequently referred by primary care, and more frequently referred by secondary health services when compared to the rest of attenders combined. This study failed to find inaccessibility of the service for minority groups relative to their proportion of the local population (Kramer, Evans and Garralda 1999).

Problems and Prospects

This chapter regarding adjustment and psychiatric disorder amongst young British Afro-Caribbeans has been constrained by the quality and range of research available. Here important methodological issues and opportunities for further research are considered. The first and most striking feature is the lack of research that specifically investigates this group of children and adolescents. Much of the available publications concern studies that are concerned with White indigenous children and a number of different ethnic minority groups which include Afro-Caribbeans (Cochrane et al., 1979; Mortimer et al., 1988; Wardle and Marsland, 1990; Hodes et al., 1996; Rona et al., 1997). The inclusion of a number of sociocultural groups means that the development and testing of specific hypotheses tends to be more limited than would be possible if the Afro-Caribbeans were the prime interest. Another limitation of these studies is that the sample sizes tend to be small.

A second issue regarding the research is an absence of a truly cultural perspective, with the lack of use of instruments that have been shown to be culturally sensitive. Generally, the instruments, categories or constructs used have originated in research with the non Afro-Caribbean community. A good example is the otherwise very impressive study of psychiatric disorder and family and background circumstances in the children of Afro-Caribbean immigrants in South London (Rutter et al., 1974; Rutter et al., 1975). The descriptions of family composition consider the number of one and two parent households, and separations from parents without clear reference to the ways in which the extended family were involved with child-rearing. This is relevant since the different organisation of Afro-Caribbean families may generate different categories to describe family composition (Smith, 1988). At the level of symptom profiles and psychiatric disorder, the teacher screening questionnaire and the parental psychiatric interview had been developed amongst White indigenous English from the Isle of Wight (Rutter et al., 1970). Thus, the Afro-Caribbean parents and children may have used terms for emotional distress not used by the White indigenous English, and their omission from these assessments contributed to the low rate of emotional symptoms (Rutter et al., 1974). It is now widely believed that the idiom for communicating distress and experience is culturally shaped, and procedures have been established for the development of culturally sensitive instruments. (Kleinman, 1988; Canino et al., 1997).

The extent to which such category problems are relevant, varies according to the type of instruments deployed. Instruments that rely on language and are concerned with affect, or certain aspects of relationships, may be more prone to these problems (Canino et al., 1997; Jenkins and Karno, 1992). By contrast, instruments that are more visual such as that used to assess maternal attitudes to children's body shape will be less prone to this kind of bias (Hodes et al., 1996). In addition the relevance of the category problem for research with this group may vary according to the length of time that the particular group of people being investigated have been in the UK, and whether they are first, second or third generation. Many children and adolescents, whose grandparents migrated to the UK decades ago, will have learnt to speak with the regional accents and speech determined by area of residence and will not be using the idioms of their grandparents.

A third issue that needs to be raised in considering the literature is the extent to which racial bias and stereotyping has contributed towards the research findings and their interpretation. This has become a particularly sensitive issue regarding the investigation of conduct disorder, antisocial behaviour, and offending amongst young Afro-Caribbean British males. For example, in assessing the level of offending, it is inadequate to know that more Afro-Caribbean adolescents have 'offended' (Smith, 1994). This could result from discriminatory policing with disproportionately more youngsters being 'stopped and searched' than their White peers. The police may be more likely to bring charges to Black than White youngsters (Smith, 1994). There may also be bias in the convictions and sentencing in the courts, in which most of the magistrates and judges are White. It has been argued that there is a greater level of offending amongst Afro-Caribbeans, over and above that occurring because of discriminatory processes, which makes this a very complex area (Smith, 1994). The problem of stereotyping and bias is not confined to the criminal justice system. Psychiatrists may also be prone to racial stereotyping (Lewis et al., 1991), although there is also evidence that this is not a crude form of racism in which the nature and extent of bias can be presumed (Littlewood, 1992). The practical relevance for the research is that checks need to be carried out to clarify whether these biases are operating within a specific field of inquiry.

The fourth methodological issue that will become increasingly important for all research with ethnic minorities, and indeed all people living in cosmopolitan cities, concerns the extent to which there is homogeneity amongst the group of people being investigated. The Afro-Caribbean region is itself heterogeneous (Smith, 1988; Hutchinson and McKenzie, 1995), and the community in the UK reflects this. In addition, there is diversity caused by different degrees of assimilation, amount of time spent in the UK, and effects associated with occupational status.

There is also very significant mixing between the Afro-Caribbean community and White and other communities (Baumann, 1995). Children of mixed Afro-Caribbean White parentage vary in the extent to which they regard themselves as Black, although many do (Tizard and Phoenix, 1993). This is reflected in significant numbers of youngsters, including those who access mental health services, not 'fitting' into the standard ethnic categories used for monitoring and service planning (Hodes et al., 1998). More sophisticated means are required for describing ethnic group membership and identity (Entwistle and Astone, 1994; Hutchinson and McKenzie, 1995).

Despite these limitations of the available literature, current findings do suggest a number of directions in which future research should be directed. Firstly, there should be adequate epidemiological studies to investigate the prevalence of the main kinds of psychiatric disorder, the level of associated impairment and mental health service utilisation by those identified as cases. Special interest should be paid to conduct disorder, depression and eating disorders in the adolescent age group. Secondly, given the reported high levels of psychotic disorders in adult Afro-Caribbeans in the UK (Jarvis, 1998), and the possibility that there are raised rates of psychosis in younger members of the community (Goodman and Richards, 1995), this should be further investigated. This should consider not only level of risk, and include family studies, but also investigate the range of psychosocial and neurodevelopmental factors associated with early onset psychosis. Thirdly, psychosocial risk, conduct disorder, intellectual functioning and scholastic attainment also require further research. It is unclear how much the situation has changed since the pioneering studies of Rutter and his colleagues (Rutter et al., 1974; 1975; Yule et al., 1975) were published, even though some have argued that rates of offending have increased (Smith, 1995). New studies also require a longitudinal perspective to clarify the factors associated with entry into, or avoidance of delinquency. It cannot be assumed that the processes identified in the previous research into offending amongst White boys in South London are the same for the Black British youngsters (Farrington, 1995). Fourthly, there should be investigation of service utilisation by those with mental health problems at the primary care level, use of specialist mental health services and child and adolescent psychiatric in-patient management. Such studies should consider patient and parent attitudes to, and satisfaction with the services. The primary goal of such a research programme would be to improve the mental health of Afro-Caribbean youngsters. However the benefits and interest in it would extend beyond this, and the research would be able to address fundamental questions regarding psychological development and mechanisms of risk and adversity.

Conclusion

The British Afro-Caribbean community has been changing rapidly over the last few decades, with a reduced number of new immigrants, and most of the youngsters have been born in the country where they grow up. The youngsters have been exposed to some of the same adversities as their parents and grandparents, including discrimination. There is a high rate of marriage and unions across the community boundary but some disillusionment regarding the possibility of integration in the dominant sections of society. This has been associated with difficulties for some youngsters, males particularly, achieving good social adjustment, including school progress. Girls seem to be more protected, and importantly, with regard to some areas such as eating attitudes and disorders, appear to be better adjusted than White British and South Asian youngsters. Although many studies make reference to the mental health of British Afro-Caribbeans, there is a need for more investigation in this area. This will expand our understanding of this community, and, by throwing light on risk and understanding of protective factors, will benefit all sections of society.

References

Akinsola, H.A. and Fryers, T. (1986), 'A Comparison Of Disability in Severely Mentally Handicapped Children of Different Ethnic Origins', *Psychological Medicine*, 16, pp. 127–33.

Alexander, C.E. (1996), *The Art of Being Black: the Creation of Black British Identities*, Clarendon Press, Oxford.

Bagley, C. (1971), 'A Comparative Study of Social Environment and Intelligence in West Indian and English Children in London', *Journal of Social and Economic Studies*, 20, pp. 420–30.

Bailey, A., Philips, W. and Rutter, M. (1996), 'Autism: Towards an Integration of Clinical, Genetic, Neuropsychological, and Neurobiological Perspectives', *Journal of Child Psychology and Psychiatry*, 37, pp. 89–126.

Bailey, D. and Garralda, M.E. (1987), 'Children attending Primary Health Care Services: a Study of Recent Life Events', *Journal of the American Academy of Child and Adolescent Psychiatry*, 26, pp. 858–64.

Balarajan, R. (1995), 'Ethnicity and Variations in the Nation's Health', *Health Trends*, 27, pp. 114–19.

Barn, R. (1990), 'Black Children in Local Authority Care: Admission Patterns', *New Community*, 16, pp. 239–63.

Barn, R. (1993), *Black Children in the Public Care System*, B.T. Batsford Ltd, London.

Baumann, G. (1995), 'Managing a Polyethnic Milieu: Kinship and Interaction in a London Suburb', *Journal of the Royal Anthropological Institute (NS)*, 1, pp. 725–71.

Bebbington, A. and Miles, J. (1989), 'The Background of Children who enter Local Authority Care', *British Journal of Social Work*, 19, pp. 349–68.

Bebbington, P.E., Hurry, J. and Tennant, C. (1981), 'Psychiatric Disorders in Selected Immigrant Groups in Camberwell', *Social Psychiatry*, 16, pp. 43–51.

Belsky, J. and Cassidy, J. (1994), 'Attachment: Theory and Evidence', in Rutter, M. and Hay, D. (eds). *Development Through Life*, Blackwell Scientific Publications, Oxford, pp. 373–402.

Bendal, P., Hamilton, M. and Holden, N. (1991), 'Eating Disorders in Asian Girls', *British Journal of Psychiatry*, 159, pp. 441.

Benson, S. (1981), *Ambiguous Ethnicity: Interracial Families in London*, Cambridge University Press, Cambridge.

Berman, S.M. and Noble, E.P. (1993), 'Childhood Antecedents of Substance Misuse', *Current Opinion in Psychiatry*, 6, pp. 382–7.

Bhugra, D., Hilwig, M., Hossein, B., Marceau, H., Neehall, J., Leff, J., Mallett, R. and Der, G. (1996a), 'First-contact Incidence Rates of Schizophrenia in Substance Misuse', *Current Opinion in Psychiatry*, 6, pp. 382–7.

Bhugra, D., Hilwig, M., Hossein, B., Marceau, H., Neehall, J., Leff, J., Mallett, R. and Der, G. (1996b), 'First-contact Incidence Rates of Schizophrenia in Trinidad and one-year follow-up', *British Journal of Psychiatry*, 169, pp. 587–92.

Blatchford, P. (1997), 'Pupils' Self-assessments of Academic Attainment at 7, 11, and 16 Years: Effects of Sex and Ethnic Group', *British Journal of Educational Psychology*, 67, pp. 169–84.

Bryant-Waugh, R. and Lask, B. (1991), 'Anorexia Nervosa in a Group of Asian Children Living in Britain', *British Journal of Psychiatry*, 158, pp. 229–33.

Burke, A.W. (1974), 'Attempted Suicide in Trinidad and Tobago', *West Indian Medical Journal*, 23, pp. 250–55.

Burke, A.W. (1976), 'Socio-cultural Determinants of Attempted Suicide among West Indians in Birmingham: Ethnic Origin and Immigrant Status', *British Journal of Psychiatry*, 129, pp. 261–6.

Canino, G., Lewis-Fernandez, R. and Bravo, M. (1997), 'Methodological Challenges in Cross-cultural Mental Health Research', *Transcultural Psychiatry*, 34, pp. 163–84.

Centres for Disease Control (1991), 'Attempted Suicide Among High School Students – United States, 1990', *Morbidity and Mortality Weekly Report*, 40, pp. 633–5.

Cochrane, R. (1997), 'Mental Illness in Immigrants to England and Wales: an Analysis of Mental Hospital Admissions', *Social Psychiatry*, 12, pp. 25–35.

Cochrane, R. (1979), 'Psychological and Behavioural Disturbance in West Indians, Indians and Pakistanis in Britain', *British Journal of Psychiatry*, 134, pp. 201–10.

Cochrane, R. and Bal, S.S. (1989), 'Mental Hospital Admission Rates of Immigrants to England: a Comparison of 1971 and 1981', *Social Psychiatry and Psychiatric Epidemiology*, 24, pp. 2–11.

Commission for Racial Equality (1990), *Annual Report*, CRE, London.

Cooper, H., Smaje, C. and Arber, S. (1998), 'Use of Health Services by Children and Young People according to Ethnicity and Social Class: Secondary Analysis of a National Survey', *British Medical Journal*, 317(7165), pp. 1047–55.

Daniel, W.W. (1968), *Racial Discrimination in England*, Harmondsworth, Penguin.

Daryanani, R., Hindley, P., Evans, C. and Fahy, P. (1998), 'Ethnicity and Service Accessibility II: a Comparative Analysis of the Ethnic Origin of Referrals with Other Referral-Based

Characteristics', poster presentation, Faculty of Child and Adolescent Psychiatry of the Royal College of Psychiatrists Annual Residential Meeting, Bristol.

DFEE (Dept for Education and Employment) News (1998), 'Permanent Exclusions from Schools in England 1996/1997 and Exclusion Appeals lodged by Parents in England (451/98)', DFEE, Darlington.

Diekstra, R.F.W., Kienhorst, C.M.W. and de Wilde, E. J. (1995), 'Suicide and Suicidal Behaviour Among Adolescents', in Rutter, M. and Smith, D.J. (eds), *Psychosocial Disorders in Young People – Time Trends and their Causes*, John Wiley and Sons Ltd, Chichester.

Dolan, B. (1991), 'Cross-Cultural Aspects of Anorexia Nervosa and Bulimia: a Review', *International Journal of Eating Disorders*, 10, pp. 67–8.

Dolan, B. Lacey, J.H. and Evans, C. (1990), 'Eating Behavior and Attitudes to Weight and Shape in British Women from Three Ethnic Groups', *British Journal of Psychiatry*, 157, pp. 523–8.

Dunn, J. (1994), 'Family Influences', in Rutter, M. and Smith, D.J. (eds), *Development Through Life: a Handbook for Clinicians*, Blackwell Scientific Publications Oxford, pp. 112–34.

Earls, F. and Richman, N. (1980), 'The Prevalence of Behaviour Problems in Three-Year-Old Children of West Indian-born Parents', *Journal of Child Psychology and Psychiatry*, 21, pp. 99–106.

Entwistle, D.R. and Astone, N.M. (1994), 'Some Practical Guidelines for Measuring Youth's Race/Ethnicity and Socio-economic Status', *Child Development*, 65, pp. 1521–40.

Fahy, T.A., Jones,, P.B., Shaw, P.C., Tokei, N. and Murray, R.M. (1993), 'Schizophrenia in Afro-Carribeans in the UK following Parental Exposure to the 1957 A2 Influenza Pandemic', *Schizophrenia Research*, P, pp. 132.

Farrington, D.P. (1995), 'The Twelfth Jack Tizard Memorial Lecture. The Development of Offending and Antisocial Behavior from Childhood: Key Findings from the Cambridge Study in Delinquent Development', *Journal of Child Psychology and Psychiatry*, 36, pp. 929–64.

Fernando, S. (1995), *Mental Health in a Multi-ethnic Society: A Multi- disciplinary Handbook*, Routledge, London.

Flory, M. (1998), 'Psychiatric Diagnosis in Child and Adolescent Suicide', *Archives of General Psychiatry*, 53, pp. 339–48.

Goldberg, D. and Hodes, M. (1992), 'The Poison of Racism and the Self-poisoning of Adolescents', *Journal of Family Therapy*, 14, pp. 51–67.

Goodman, R. and Richards, H. (1995), 'Child and Adolescent Psychiatric Presentations of Second-generation Afro-Caribbeans in Britain', *British Journal of Psychiatry*, 167, pp. 362–9.

Goodyer, I., Wright, C. and Altham, P. (1990), 'The Friendships and Recent Life Events of Anxious and Depressed School Age Children', *British Journal of Psychiatry*, 156, pp. 689–98.

Gould, M.S., King, R., Greenwald, S., Fisher, P., Schwab Stone, M., Kramer, R., Flisher, A.J., Goodman, S., Canino, G. and Schaffer, D. (1998), 'Psychopathology associated with Suicidal Ideation and Attempts among Children and Adolescents', *Journal of the American Academy of Child and Adolescent Psychiatry*, 37, pp. 915–23.

Graham, J. and Bowling, B. (1995), *Young People and Crime*, Home Office Research Study 145, Home Office, London.

Graham, P. J. and Meadows, C.E. (1967), 'Psychiatric Disorder in the Children of West Indian Immigrants', *Journal of Child Psychology and Psychiatry*, 8, pp. 105–16.

Haskey, J. (1996), 'Population Review: (6) Families and Households in Great Britain', *Population Trends*, 85, pp. 7–24.

Haskey J. (1997), 'Population Review: (8) The Ethnic Minority and Overseas-born Populations of Great Britain', *Population Trends*, 88, pp. 13–30.

Hawton, K. and Fagg, J. (1992), 'Deliberate Self-Poisoning and Self-Injury in Adolescents. A Study of Charactersitics and Trends in Oxford, 1976–89', *British Journal of Psychiatry*, 161, pp. 816–23.

Hill, A.J., Weaver, C. and Blundell, J.E. (1990), 'Dieting Concerns of 10-year-old Girls and their Mothers', *British Journal of Clinical Psychology*, 29, pp. 346–8.

Hodes, M., Creamer, J. and Walley, J. (1998), 'The Cultural Meanings of Ethnic Categories', *Psychiatric Bulletin*, 22, pp. 20–24.

Hodes, M., Jones, C. and Davis, H. (1996), 'Cross-Cultural Differences in Maternal Evaluation of Children's Body Shapes', *International Journal of Eating Disorders*, 19, pp. 257–63.

Holden, N. and Robinson, P.H. (1988), 'Anorexia Nervosa and Bulimia Nervosa in British Blacks', *British Journal of Psychiatry*, 152, pp. 544–9.

Home Office (1991), *Statistical Bulletin*, 21 May, London: Home Office.

Hutchinson, G. and McKenzie, K. (1995), 'What is an Afro-Caribbean? Implications for Psychiatric Research', *Psychiatric Bulletin*, 19, pp. 700–2.

Jenkins, J. and Karno, M. (1992), 'The Meaning of Expressed Emotion: Theoretical Issues Raised by Cross-cultural Research', *American Journal of Psychiatry*, 149, pp. 9–21.

Jarvis, E. (1998), 'Schizophrenia in British Immigrants: Recent Findings, Issues and Implications', *Transcultural Psychiatry*, 35, pp. 39–74.

Kramer, T., Evans, N. and Garralda, M.E. (1999), 'Ethnic Diversity among Child and Adolescent Psychiatric (CAP) Clinic Attenders', *Child Psychology and Psychiatry Review*, in press.

Kleinman, A. (1988), *Rethinking Psychiatry. From Cultural Category to Personal Experience*, The Free Press, New York.

Lacey, J.H. and Dolan, B.M. (1988), 'Bulimia in British Blacks and Asians. A Catchment Area Study', *British Journal of Psychiatry*, 152, pp. 73–9.

Lewis, G., Croft-Jeffreys, C. and David, A. (1990), 'Are British Psychiatrists Racist?', *British Journal of Psychiatry*, 157, pp. 410–15.

Littlewood, R. (1992), 'Psychiatric Diagnosis and Racial Bias: Empirical and Interpretative Approaches', *Social Science and Medicine*, 34, pp. 141–9.

Littlewood, R. (1995), 'Psychopathology and Personal Agency: Modernity, Culture Change and Eating Disorders in South Asian Societies', *British Journal of Medical Psychology*, 68, pp. 45–63.

Mabey, C. (1981), 'Black British Literacy: a Study of Reading Attainment of London Black Children from 8–15 Years', *Educational Research*, 23, pp. 83–95.

MacCormack, C.P. and Draper, A. (1987), 'Social and Cognitive Aspects of Female Sexuality in Jamaica', in Caplan, P. (ed.), *The Cultural Construction of Sexuality*, Routledge, New York, pp. 143–65.

Mackintosh, N.J. and Mascie-Taylor, C.G.N. (1985), 'The IQ Question, in Department of Education and Science', *Education for All*, Chapter 3, Annexe D, HMSO, London.

Markantonakis, A. (1990), 'Anorexia Nervosa in People of Asian Extraction', *British Journal of Psychiatry*, 157, pp. 783.

Maughan, B. and Rutter, M. (1985), 'Black Pupils' Progress in Secondary Schools: II. Examination Attainments', *British Journal of Developmental Psychology*, 4, pp. 19–29.

Maughn, B., Dunn, G. and Rutter M. (1985), Black Pupils' Progress in Secondary School:1. Reading Attainment between 10 and 14', *British Journal of Developmental Psychology*, 3, pp. 113–22.

Merril, J. and Owens, J. (1987), 'Ethnic Differences in Self-poisoning – a Comparison of West-Indian and White Groups', *British Journal of Psychiatry*, 150, pp. 765–8.

Midence, K., McManus, C., Fuggle, P. and Davies, S. (1996), 'Psychological Adjustment and Family Functioning in a Group of British Children with Sickle Cell Disease: Preliminary Empirical Findings and a Meta-analysis', *British Journal of Clinical Psychology*, 35, pp. 439–50.

Mortimer, P., Sammons, P., Stoll, L., Lewis, D. and Ecob, R. (1988), *School Matters – The Junior Years*, Paul Chapman Publishing, London.

Mukai, T., Crago, M. and Shisslak, C.M. (1994), 'Eating Attitudes and Weight Preoccupation among Female High School Students in Japan', *Journal of Child Psychology and Psychiatry*, 35, pp. 677–88.

Nasser, M. (1997), *Culture and Weight Consciousness*, Routledge, New York.

Neehal, J. and Beharry, N. (1994), 'Demographic and Clinical Features of Adolescent Parasuicides', *West Indian Medical Journal*, 43, pp. 123–6.

Nicol, A.R. (1971), 'Psychiatric Disorder in the Children of Caribbean Immigrants', *Journal of Child Psychology and Psychiatry*, 12, pp. 273–81.

Patton, G.C., Johnson-Sabine, E., Wood, K., Mann, A.H. and Wakeling, A. (1990), 'Abnormal Eating Attitudes in London Schoolgirls: a Prospective Epidemiological Study: Outcome at 12 Month Follow-up', *Psychological Medicine*, 20, pp. 383–94.

Peach, C. (1996), *Ethnicity in 1991 Census: the Ethnic Minority Populations of Great Britain*, Volume 2, Office for National Statistics, HMSO, London.

Peach, C. (1998), 'Trends in Levels of Caribbean Segregation, Great Britain, 1961–91', in Chamberlain, M. (ed.), *Caribbean Migration: Globalized Identities*, Routledge, London.

Puri, B.K., Lambert, M.T. and Cordess, C.C. (1995), 'Characteristics of Young Offenders Detained Under Section 53(2) at a Young Offenders Institution', *Medicine Science and Law*, 35, pp. 69–76.

Quinton, D. (1994), 'Cultural and Community Influences', in Rutter, M. and Hay, D. (eds), *Development through Life: a Handbook for Clinicians*, Blackwell Scientific Publications, Oxford, pp. 112–34.

Reiss, D. (1996), 'Abnormal Eating Attitudes and Behaviours in Two Ethnic Groups from a Female British Urban Population', *Psychological Medicine*, 26, pp. 289–99.

Robins, L.N. and McEvoy, L. (1990), 'Conduct Problems as Predictors of Substance Abuse', in Robins, L. and Rutter, M. (eds), *Straight and Devious Pathways from Childhood to Adulthood*, Cambridge University Press, Cambridge, pp. 182–204.

Robinson, P.H. and Andersen, A. (1985), 'Anorexia Nervosa in American Blacks', *Journal of Psychiatric Research*, 19, pp. 183–8.

Rona, R.J., Li, L. and Chinn, S. (1997), 'Determinants of Nocturnal Enuresis in England and Scotland in the '90s', *Developmental Medicine and Child Neurology*, 39, pp. 677–81.

Rutter, M. (1987), 'Psychosocial Resilience and Protective Mechanisms', *American Journal of Orthopsychiatry*, 57, pp. 316.

Rutter, M. (1994), 'Continuities, Transitions and Turning Points in Development', in Rutter, M. and Hay, D. (eds), *Development through Life: a Handbook for Clinicians*, Blackwell Scientific Publications, Oxford, pp. 1–25.

Rutter, M., Tizard, J. and Whitmore, K. (1970), *Education, Health and Behaviour*, Longmans, London.

Rutter, M., Yule, W., Berger, M., Yule, B., Morton, J. and Bagley, C. (1974), 'Children of West Indian Immigrants – I. Rates of Behavioural Deviance and of Psychiatric Disorder', *Journal of Child Psychology and Psychiatry*, 15, pp. 241–62.

Rutter, M., Yule, B., Morton, J. and Bagley, C. (1975), 'Children of West Indian Immigrants. III. Home Circumstances and Family Patterns', *Journal of Child Psychology and Psychiatry*, 16, pp.105–23.

Scarr, S., Caparulo, B.K., Ferdman, B.M., Tower, R.B. and Caplan, J. (1983), 'Developmental Status and School Achievements of Minority and Non-minority Children from Birth to 18 years in a British Midlands Town', *British Journal of Developmental Psychology*, 1, pp. 31–48.

Shaffer, D., Gould M.S., Fisher, P., Trautman, P., Moreau, D., Kleinman, M. and Flory, M. (1998), 'Psychiatric Diagnosis in Child and Adolescent Suicide', *Archives of General Psychiatry*, 53, pp. 339–48.

Shaffer, D. and Piacenti, J. (1994), 'Suicide and Attempted Suicide', in Rutter, M., Taylor, E. and Hersov, L. (eds), *Child and Adolescent Psychiatry, Modern Approaches*, Blackwell Scientific Publications, Oxford, pp. 407–24.

Smith, D.J. (1994), 'Race, Crime and Criminal Justice', in Maguire, M., Morgan, R. and Reiner, R. (eds), *The Oxford Handbook of Criminology*, Clarendon Press, Oxford, pp. 1041–118.

Smith, D.J. (1995), 'Youth Crime and Conduct Disorders', in Rutter, M. and Smith, D.J. (eds), *Psychosocial Disorders in Young People – Time Trends and their Causes*, John Wiley and Sons Ltd, Chichester.

Smith, R.T. (1988), *Kinship and Class in the West Indies*, Cambridge University Press, Cambridge.

Soni Raleigh, V. (1992), 'Suicide Levels and Trends among Immigrants in England and Wales', *Health Trends*, 24, pp. 91–4.

Soni Raleigh, V. (1996), 'Suicide Patterns and Trends in People of Indian Subcontinent and Caribbean Origin in England and Wales', *Ethnicity and Health*, 1, pp. 55–63.

Striegel-Moore, R.H. (1993), 'Etiology of Binge Eating: a Developmental Perspective', in Fairburn, C.G. and Wilson, G.T. (eds), *Binge Eating. Nature, Assessment, and Treatment*, Guilford Press, New York and London, pp. 144–72.

Swann Report (1995), *Education For All: the Report of the Committee of Enquiry into the Education of Children from Ethnic Minority Groups*, HMSO, London.

Tizard, B. and Phoenix, A. (1993), *Black, White or Mixed Race? Race and Racism in the Lives of Young People of Mixed Parentage*, Routledge, London.

Tomlinson, S. (1983), *Ethnic Minorities in British Schools: a Review of Literature, 1960–1982*, Heinnemann Educational, London.

Vandereycken, W. and Hoek, H.W. (1992), 'Are Eating Disorders Culturebound Syndromes?', in Halmi, K.A. (ed.), *Psychobiology and Treatment of Anorexia Nervosa and Bulimia Nervosa*, American Psychiatric Press, Washington. DC, pp. 19–36.

Wardle, J. and Marsland, L. (1990), 'Adolescent Concerns about Weight and Eating; a Social-developmental Perspective', *Journal of Psychosomatic Research*, 34, pp. 377–91.

Werner, E.E. (1992), *Overcoming the Odds; High Risk Children from Birth to Adulthood*, Cornell University Press, Ithaca, NY.

Werry, J.A. and McClellan, J.M. (1992), 'Predicting Outcome in Child and Adolescent Schizophrenia and Bipolar Disorder', *Journal of the American Academy of Child and Adolescent Psychiatry*, 32, pp. 147.

Whitmarsh, A. and Harris, T. (1996), *Social Focus on Ethnic Minorities*, HMSO, London.

Wing, L. (1979), 'Mentally Retarded Children in Camberwell (London)', in Hafner, H. (ed.), *Estimating Needs for Mental Health Care*, Springer Verlag, Berlin.

Yule, W., Berger, M., Rutter, M. and Yule, B. (1975), 'Children of West Indian Immigrants II. Intellectual Performance and Reading Attainment', *Journal of Child Psychology and Psychiatry*, 16, pp. 1–17.

Zigler, E. and Levine, J. (1981), 'Age on First Hospitalization of Schizophrenia', *Journal of Abnormal Psychology*, 90, pp. 458–67.

Chapter 9

Mental Health Problems in Black Refugees

Ros Ramsay and C. Gorst-Unsworth

Introduction

Definition of a Refugee

According to Article 1 of the 1951 United Nations Geneva Convention, a refugee is someone who 'owing to a well founded fear of being persecuted for reasons of race, religion, nationality, membership of a particular social group or political opinion' has left his or her country and is unable to return there. Many governments also recognise as refugees people who are not targets of persecution but are victims of war, violence, and other social and political disasters. The 1967 United Nations High Commission on Refugees (UNHCR) Protocol Relating to the Status of Refugees extended the definition so that individuals would be eligible for assistance and protection based on the principle of nonrefoulment (nonreturn) to their home country (Marsella et al., 1994). Within Africa according to the Organisation for African Unity's 1969 Accord, the term refugee applies not only to those persecuted as defined in the 1951 convention but also to 'every person who, owing to external aggression, occupation, foreign domination or events seriously disturbing public order is compelled to leave his place of habitual residence in order to seek refuge'. The emphasis has shifted from an individual's personal fear to include other difficulties in the conditions in country of origin (Leopold and Harrell-Bond, 1994). Some refugees are people who have been forced to move within their own country and are internally displaced persons. Within the UK the term is generally used to include:

- refugees who have been granted asylum;
- asylum seekers who are applying for political asylum or refugee status in the UK and who have been granted temporary admission by the immigration service while their applications are considered;

- those granted Exceptional Leave to Remain (ELR). They must apply for renewal periodically, the delay between application and hearing a decision varying from less than several months to several years, with a further delay before families are allowed to join applicants.

Refugee Numbers

The UN High Commission on Refugees estimates there are 20 million refugees throughout the world. The number of internally displaced people is harder to estimate, but may be between 15 and 25 million, giving a total of around 40 million forced migrants in the world (Medical Foundation for the Care of Victims of Torture, 1994; Leopold and Harrell-Bond, 1994).

Refugees in Africa

The majority of current international refugees are from developing countries and are forced to relocate in developing countries. Leopold and Harrell-Bond (1994), citing information from the 1991 International Council for Voluntary Agencies, suggest that a third of the world's international refugees and half the internally displaced people may be in Africa. This equates with the 1992 United States Committee for Refugees (USCR) estimate of 5.3 million international refugees in Africa.

Over recent years there has been a spread of democracy and moves to resolve some long-standing conflicts within Africa, for example, in Angola, Ethiopia, Mozambique and South Africa. However, new conflicts have also arisen. Refugees have gone from Liberia to Guinea, Sierra Leone, Cote d'Ivoire and other west African states. There is now a large refugee population in the Horn, with people coming first from Ethiopia and Eritrea, then Somalia; and in Rwanda. The situation in other parts of Africa remains unstable.

People have left their homes for a variety of reasons, including political and economic causes. The destination of the refugees varies. There are large groups of rural refugees who cross the borders of their country of origin and seek asylum in a neighbouring area, which is often similar to their home environment, including from a cultural and ethnic point of view. Some people may self settle among the host population, while others live in organised rural settlement areas or in the growing number of refugee camps. There are also small, scattered groups with a fairly high educational level from an urban background, who tend to congregate in African capital cities, particularly the politically more important capitals (Peltzer, 1989).

Black African Refugees in the UK

A much smaller number of refugees, less than 5 per cent of the number worldwide, come to Europe. The Refugee Council estimates there may be about 360,000 refugees and asylum seekers in the UK, with about 80 per cent living in London. This group includes about 65,000 children, some of them unaccompanied minors (A. Thomas, personal communication). Accurate figures about the size of the refugee population are not available. Refugee populations tend to be mobile and change with the continuing influx of asylum seekers. Refugee community organisations can estimate the numbers of people, using their services, or with whom they have some contact. Some local authority housing departments may have data about numbers of refugees housed within the borough.

More specifically, the Home Office provides information about applications for asylum status (Watson and Danzelman, 1998). Between 1988 and 1993, the number of applications increased fivefold (Jacobs, 1995). Reviewing the six years, 1992–97, the number of applications for asylum in the UK for people from Africa was highest in 1995 (approximately 23,000), falling to about 10,000 in 1996 and 1997. In July 1998, the Refugee Council estimated that 52,000 asylum seekers were waiting for a decision on their asylum claim and a further 21,000 were waiting for appeal verdicts (Refugee Council Briefing, 1998).

Refugees come from a number of different countries in Africa, including Algeria, Angola, Ethiopia, Gambia, Ghana, Ivory Coast, Kenya, Liberia, Nigeria, Sierra Leone, Somalia, Sudan, Tanzania, Togo, Uganda and Zaire (Watson and Danzelman, 1998). Applications from Africa accounted for about 30 per cent of all applications in 1997. Eight per cent of all applicants came from Somalia, including 122 unaccompanied children. Only about one in five of all asylum seekers were granted refugee status or exceptional leave to remain in 1997. A quarter of all grants of asylum status and a third of all grants of exceptional leave to remain came from Somalia. Forty per cent of all refusals in 1997 came from Africa, with the highest number from Nigeria and Ghana (Watson and Danzelman, 1998). In 1995 the Refugee Council reported that the majority of immigration detainees come from Africa, in particular, Algeria, Ghana, Nigeria and Zaire (Refugee Council Factsheet no. 3, 1995).

Refugee Needs

Migration, including forced migration, has a long history. It includes the 'extracted migration' of around 40 million Africans forced to work as slaves in the west. Leopold and Harrell-Bond (1994) argue that not only is the current refugee problem the biggest in size and scope in human history, but there has also been a significant change in attitude towards refugees. Governments in the west have introduced immigration and asylum rules in an attempt to limit the arrival of members of refugee groups. There have been attempts to return large refugee populations to their home countries and UNHCR declared 1992 the Year of Voluntary Repatriation.

Refugees are a heterogeneous group with diverse and complex needs. Many have experienced torture, rape, brutality and deprivation. There are likely to be further stresses over their flight. In the refugee camps resources are scarce and the people's futures unknown. Marsella et al. (1994) report some of the problems encountered in living in a refugee camp: a sense of loss, uncertainty, distrust, scepticism, helplessness, vulnerability, powerlessness, overdependency, violence, crime and social disintegration. The mortality rate is high in the acute phase of displacement, especially among the displaced populations in northern Ethiopia and Southern Sudan (Jablensky et al., 1994; de Girolamo, 1994). The tendency in the camps is for governments to make a priority of human survival and to concentrate on providing food, shelter and attempts to manage life-threatening diseases, neglecting any less immediate needs.

There are further stresses on arrival in the host country and with any subsequent migration and resettlement. There is often prolonged uncertainty about refugee status, with some asylum seekers spending time on arrival in a detention centre. Refugees and asylum seekers living in the community have to deal with problems of acculturation, racism, language, unemployment, housing and health, against the background of their multiple losses of family and friends, home and culture as well as the torture, persecution and imprisonment they may have experienced.

Eighty per cent of refugees are women and children (Forbes Martin, 1994). Desjarlais et al. (1995) recognise women, children and the elderly as being particularly vulnerable. The special needs of women are related to their lack of power in relations with men, making them at increased risk of certain forms of violence, such as rape. They also have poorer access to resources and are more dependent and isolated following resettlement. The special needs of children are related to the difficulties they experience at a stage when they are still developing. Unaccompanied children are at most risk. Elderly people may also have less access to resources and may be more isolated.

Although asylum seekers are entitled to access the health service, the Asylum and Immigration (Appeals) Act, 1993, and the Asylum and

Immigration Act, 1996, have limited their access to permanent local authority accommodation, even if a person fits the criteria for being in priority need, and many face homelessness or bed-and-breakfast accommodation (Jacobs, 1995). In 1994, 1,345 households applied for rehousing under the homelessness legislation in London and were refused assistance on the grounds that they were asylum seekers, on average 42 households per borough (Pleace and Quilgars, 1996). Changes in social security regulations in 1987 restricted asylum seekers entitlement to income support while the Asylum and Immigration Act, 1996, denies in-country asylum seekers, and those appealing against a negative decision, any access to benefits.

Against this background of increasing difficulties faced by asylum seekers the Refugee Council (Factfile no. 1, 1997) has reported a growing number of suicides, particularly among young men from the Horn of Africa.

Children have their own difficulties. Many have had their education interrupted, speak little or no English and may be living in temporary accommodation, not necessarily in their own family. They may experience bullying, or isolation on arrival at school. They may have no rights to further education because of their immigration status or lack of access to benefits (Refugee Council Factfile no. 6, 1997).

Several health authorities have commissioned surveys of the needs of local refugee populations in London. Gammell et al. (1993) worked with local refugee communities in Newham and trained field workers from different communities to carry out a household survey. One thousand one hundred and fifty-one questionnaires were completed, including 186 from Somali refugees and 146 from refugees from Zaire. The respondents had high indices of deprivation: high unemployment, overcrowding and living in rented accommodation. Only half the refugees had been in the UK for more than two years, and many had spent their first year unable to communicate in English. Similarly, a survey of 59 attenders at the Somali Counselling Project in East London reported considerable employment and housing difficulties (British Red Cross, 1992). The Day-care Trust (1995), studying the needs of refugees and their families, interviewed 71 parents from Eritrea, Ethiopia and Somalia. Many of the refugees experienced isolation and insecurity and language barriers prevented them from communicating easily outside their own communities. Refugees' 'past experiences combined with their present situation to create a pervasive sense of fear within refugee families, including among the children'.

Mental Health of Refugees

Psychiatric Morbidity in Refugee Populations: Review of the Research Evidence

In recent years there has been much interest in trauma as a major factor in psychiatric morbidity. The diagnosis of post traumatic stress disorder (PTSD) is widely used and cases have been reported following exposure to a range of adverse experiences from minor accidents to natural disasters.

Several well designed studies have established a clear link between major traumatic events and psychiatric morbidity (Rosser et al., 1991; Weisaeth, 1989; Green, 1994; Wilson and Raphael, 1993; McFarlane, 1987). The question of aetiological factors has been investigated. The 'dose' of trauma, proximity to the traumatic event, threat to life, locus of control, personality factors such as previous vulnerability, attributional style, post trauma support, social stresses and timing of help or treatment are all thought to be important in the severity of reaction.

Most of the published work relates to a single distinct traumatic event. However, a refugee in exile presents a particularly complex situation, often reporting several episodes of trauma and associated losses. Well designed empirical research on refugee groups is in relatively early stages (for instance, little appears on the Cochrane database and no systematic reviews have been carried out). There are several studies demonstrating that the refugee experience, particularly if involving torture, causes considerable psychological sequelae in some survivors. The rates of psychiatric morbidity vary from 14 per cent to 71 per cent for depression (Hauf and Vaglum, 1995; Mollica et al., 1987); and 3 per cent to 58 per cent for PTSD (Yehuda and McFarlane, 1995).

There is a compelling argument that the term PTSD has been diluted or discredited by its wide use and that caution must be applied when using this diagnosis. The trauma model is essentially a Western concept and may represent an adaptive reaction to an abnormal political situation. The survivor's reaction should be seen within the appropriate cultural frame work and not automatically labelled as dysfunctional. However, there is no doubt that refugees in exile can present with symptoms of distress and/or problems in functioning which may relate to different aetiological factors (Summerfield, 1995, 1996, 1997).

Several authors have now begun to look at the reasons for variation in rates of morbidity, in particular, factors connected with the trauma itself and the factors connected with the exile experience. A four-dimensional model has been put forward in order to understand the different elements of the reaction particularly in refugees who have experienced torture (Turner and Gorst-Unsworth, 1990). The four dimensions are:

1 re-experiencing phenomena and problems in processing the experience (akin to the PTSD reaction).
2 depressive reactions (thought to be related to the associated losses).
3 somatic symptoms (sometimes directly related to the physical torture but often an expression of psychological distress).
4 the existential dilemma (enduring changes in attitudes to priorities and values such as religion, family life, relationships, career etc.).

Since this model was proposed there have been attempts to test its validity and the hypothesis that the different elements are associated with different aetiological factors. Ramsay, Gorst-Unsworth and Turner (1993) examined 100 survivors of torture from different countries and found that a PTSD diagnosis had the strongest association with severity of torture experience and there was a weaker association between torture experience and diagnosis of depression. Gorst-Unsworth et al. (1993) reported that reactions described under the existential dilemma were common in survivors of torture and these changes were more likely when there was a low expectation of torture, or in previously highly religious people. A later study found a significant association between sexual torture and the avoidance symptom cluster within the PTSD criteria (Van Velsen et al., 1996).

Hauf and Vaglum (1995) studied 145 Vietnamese refugees in Norway in relation to several social factors in exile. They found that after three years of resettlement there remained similar levels of psychological distress to that on arrival. Female gender, extreme traumatic experience, negative life events in Norway, lack of a close confidant and chronic family separation, were identified as predictors of psychopathology. In the same year, Sundquist (1995) compared a large group of Latin-American refugees in Sweden with a group of Finnish migrants and South European labour migrants, and a control group of Swedish nationals. He found that ethnicity was a strong independent variable as well as social class in relation to self-rated illness.

Lavik et al. (1996) examined 231 refugees, 12 per cent of whom were from Africa. They concluded that refugees constitute a population at risk from mental disorder and that traumatic stressors and social factors in exile constitute independent factors, but for psychotic symptoms, separate factors exist.

Pernice and Brook (1996) examined 129 Southeast Asian refugees in New Zealand. They compared this group to 57 Pacific Island immigrants and 63 British immigrants. Anxiety and depression scores were affected by post-immigration factors such as experiencing discrimination in New Zealand, not having close friends, being unemployed and spending most of one's time with one's own ethnic group. In 1997, Silove et al. in Sydney, Australia, interviewed 40 asylum seekers from several different countries and found that psychiatric morbidity was associated with several factors, in addition to the premigration trauma e.g. poverty, conflict with immigration officials, delays in processing refugee applications, unemployment and racial discrimination.

In 1998, a study of 84 male asylum seekers from Iraq (Gorst-Unsworth and Goldberg, 1998) found that social factors in exile, particularly the level of 'affective' social support, proved important in determining the severity of both post traumatic stress disorder and depressive reactions. Poor social support was a stronger predictor of depressive morbidity than trauma factors.

Although our understanding of different risk factors is increasing, it is important to remember that the rates of psychiatric diagnosis, with an emphasis on mental state phenomena, may not correlate with ability to function, and do not necessarily imply a need for psychiatric treatment (Summerfield, 1996). Rooke (1995), describing his experience in a refugee camp for Rwandan refugees, comments on the surprising lack of 'psychiatric cases', and the resilience of both adults and children alike.

Most research so far has not sought to separate black refugees from other ethnic groups. There are only a few reports relating to specific groups from Africa, the majority being merely descriptions of various physical and psychological symptoms given by survivors of various traumatic events. However, Shisana and Celentano (1987) examined 88 Namibian refugees and measured social support, coping style, as well as traumatic events and health status. They found that social support and coping style could mediate in the relationship between traumatic experience and health outcome.

There does not appear to be any evidence at present to suggest that black refugees present different problems to those of other refugees, but rather that cultural loss and social support and networks are equally important in terms of recovery in exile.

Specific Difficulties associated with Detention

For many years it has been the practice of the UK immigration authorities to detain certain asylum seekers, either on their entry to Britain, or prior to forced deportation. Asylum seekers are held sometimes in a special immigration detention centre, or occasionally in prisons such as Pentonville, Rochester or Reading.

Such detention, particularly in a criminal establishment, has caused concern among the medical profession as well as immigration lawyers and community groups. A letter to *The Lancet* in 1991 described a particular survivor of torture from Zaire who had been detained in Pentonville prison and was found to be depressed, suicidal and with features of post traumatic stress disorder triggered by the conditions in Pentonville, which reminded him of his original detention and torture in Zaire. The six authors of the letter cited detention of torture survivors as 'cruel, degrading and fundamentally unsound' (Summerfield et al., 1991). In the same year, following the death of a Zairian asylum seeker in Pentonville, various bodies, including the Royal College of Psychiatrists, the BMA and the Medical Section of Amnesty International, made supportive statements to the condemnation of the government practice of detaining asylum seekers (Gorst-Unsworth et al., 1991).

In the psychiatric literature, 10 cases of detained asylum seekers were documented in detail. All were male and six were from African countries. All reported torture in their countries of origin. There was a high level of psychiatric morbidity on examination, with all of the sample reporting depressed mood, and nine saying they felt completely hopeless about the future. Definite suicidal ideation was reported by four and two had made previous suicide attempts (Bracken and Gorst-Unsworth, 1991).

Although the Home Office do not publish official figures, it was reported in 1997, in the *BMJ*, that over 700 asylum seekers were being detained in British prisons at the time (Bunce, 1997). It is possible that black asylum seekers are more likely to be detained than other ethnic groups. Of 606 detainees on June 22, 1994 the majority were from Africa (Refugee Council Factsheet no. 3, 1995) and the reasons for detention appeared arbitrary. In 1997, 221 asylum seekers in detention were later found to be refugees or given ELR by the Home Office (Refugee Council Briefing, 1998).

Psychiatric Problems in Refugee Children: Review of the Research Evidence

Although many adult refugees will have to leave their children behind when fleeing persecution, others may be successful in bringing their family to the UK, either initially, or after several years under the Rights of Family Reunion.

Some children arrive in the UK as unaccompanied minors, sent by their family alone to escape violence and threats in their own country and with the hope of better opportunities.

Refugee children in a western country of exile have many tasks of adaptation. If alone, they may have to adapt to a new environment, a new family and new friends. Later they may have to re-integrate into a family from whom they have been separated for a long time. The success of adaptation to a new culture may depend on the proximity of families and children with the same language and culture to whom they can relate (Kinzie et al., 1986).

Much of the published work on refugee children is qualitative rather than empirical. There is more written about children in countries of conflict, or direct victims of war, rather than about the refugee experience. Examples of situations in which children have been chronically exposed to violence during their development, and even actively recruited into armed struggle, are well described in South Africa and Mozambique. RENAMO, the rebel military movement in Mozambique, is known to have abducted boys at an early age and subjected them to dehumanising experiences, including forced killings of their own families in order to transform them into hardened soldiers (Boothby et al., 1991). Melzak (1996) states that many different factors will influence how a child reacts and adapts to a traumatic experience. The age, extent of violence, relationship of the child to the perpetrator, the meaning of the violence to the child in the short and long term, the extent to which the violence is connected with loss and change, and whether or not the child generalises his or her understanding of the world from specific experiences of violence, are all crucial factors. Richman (1993), in a comprehensive review on children in situations of political violence, discusses the problems in studying this group. She states that one must be careful in generalising from one population to another.

Clearly the problems of children in the midst of conflict in their own country, those in refugee camps in developing countries, and those in exile in a developed country will all have different problems and needs. Methods of investigation are also problematic, some being common to the study of adults, such as cultural differences, use of interpreters and the mobility of the population. However, there are also specific difficulties in working with children, for example, information based on straightforward questionnaires alone is not reliable, and explorative interviews are better, but time consuming. The functioning of a child within his or her social context should also be taken into account.

Another review of research into child victims of war points out that a recurring difficulty has been the heavy use and reliance on clinical samples, from which inferences have been drawn to the larger population (Jensen and Shaw, 1993).

Studies of children after disasters have established typical reactions which include sleep disturbance, difficulties in concentration, loss of developed mental skills, flashbacks, anxiety and panic associated with reminders of the event, depressed mood, conduct difficulties, lack of confidence in the future and re-enactment of the events in play (Udwin, 1993; Lonigan et al., 1991; Yule et al., 1990).

Some studies suggest that symptoms of PTSD in refugee children can be long lasting. In a study of 50 Iranian refugee children in Sweden, PTSD was diagnosed in 21 per cent after the event while two and a half years later the prevalence of PTSD was 23 per cent (Almqvist and Brandell-Forsberg, 1997).

Richman et al. (1993) studied 50 children in Mozambique who had been exposed to organised violence and found that a quarter were highly distressed according to their symptoms, although they were functioning reasonably well within their situation. Boothby (1994) studied 42 former boy soldiers from RENAMO camps in Mozambique and found that time spent in the camp, rather than personal involvement in violence, was important in later adjustment. Boys who spent less than six months in the camp emerged with their basic trust and values intact. Even in those who had spent longer, and were exhibiting aggressive behaviours, after three months in a refugee centre they showed a softening of attitude, increased attachment behaviour, positive feelings towards their caretakers and interest in social activities.

Wolff et al. (1995) studied Eritrean children and compared a group of 74 living in an orphanage with an equal number living with their families in a refugee camp. Surprisingly there were relatively few clinically significant differences between the comparison groups. The orphans showed more behavioural symptoms of emotional distress but performed better on cognitive and language performance measures. The researchers concluded that 'when group care is child centred it can, under some circumstances, be a viable solution for unaccompanied children in countries where adoption and foster care are not realistic alternatives'.

Some studies give conflicting results, suggesting that family relationships and, in particular, maternal health is a stronger predictor of morbidity in children than the level of trauma exposure. A study of 58 Guatemalan Mayan Indian children in Mexican refugee camps, found minimal evidence of psychiatric morbidity. There was a strong association between depressive symptoms in girls and poor health status of their mothers (Miller, 1996).

In summary, there are many methodological difficulties in studying refugee children in exile and it is important that studies are carried out by those well trained and experienced in interviewing children under stress. In spite of these drawbacks it does seem that a refugee child may suffer great difficulty in adapting to a new situation and assimilating experiences from the past. There are many factors that influence the nature of a child's reaction and some protective factors. It appears that in certain circumstances children can be more resilient than expected and can be helped to develop a relatively normal life. Rutter (1985), in his review of adversity and resilience, points out that 'coping with stress situations can be strengthening and ... the quality of resilience resides in how people deal with life changes and what they do about their situations'.

Treatment and Training Issues

Given that refugees may have suffered various different traumas and losses before and during their exile, how do we rationally go about offering appropriate treatment and management to this group? The literature has many descriptions of different treatment strategies employed for refugees. Many of the accounts are purely descriptive in nature based on the particular professional's background, training and personal ideas of the best way to work with traumatised groups. The PTSD model of treatment is applied by many workers in the field with apparent success (Friedman and Jaranson, 1994). Based on the western PTSD model, different therapeutic methods have been described. Many of these accounts do not attempt to evaluate the evidence for effectiveness of treatments but it is widely assumed that a number of psychological methods can be helpful.

These methods include:

- Individual psychotherapeutic approaches and counselling techniques aimed at helping the individual to bear witness and ventilate feelings around the experience. Some have called this approach 'the testimony method' (Agger et al., 1990), but most of the techniques generally involve retelling the trauma story in some way (Blackwell, 1997; Landry, 1989; Schlapobersky, 1993; Peltzer, 1989; Schreibeer, 1995).
- Family therapy methods and in particular healing rituals taking into account the cultural background of the families (Jaffa, 1993; Woodcock, 1995).
- Group work aimed at regaining the sense of inclusion and identity and sense of shared purpose (Shackman and Tribe, 1989; Woodcock, 1997).

- Movement psychotherapy which recognises the body mind continuum using interpretation of bodily postures and movements to facilitate a relationship between therapist and patient. This can be particularly useful if there have been physical consequences of torture or if the patient finds a western model of talking therapy difficult to work with (Callaghan, 1993).
- Specialised physiotherapy, a hands-on therapy sometimes well accepted by cultures where touch is a more frequent communication than in western cultures. It can also be particularly helpful in the hyperventilation syndrome (Hough, 1992).

Empirical study is more likely to have been done in the field of pharmacotherapy and behaviour therapy. However, comparison of different treatment options has not been well investigated and most of the work chooses populations with a history of single trauma, very few studies having been done specifically on refugee populations.

There is some evidence to support the efficacy of a wide range of psychotropic drugs in relieving some or all of the symptoms of PTSD. Those studied and recommended have included the: SSRIs fluo (Van der Kolk et al., 1994); tricyclic antidepressants (Davidson et al., 1997; Boehnlein et al., 1985); MAOIs (De Martino et al., 1995; Davidson, 1997). Other authors have investigated newer psychotropics such as brofaromine (a combined MAO-A inhibitor and 5HT transport inhibitor) (Katz et al., 1994). Benzodiazepines do not have a place, due to problems with tolerance and withdrawal.

Some empirical studies have examined with quantitative techniques the efficacy of various psychological cognitive and behavioural techniques, such as eye-movement desensitisation (Pitman et al., 1996; Rothbaum, 1997), cognitive behavioural therapy (Chemtob et al., 1997), exposure techniques (Richards et al., 1994; Basoglu, 1992) and brief trauma-focused psychotherapy (Goenjian et al., 1997).

Unfortunately most of these studies have involved small numbers with some methodological flaws. It is likely that improvements in many cases may be due to the non-specific effects of a close therapeutic relationship, rather than the particular technique described.

Many authors advocate combined use of pharmacotherapy and psychological or social treatments (Dow and Kline, 1997; Soloman et al., 1992; Turner and Gorst-Unsworth, 1993).

Most accounts of treatment fail to address the broader framework, and in particular ignore the social world of the survivor, which may be the most important factor in determining how well the refugee will cope over time.

In his advice to non-governmental organisations (NGOs) setting up in war zones, Summerfield (1996) points out that the western model of trauma work is based on several false assumptions. These include the idea that:

- Adverse events are bound to cause psychological injury. We need to be clear about the target group and understand that distress or suffering is not the same as psychological disturbance.
- There is a universal human response to stressful events. Questionnaires are often devised to identify 'caseness' for traumatic damage but the meaning of symptoms and the impact of those symptoms on a person's daily life is a highly individual measure.
- Large numbers of victims will need professional help. Some authors have assumed that refugees need to be 'sensitised' to mental health issues in order to accept the help that is on offer. Many refugees, however, have far more pressing issues to deal with than their psychological symptoms. There will be a minority with clear cut problems or frank mental illness, but sufferers, their relatives, friends or neighbours are usually well aware if this is the case.
- Victims do better if they ventilate their emotions and talk through their experiences. Western talking therapies have been largely unsuccessful in unstable and impoverished settings such as war zones. Some professionals are convinced that even when survivors of trauma are coping well and reassembling their lives that the real problem lies 'hidden'. Many post-disaster services are being initiated on very little objective evidence of the effectiveness of psychological debriefing (Raphael et al., 1995). Non-western cultures often see no place for the revelation of intimate material outside the close family circle.
- There are vulnerable groups and individuals who need to be specifically targeted for psychological help. Some workers have argued that certain types of survivor are particularly vulnerable, for example, children and adolescents, women who have been raped, the elderly etc. Women in Bosnia who had been raped were targeted after much media coverage. However, some of the Bosnian Muslim women spoke out and put their rape in the context of an assault on their culture and ethnic identity, not as an individual trauma. Butonese women who have been raped reported that their overriding concern was the lack of school for their children in the refugee camps, not their own trauma of the rape experience.

It is clear that if we are to offer rational treatment to refugees we should be fully aware of the debates regarding post trauma treatment and also that we should listen to what the survivor is telling us and not assume that the professional knows best. It is likely that psychological treatment comes low down in the hierarchy of need well below basic social needs such as housing, financial issues, general health issues and family or social support.

Mental Health Service Needs of Refugees

Refugees in flight and in refugee camps have wide-ranging needs. They may be the focus of humanitarian concern, seen to be in need of services and protection. The UNHCR has a formal mandate to ensure the legal protection of those under its care. It is now increasingly involved in co-ordinating assistance to refugees. A number of other UN organisations, voluntary organisations or NGOs as well as the host government may also provide care. Much more limited help is available to internally displaced people. In Africa, most assistance is given to the Horn and Southern Africa, and the least to West Africa (Leopold and Harrell-Bond, 1994).

As the number of refugees in the world has grown there has been a tendency to label refugees as a problem. Relief programmes have limited funds and will focus on the most pressing problems in the camps: malnutrition, crowding, poor water supply and hygiene as well as physical trauma and psychosocial stress. A high proportion of the morbidity of refugees in camps is seen and managed in the primary health care setting as refugees attend local primary health care centres. This may be most helpful for refugees who express their psychological distress in somatic terms or who would feel stigmatised attending a mental health facility (de Girolamo, 1994).

For refugees arriving in the UK, there is a tendency for health care professionals to ignore the social context, instead focusing on their limited brief of treating any disorder. Although some refugee groups have indigenous support groups in place, others are more isolated (Ramsay and Turner, 1993). Work with children is time consuming and may again involve consultation with several different agencies and sometimes with interpreters. Some GPs may not wish to accept refugees onto their practice lists (Gammel et al., 1993). At an organisational level, refugees are rarely included in any ethnic monitoring exercise (Summerfield, 1995). Failure to plan and coordinate service provision between different statutory and non-statutory services leads to patchy provision, and there may be a lack of information for professionals about what is available in the locality (Ramsay and Turner, 1993).

Refugees' Difficulties in Accessing Services

Uptake of statutory mental health services may be low (Gammel et al., 1993; Grant and Deane, 1995; Jacobs, 1995, Refugee Council Factfile no. 2, 1997). Refugees may feel ashamed to reveal their experiences to other members of their family or community (Schreiber, 1995). There may be a cultural reluctance for them to approach mental health professionals. Out of respect, or due to feelings of shame, refugees may not admit to health professionals that they are experiencing adjustment problems (ibid.). Refugees may not make a clear distinction between psychological and physical problems and may seek help more readily for physical rather than psychological problems (Boehnlein, 1987). Some refugees may prefer to consult with a traditional healer (Schreiber, 1995). Refugees may also be wary of statutory services because of experiences of dealing with government organisations in their country of origin and while applying for asylum. They may be suspicious of mental health workers as authority figures and fear that disclosing their mental health problems could affect their status or application for asylum (Wilson, 1993).

Refugees who wish to access services may experience difficulties in knowing how to do so, particularly if they need to contact a number of different organisations (Atkin and Rollings, 1993; Gammel et al., 1993). Language barriers may be present, the lack of adequate interpreting services preventing refugees making contact with mental health services (Ramsay and Turner, 1993).

Health Service Provision

In the refugee camps, de Girolamo (1995) has emphasised the importance of decentralised primary health care, undertaken by non-specialised general health workers, collaborating with government and non-government sectors, and also requiring the active participation of the community and family. This was seen as the way to achieve WHO's objective 'Health for All by the Year 2000'. In the absence of specialised mental health facilities, WHO and UNHCR have introduced a training manual ('Mental Health of Refugees', 1996) for relief workers about how to identify and manage the most common psychological and psychosocial problems found in refugee camps. The manual includes a section on psychosis and on helping people who have been raped or tortured.

In the UK, due to the multiple needs of refugees, easy access to services without unnecessary institutional barriers is essential (Atkin and Rollings, 1993). It is helpful if services are integrated as far as possible: within the health field and more broadly between health and education, training, language services, employment, social services, justice and other services (Boehnlein, 1987). Some have suggested integrating western health services with traditional healing (Schreiber, 1995).

The Refugee Council has found evidence that many refugee community groups provide essential services for their community members. For example, they may offer interpreters, advisors and advocates who mediate between mainstream providers and an individual refugee, as well as providing a place to go and meet others, receive informal counselling, support and social activities (Jacobs, 1995). Many of these groups are voluntary and receive little or no statutory funding. Although refugees need targeted services it is important to prevent the segregation of refugees from the rest of the community and local services.

There are examples of good practice, with a speedy, clearly co-ordinated and planned response to managing the health needs of a newly arrived refugee group. For example, following the arrival of refugees from Somalia, in Cardiff, a GP was the first to alert the establishment to a specific health need and the first to respond (Ruddy, 1992).

Conclusions

There is a large number of black refugees worldwide. Many remain in Africa, and less than 5 per cent come to Europe, including the UK. Among detained people seeking asylum in the UK, the highest number come from Algeria, Nigeria, Sierra Leone, Somalia and Zaire, with those most frequently granted asylum coming from Somalia (Watson and Danzelman, 1998).

Refugees have complex needs, crossing the traditional boundaries of health care and other agencies. Very little is known about social and cultural needs, with only marginally more known about health needs. In the immediate transition phase, physical needs are most obvious, and high rates of mortality have been reported in northern Ethiopia and southern Sudan. Workers in the refugee field point to the high level of need of all refugees, but we lack high quality evidence about this need. Against this background of poorly researched need there is also a compelling argument that we may be overmedicalising some of the problems that refugees report (Summerfield, 1996). For example, Jacobs (1995) quotes one mental health worker: 'Psychiatrists seem to diagnose all Somalis with paranoid schizophrenia.' At present, mental health professionals know little about cultural attitudes to trauma in black refugees.

Earlier work on refugee populations focused on symptom profiles, but there is now more interest in understanding the social factors related to exile. Factors such as lack of housing, unemployment, and fear of deportation may be as difficult for a refugee to deal with as the original trauma (Wilson, 1993).

More is known about the cultural needs of refugees from other parts of the world. For example, the needs of southeast Asian refugees in the USA and Australasia have been researched. In response to research findings it has been possible to develop culturally sensitive services for these populations.

Services have grown up piecemeal in different places, sometimes in the voluntary sector (Jacobs, 1995). We do not know the most appropriate way to organise them, to ensure that they are responsive to the refugees' needs, but do not become marginalised by health planners. In some countries, such as Australia, the Netherlands and in Scandinavia there have been more attempts to include refugee health programmes as part of the governments health plans, and this approach may reduce the adverse social factors refugees face (Hauf and Vaglum, 1995; Silove et al., 1997; Van de Wijngaart, 1997).

Recommendations

More information is needed specifically about the black refugee population, both their mental and physical health needs, and also about their cultural background, including their approach to dealing with traumatic events and seeking help from health professionals. Although there are anecdotal reports about therapeutic work with refugees, we need more controlled studies into the effectiveness and acceptability of different treatment approaches.

Health workers are limited in what they can offer to refugees and need to recognise the symptoms within the context of wide ranging social disruption. Changes in government policy may have more impact in meeting the wider needs of refugee populations particularly in relation to detention of newly arrived asylum seekers, family reunion, and housing and benefits policy.

Acknowledgement

We are grateful for the helpful comments made by Dr Derek Summerfield made on an earlier draft of this chapter.

References

Atkin, K. and Rollings, J. (1993), *Community Care in Multi-racial Britain. A Critical Review of the Literature*, HMSO, London.

Boehnlein, J.K. (1987), 'A Review of Mental Health Services for Refugees between 1975 and 1985 and a Proposal for Future Services', *Hospital and Community Psychiatry*, 38, pp. 764–8.

British Red Cross (1992), 'Health Situation of Refugees and Asylum Seekers in the United Kingdom', Paper 2, The Somalis, British Red Cross, London.

Desjarlais, R., Eisenberg, L. Good, B. and Kleinman, A. (1995), *World Mental Health: Problems and Priorities in Low-income Countries*, Oxford University Press, Oxford.

Forbes Martin, S. (1994), 'A Policy Perspective on the Mental Health and Psychosocial Needs of Refugees', in Marsella, A.J., Bornemann, T., Ekblad, S. and Orley, J. (eds), *Amidst Peril and Pain: the Mental Health and Well Being of the World's Refugees*, American Psychological Association, Washington, DC.

Gammell, H., Ndahiro, A., Nicholas, M. and Windsor, J. (1993), 'Refugees (Political Asylum Seekers) Service Provision and Access to the NHS. A Study by the College of Health for Newham Health Authority and Newham Healthcare', College of Health, London.

de Girolamo, G. (1994), 'Primary Health Care of Refugees', in Marsella, A.J., Bornemann, T., Ekblad, S. and Orley, J. (eds), *Amidst Peril and Pain: the Mental Health and Well Being of the World's Refugees*, American Psychological Association, Washington, DC.

Grant, C. and Dean, J. (1995), 'Brixton Refugee Health Project. Factors which influence Uptake and Provision of Primary Health Services for Refugees', Brixton Challenge, London.

Jablensky, A., Marsella, A.J., Ekblad, S., Jansson, B., Levi, L. and Bornemann, T. (1994), 'Refugee Mental Health and Well-being: Conclusions and Recommendations', in Marsella, A.J., Bornemann, T., Ekblad, S. and Orley, J. (eds), *Amidst Peril and Pain: the Mental Health and Well Being of the World's Refugees*, American Psychological Association, Washington, DC.

Jacobs, C. (1995), 'Services for Refugee Communities', in Harding, C. (ed.), *Not just Black and White: an Information Pack about Mental Health Services for People from Black Communities*, Good Practices in Mental Health, London.

Leopold, M. and Harrell-Bond, B. (1994), 'An Overview of the World Refugee Crisis', in Marsella, A.J., Bornemann, T., Ekblad, S. and Orley, J. (eds), *Amidst Peril and Pain: the Mental Health and Well Being of the World's Refugees*, American Psychological Association, Washington, DC.

Marsella, A.J., Bornemann, T., Ekblad, S. and Orley, J. (1994), 'Introduction', in Marsella, A.J., Bornemann, T., Ekblad, S. and Orley, J. (eds), *Amidst Peril and Pain: the Mental Health and Well Being of the World's Refugees*, American Psychological Association, Washington, DC.

Medical Foundation for the Care of Victims of Torture (1994), *A Betrayal of Hope and Trust. Detention in UK Survivors of Torture*, Medical Foundation for the Care of Victims of Torture, London.

Peltzer, K. (1989), 'Assessment and Treatment of Psychosocial Problems in Refugees in Zambia', *International Journal of Mental Health*, 18, pp. 113–21.

Pleace, N. and Quilgars, D. (1996), *Health and Homelessness in London*, Centre for Housing Policy, University of York.

Ramsay, R. and Turner, S. (1993), 'Refugees Health Needs', *British Journal of General Practice*, 43, pp. 480–81.

Refugee Arrivals Project (1994), 'Refugee Arrivals Project Annual Report', Room 2005, 2nd floor, Queen's Building, Heathrow Airport, Middlesex.

Refugee Council (1995), 'Refugee Council Factsheet No. 3, February 1995. Detention of Asylum Seekers in the UK', Refugee Council, London.

Refugee Council (1997), 'Refugee Council Factfile No. 1, June 1997. The Health Concerns of Asylum Seekers and Refugees', Refugee Council, London.

Refugee Council (1997), 'Refugee Council Factfile No. 2, June 1997. Access to the National Health Service', Refugee Council, London.

Refugee Council (1997), 'Refugee Council Factfile No. 6, October 1997. The Education, Training and Employment of Asylum Seekers and Refugees', Refugee Council, London.

Refugee Council (1998), 'Briefing on the Government's Immigration and Asylum White Paper, July 1998', Refugee Council, London.

Ruddy, B. (1992), 'Any Port in a Storm', *Health Service Journal*, 102, p. 29.

Schreiber, S. (1995), 'Migration, Traumatic Bereavement and Transcultural Aspects of Psychological Healing: Loss and Grief of a Refugee Woman from Bagameder County in Ethiopia', *British Journal of Medical Psychology*, 68, pp. 135–42.

Summerfield, D. (1995), 'Addressing Human Response to War and Atrocity. Major Challenges in Research and Practices and the Limitations of Western Psychiatric Models', in Kleber, R.J., Figley, C.R. and Gersonsm, B.P. (eds), *Beyond Trauma: Cultural and Societal Dynamics*, Plenum Press, New York.

Watson, M. and Danzelman, P. (1998), 'Asylum Statistics UK 1997', *Home Office Statistical Bulletin*, issue 14, Government Statistical Service, London.

Wilson, M. (1993), *Mental Health and Britain's Black Communities*, King's Fund Centre, London.

World Health Organisation (1996), *Mental Health of Refugees*, WHO and UNHCR, Geneva.

Chapter 10

Substance Abuse in Black People of African Descent

Zelpha Kittler

Introduction

Race is a social invention. In genetic terms the physical or biological differences between groups defined as 'races' are negligible, and there has been as yet no persuasive evidence for ascribing psychological, intellectual, or moral capacities to individuals on the basis of either skin colour or physiognomy. Yet, the existence of inequalities, not only in education, employment, and income in relation to race and ethnicity, but also in health and healthcare remains an incontrovertible fact. Raj Bhopal (*BMJ*, 1997) in reviewing a number of research studies showing that Black Americans receive less healthcare than white Americans concluded that these differences were not entirely accounted for by variations in socio-economic circumstance.

The history of the last two centuries is littered with examples of the use of dubious 'scientific' theory to bolster the prevailing ethos of the racial superiority of the White European. These putative racial differences were assumed to be biological and thus propounded to justify policies subordinating 'coloured' groups which included slavery, eugenics and the inequitable practice of medicine. Campaigns in the United States exploited the country's endemic racism and xenophobia, fuelling the prohibition movement with hysterical language and racial stereotyping. Woodiwiss in his book *Reform, Racism and Rackets: Alcohol and Drug Prohibition in the United States* illustrates this point with quotations from two leading politicos of the day. In 1914, Richard Pearson Hobson, an elected Representative of Alabama, introduced the idea of alcohol prohibition to the House of Representatives using the following arguments:

> Liquor will actually make a brute out of a Negro, causing him to commit unnatural crimes ... the effect is the same on the white man, though the white man being further evolved, it takes longer time to reduce him to the same level.

In similar ways anti-black sentiment was used to fuel arguments for the prohibition of cocaine. In 1910, Dr Hamilton Wright, the man responsible for the Report on the International Opium Commission, concluded that:

> ... this new vice, the cocaine vice, the most serious to be dealt with, has proved to be the creator of criminals and unusual forms of violence, and it has been a potent incentive in driving the humbler Negroes all over the country to abnormal crimes.

The fact that those in positions of power and authority successfully deployed the 'race card' in their onslaught against the twin evils of drugs and alcohol is perhaps not surprising, given the overt racist attitudes of the time. It is more disquieting that in this present era, myths and stereotypes about the nature and extent of drug use among African Americans continue unabated. Approximately 400 individuals in Washington, DC were asked to describe typical drug-users; more than 95 per cent envisaged a black individual (Watson and Jones, 1989).

Terminology

In the United States 'black' is typically understood to mean people of African ancestral origins that fall into the racial group referred to as 'Negroid' in the nineteenth century. In Britain the term 'black' has been used more broadly to refer to people of African-Caribbean and South Asian descent. This usage has historical antecedents with both groups sharing experiences of discrimination by the majority community based on their 'non-whiteness', coupled with the successful usurpation of the term from the American Black Power Movement by political activists in Britain in the 1960s and 1970s as a unifying symbol of racial pride and assertive group identity. Atvar Brah, writing in *Race, Culture and Difference*, highlights the difficulties inherent in 'ethnicism' – defining ethnic difference as the primary modality around which social life is constructed, and discounting other experiences centred around class, gender, or sexuality. A group defined as culturally different is assumed to be internally homogenous. He argues that ethnicism often fails to differentiate between the term 'black', as a political adage adopted by subordinate groups to symbolise resistance to racial oppression, and the use of the same term by some local authorities as a basis for the allocation of resources. He argues that a broad definition of 'black' may conceal the cultural needs of groups other than those of African-Caribbean origin. While acknowledging the debate surrounding the usage of the term black with its differing cultural and political meanings, for the purposes of reducing what would otherwise be a Herculean task to manageable proportions, the focus of this chapter will be substance use among members of the black community in US/Europe, defined narrowly as those with African ancestral origin and focusing on epidemiological issues and treatment needs.

Search

A literature search was conducted using the databases Medline and Embase, covering the years 1994 to 1998, exploring the terms 'substance related disorder' and 'black', and combining the two searches, resulting in a total of 160 papers. The abstracts were then viewed and distilled down to a final selection of 12, excluding a large number relating primarily to adolescent substance misuse, alcohol related disorders, HIV infected drug users, and pregnant users. Also excluded were small studies with limited numbers of black subjects. The focus was on broad based large-scale or epidemiological studies, plus studies examining cultural issues and treatment outcomes among ethnic groups of African ancestry. Recent editorials and papers on controversies surrounding ethnicity in research were retrieved from the *British Medical Journal* computer file. A literature search was also conducted, using the database of the Institute for the study of Drug Dependency using the keywords 'drug use in black communities UK/US 1995 to 1998'. The ISDD library is one of the world's most comprehensive, multidisciplinary libraries on drugs with over 60,000 documents from the UK and around the world. This search yielded 86 documents from which 20 were selected, including chapters from four books: *Psychiatric Disorders in the US, Race, Culture and Difference, Reform, Racism and Rackets: Alcohol and Drug Prohibition in the United State*s and *Race, Drugs, Europe: Specialist Drug Services and Managing Change to Meet the Needs of Black and other Visible Minority Drug Users: Volume1: England, France, the Netherlands, Portugal*. Where appropriate, a select number of articles was retrieved via the reference lists from the original subset of documents studied.

Epidemiological Studies

While epidemiological studies comprising aggregate data on large segments of disparate populations can be misleading re-specific segments of the population, they nonetheless are of use in the planning of public health strategies. To date, the most comprehensive information on substance use disorders is provided by four surveys: the Epidemiological Catchment Area study (Robins and Regier, 1991), the National Co-morbidity Survey (Anthony et al., 1994; Kessler et al., 1994; Warner et al., 1995), the National Household Survey on Drug Abuse (SAMSA, 1995d) and the CARDIA study (Braun, 1996).

The ECA study (Robins and Regier et al., 1991) was conducted from 1980 to 1984, prior to the striking decline in the prevalence of drug use in the population, and obtained diagnoses based on DSM III diagnostic criteria (American Psychiatric Association, 1980). The ECA had an unrestricted age range and was based on a sample of five local areas; it also included supplemental samples of the institutionalised population. Six classes of drugs were covered in the survey: cannabis, stimulants, sedatives, cocaine, opioids and hallucinogens. Case definition of drug abuse and drug dependence required a pattern of pathological abuse leading to impaired functioning and symptoms of tolerance/withdrawal respectively. Prevalence rates for lifetime history of illicit drug use did not differ significantly between the 'black' respondents compared with white/other respondents for all age groups. However, there was a higher life-time prevalence of illicit drug use in the 18–20 age group among the 'white/other' category (63 per cent) compared with the 'black' category (53 per cent), and also in the 30–44 years group with again a higher life-time prevalence rate of drug use among white compared with black respondents. More importantly, these figures were also reflected in higher life-time prevalence rates of drug abuse/dependence among white subjects compared with black subjects for both age groups (14 per cent of white subjects compared with 11 per cent of black subjects in the younger age group, and 7 per cent compared with 5 per cent in the older age-group respectively). There were higher prevalence rates among men compared with women among both ethnic groups. It is of interest that among those receiving a lifetime diagnosis of abuse/dependence there was a higher proportion of white females qualifying for a dependency diagnosis compared with their black female counterparts (53 per cent cf. 35 per cent). These differences are less marked among white males compared with black males. These figures are for the 18–29 age group as the numbers are too small to make worthwhile comparisons among other age groups. Though the prevalence figures are lower for blacks than whites, these differences are not statistically significant.

The National Household Survey on Drug Abuse (Kandel et al., 1997; SAMHSA, 1995d) a national survey of drug use patterns in the general population aged over 12 was initiated in 1972 and has been conducted every

2–3 years until 1988 and annually thereafter. Individuals in the ages of highest risk (12–34) and ethnic minorities are over-sampled. While the survey focuses on patterns of use among 12 classes of drugs, questions have also been asked pertaining to symptoms of dependence approximating to DSM IV criteria. A recent paper examined data on drug-related symptoms of dependence from the three most recent surveys to ascertain prevalence of substance dependence among four drugs (alcohol, marijuana, nicotine and cocaine) among adolescents and adults, and to examine last year conditional dependence as a function of age, gender and ethnicity, controlling for other demographic variables. In the total population, significantly more men than women in each ethnic group (White, Black, Hispanic and Other) were using the four substances, in particular the two illicit substances. White men had a significantly higher prevalence of alcohol use compared with black men and white women had higher prevalence of alcohol use than black and Hispanic women across all age groups. For cocaine, Hispanics and black individuals had higher rates of use than whites. These differences were statistically significant (4.6 per cent, cf. 3.2 per cent). Those individuals reporting use of cocaine in the last year were more likely to report dependent use in the black population compared with the white population (22.1 per cent, cf. 9.8 per cent); among black women who had used cocaine, a higher percentage were dependent in the past year compared with black males. In contrast, white women cocaine users were as likely as white male users to report last year's dependence. According to this study, blacks were more likely than whites to be dependent on alcohol, however this difference disappeared when socio-demographic factors were taken into account.

The National Co-morbidity study, Warner et al. (1995), aimed to analyse nationally representative data on life-time and 12-month prevalence of use and dependence on illegal drugs (marijuana, cocaine/crack, heroin and hallucinogens), non-medical prescription drugs and inhalants. The 15–54 age group (non-institutionalised) were interviewed, and diagnoses made according to DSM IIIR criteria. Prevalence rates of lifetime drug use, dependence and 12-month dependence were examined among the four ethnic groups: white, Black, Hispanic and other. The results show that whites are significantly more likely than non-whites to use drugs at some time in their lives, and among lifetime users there was no significant association between race and dependence. However, among respondents with a lifetime history of dependence, blacks were significantly more likely than whites to report recent dependence, i.e. in the previous 12 months.

The CARDIA (Coronary Artery Risk Development in Young Adults) Study (Braun et al., 1996) was a longitudinal cohort study whose goal was to identify and monitor the distribution of coronary heart disease risk factors (including illicit drug use) in a randomly sampled cohort of men and women (white and African American) aged between 20 and 32 years of age in 1987. Data from the study (using self-administered questionnaire) was utilised to examine the relationship between sociodemographic factors and use of other illicit substances for cocaine use over a five-year period. Self-reported current cocaine use declined across all ethnicity-sex groups between 1987 and 1992, with a greater decline among white compared with black subjects and higher proportions of current cocaine users being black and male (8.4 per cent black males, cf. 2.1 per cent white males) in 1992. However, among those who had never used cocaine there was a higher proportion of black subjects compared with white (58.6 per cent, cf. 47.5 per cent). Other important risk factors for cocaine use were: being unemployed, single, male, in the older half of the cohort and higher levels of alcohol, marijuana, and other illicit substances.

The OPCS (Office of Population Censuses and Surveys) Surveys of Psychiatric Morbidity in Great Britain was carried out between April 1993 and August 1993 with the aim of establishing prevalence rates for psychiatric disorders among adults aged 16 to 64 years in Great Britain. The main focus of the study was psychopathology as measured by the Clinical Interview Schedule but an attempt was also made to measure drug and alcohol dependence. Private households were sampled using postal sectors that were stratified by socio-economic group within Regional Health Authorities and achieved an 80 per cent response rate. Individuals were asked to define their ethnic grouping with reference to a list of nine possible classifications which were later collapsed into four categories: White, West Indian or African, Asian or Oriental, and Other. Drug dependence was assessed via a self-completed questionnaire using questions from the ECA study. Five questions measured drug dependence from a list of ten types of drug: frequency of use stated dependence, inability to cut down, need for larger amounts, and withdrawal symptoms. A positive response to any statement was used to indicate drug dependence. The results showed that although those in the self-designated group 'Asian/Oriental' were significantly less likely to score for alcohol dependence compared with White subjects there were no significant ethnic differences in those scoring under the rubric 'drug dependence'.

Methodological Limitations

The findings from the above epidemiological studies show that although black individuals are less likely than whites overall to experiment with most drugs, they are more likely to persist in their drug use. It is important to bear in mind that though prevalence rates may differ among ethnic groups this does not necessarily imply a causal association or a biological predisposition to dependency among one or other ethnic group. Both the ECA and NCS are descriptive, based on statistical analyses that do not control for potentially confounding variables such as urbanicity, low-income, unemployment etc. among the different racial groups. As a result, these basic comparisons can reinforce racial prejudices and draw public attention away from community characteristics or other factors that may better explain differential patterns of drug use.

The NHSDA undertook more complex statistical analysis in an attempt to control for confounding socio-demographic variables among their sample, but still came to the conclusion that life-time rates of crack cocaine use were higher among blacks compared with whites. More detailed re-analysis (by Lillie-Blanton et al.) of the original data from the NHSDA study, grouping the respondents into neighbourhood clusters (i.e. racially mixed neighbourhoods with at least one crack cocaine user), showed that life-time rates of crack use did not differ between whites and blacks.

As further evidence of the importance of social environment in rates of drug use among the black American population, in a paper by Emsminger et al. (1997), a subset of the Woodlawn Cohort, a longitudinal epidemiological study of a cohort of African Americans who spent some or all of their childhood in a deprived inner city neighbourhood, were compared to a matched sample (age, urbanicity and ethnicity) from the NHSDA. The results showed that though the majority were non-drug users, respondents from the Woodlawn cohort had past year rates more than twice that of the matched sample of NHSDA respondents for crack cocaine, and more than twice the rate of heroin use. Those incarcerated Woodlawn respondents reported disproportionately high rates of drug use. Reports of drug-trafficking also differed according to residential area, with 61 per cent of those living in Woodlawn reporting heavy trafficking compared to 13 per cent of those living in the Chicago suburbs. This underlines the importance of drug availability among inner-city neighbourhoods where most residents do not have the social and economic resources to protect their neighbourhood from encroachment by drug dealers. The information that ethnic differences are confounded by social factors need not affect the use of ethnic group as an indicator of risk per se. Its importance lies in identifying a population at especially high risk and is salient therefore in decisions about allocation of resources and concentration of attention on this particular group. When exploring the causes of drug abuse, however, we need no longer consider causes that are specifically connected with ethnicity. The ethnic difference provides no clues as to aetiology; in terms of global strategies to tackle drug abuse. Research suggests that individual governmental policies may need to concentrate more on social and environmental factors as significant in the genesis of drug abuse.

The CARDIA study also adopted multivariate statistical techniques to adjust for socio-demographic differences amongst the two groups as well as a sampling technique that provided adequate representation by sex and ethnicity. The follow-up results of a differential pattern of cocaine use among black participants compared with white need to be interpreted with some caution as the retention rate though high (80.6 per cent) may obscure a differential loss to follow-up among the two ethnic groupings, as although the authors examined loss to follow-up in terms of cocaine use status at recruitment and concluded there was no difference between the follow-up and drop-out group on this variable, they did not however comment on other relevant socio-demographic variables such as ethnic group among the retained and drop-out group.

The findings from the OPCS Survey of Psychiatric Morbidity in Great Britain (Meltzer et al., 1995) on prevalence rates of drug dependence amongst different ethnic groupings are difficult to interpret for a number of reasons. Firstly, only 4 per cent of the sample identified themselves as belonging to one of the ethnic minority groupings, thus making any meaningful comparisons in terms of age/sex or regional variations within the ethnic subgroups impossible, as well as obscuring any elevated levels of dependence within these sub-sections. Secondly, though the questions relating to drug dependence were based on those from the ECA sample, the threshold required for assigning someone to the dependence category within the British study was far less stringent compared to the ECA study, which required the subject to have experienced either tolerance/withdrawal phenomena to fulfil a diagnosis of 'dependence'. Within the OPCS, sample frequency of drug use by itself (at least two or more weeks of daily drug use in last 12 months) could theoretically suffice an individual to qualify, thus making comparison of British prevalence rates with other large-scale epidemiological studies problematic. Though the study attempted to examine sex and age distribution among non-responders and adjust the results accordingly, it is not known whether there was a differential non-response rate among members of particular ethnic groupings which also could have affected the final results.

Reliability and Validity of Substance Use Disorder: Cross-cultural Issues

The issue of using self-reported drug use is a problem inherent to all large-scale community studies due to participants reluctance to admit to a socially proscribed activity and hence the reliability and validity of self-reported substance use data has been questioned. Harrison et al. (1993), in an endeavour to assess the reliability of self-report data on marijuana and cocaine use examined consistency of reports across birth cohorts by examining prevalence rates for multiple years of the National Household Survey of Drug Abuse (NHSDA). They also analysed longitudinal inconsistencies in self-report drug use between two waves of the National Household Survey Youth Cohort (NSL-Y). A comparison was made between 1985 and 1990 NHSDA surveys by analysing data within five year birth cohorts; this revealed inconsistencies between 1985 respondents and their birth cohorts in 1990 with the Hispanic sample most likely to report consistently and the White sample least likely. Approximately one-fifth of subjects who had admitted using marijuana or cocaine in the 1984 survey (NSL-Y) subsequently denied ever using in 1988. Predictors of inconsistently denying use were frequency of use (less than 10 times in past year) and being of African-American ethnicity. The results of the study are consistent with other reports showing that sporadic drug users are less likely to report their drug use consistently than regular users. Hence it is more difficult to reach an accurate estimate of prevalence rates for infrequent drug users.

From a public health perspective, the finding that frequent drug users provide consistent drug reports is more reassuring and although test-retest reliability is no measure of validity, nevertheless it serves to boost confidence in the data as being a reasonable estimate of problematic drug use. From a review of the literature, the authors (Harrison et al.) conclude that in general, surveys using face-to-face interviews report lower prevalence rates of substance use compared with self-administered questionnaires. The CARDIA Study using a self-administered questionnaire which defined current use as one or more days cocaine use in the last month may give more reliable estimates of cocaine use but is limited in being unable to differentiate problematic or dependent users from recreational users. The World Health Organisation funded a large cross cultural study examining the applicability of substance use disorder diagnosis and assessments in different cultural settings using a variety of qualitative and quantitative methods (Room et al., 1997). The aim of the Cross-Cultural Applicability Research study (CAR) was to ascertain whether Eurocentric-based concepts of addiction, incorporated in terms such as 'dependence syndrome', 'withdrawal state' and 'harmful' are recognised as such in other cultural settings with differing social attitudes and perceptions of alcohol and drug use. In each of nine settings (ranging from Ankara to Seoul), data was collected for both alcohol and one other drug prevalent in that area, and instruments translated into the local dialect using bilingual experts. Interviews were conducted with local individuals from both lay and professional constituencies who had involvement in either drug or alcohol work.

Using semi-structured interviewing techniques, and focus group discussion to tap into local concepts of what constitutes normal and abnormal use of a substance, the meanings of various diagnostic terms relating to alcohol/drug dependence and similarities and differences between alcohol and drug abuse and addiction were explored. The findings of the study overall supported the feasibility of translating diagnostic instruments into a diversity of languages in diverse cultural settings and receiving meaningful answers. However, the study threw up a number of caveats: an over-arching finding was the fact that certain concepts common in Western world-view which assumed self-consciousness about feelings were alien to the folk-tradition of some cultures. For example, in Kannada, a dialect used in Bangalore (India), there is no equivalent term for 'feeling' used in an emotional sense; 'feel' after drinking was translated with a word which also means experience. Hence, positive and negative feelings were translated as good/pleasant and bad/negative experiences. As finally adopted, the ICD-10 Dependence Syndrome has six criteria, three of the following of which are necessary to make a diagnosis: strong desire or compulsion to take substance, impaired capacity to control, withdrawal/use to relieve withdrawal, tolerance, neglect of alternative pleasures and activities, harmful use (use despite physical or psychological harm) and narrowing of repertoire. In all sites, except Bangalore, there was a tendency to see drug use in more clinical terms than alcohol use. In several sites tolerance was understood in its technical meaning for the drug type included in the study but not for alcohol. Craving and compulsion were recognised in most sites but the meaning was often not differentiated from loss or impairment of control or from dependence more generally. In lay usage there was little distinction in any place between 'harmful use' and 'abuse'. Harmful use was understood to include social, economic and family problems as well as physical and psychic health problems; the intention in ICD-10 was to confine the term harm to health. For illicit drugs, many sites reported that lay respondents made no distinction between use and abuse and harmful use, no doubt reflecting a generally greater social condemnation of illicit drug compared with alcohol use. More significantly, there were substantial variations in thresholds for identifying and defining dependence or addiction, especially relating to alcohol use in cultural drinking was socially proscribed, and respondents who were drinking relatively insignificant levels of alcohol nevertheless viewed themselves as dependent and a mechanistic application of scoring algorithms for dependence would have resulted in inappropriate diagnosis. Hence, an epidemiological study that may yield reliable answers to interview items on a questionnaire in a culture that does not accept the diagnostic coding system as understood by the researchers is likely to yield diagnoses that would be seen as inappropriate or wrong within that society.

The CAR study findings pose nosological questions pertaining to the most appropriate way to diagnose dependence in different cultures. The authors suggest a number of possible solutions to this dilemma: a return to a culturally differentiated definition of dependence, as in the earliest World Health Organisation definition of alcoholism, as use going beyond 'the social drinking customs of the whole community concerned', or alternatively undertaking a search for new criteria that would be universally validated as diagnostic of dependence. The study reminds us of the need to be cautious in imposing our own view of drug dependence or misuse on cultural or ethnic groups which may accommodate certain forms of drug use within their own community without it being viewed as problematic, for example marijuana use among members of the Rastafarian community or Khat use among the Sudanese community. The study highlights the need for a sound understanding of cultural norms within differing ethnic groups, especially recent immigrant groups or those who have not been fully assimilated into the majority culture. It also underlines the need for careful validation of diagnostic instruments within diverse communities using a variety of qualitative and quantitative methods.

Substance Abuse Treatment

Howard et al. (1996), in a review of substance abuse treatment programmes comparing outcomes between different ethnic groups conducted in the 1970s and 1980s, summarises studies showing that black clients were less likely to stay in methadone maintenance treatment compared with their white counterparts, and had higher levels of continuing illicit drug misuse while in treatment compared with their white counterparts. Howard quotes a study by Brown et al. in 1985, based on more than 27,000 substance misusers, in differing treatment modalities which showed that black clients were more likely than white clients to be discharged from treatment with the majority group being retained in treatment longer, regardless of ethnicity. Howard et al. have criticised these and other studies for failure to apply multivariate analysis or adequate controls to account for differences in outcome. They point to the need to examine differences in treatment modalities in terms of intensity of service delivery, programme selection of clients and ethnicity of staff composition. Even in studies that have addressed race or ethnicity specifically, the majority has taken a short-sighted view of the impact of social and economic conditions as they affect these clients and their treatment effectiveness.

In order to address these, and other limitations in previous research which had concluded that being of black ethnicity was associated with poorer outcomes, Howard et al. conducted a national survey of non-methadone out-patient based substance misuse treatment organisations. A stratified random sample of substance misuse treatment organisations was surveyed by telephone in 1990, with a high response rate. Non-methadone treatment organisations were analysed to ascertain if black ethnicity was a significant determinant of treatment outcome in terms of completing treatment and achieving abstinence when the following factors were controlled for: socioeconomic deprivation, substance user profile, organisational characteristics and treatment practices. When indicators of the social environment in which the treatment organisation operates were taken into consideration the proportion of black clients attending a service was not a determinant of treatment outcome. Organisations located in poor, urban areas had substantially worse treatment outcome rates compared with organisations in rural, non-poor areas; these factors superseded race as a predictor of treatment success. Hence, poorer treatment outcomes in deprived areas are more likely to relate to the inherent difficulty of remaining drug-free in an impoverished environment with little self-esteem enhancing opportunities and a cue-rich drug-ubiquitous habitat. These findings suggest that a viable treatment approach would be one that places more emphasis on socio-enviromental influences to which the client is exposed and less emphasis on a client's race.

Culturally Specific Programmes

Numerous recommendations have been made regarding separate, culturally specific programmes for African-Americans. There is evidence from Brown et al.'s multi-modality study that the majority group were retained longer in treatment regardless of ethnicity, which would imply that the minority group attending a particular treatment programme may feel alienated and therefore intuitively it would make sense to resource separate services for the main ethnic minority groups. Recent years have witnessed a burgeoning of culturally specific treatment programmes aimed at African American and Hispanic drug-users. According to Bell (1990), the rationale for these programmes has been based on the premise that many African-Americans have race-related problems in dealing with self-concept and that denial of racial and cultural differences within the treatment setting hampers the therapeutic effectiveness of chemical dependency services available to African-American people (Institute of Black Chemical Abuse). The IBCA model provides culturally specific chemical dependency services to the black community via a combination of primary preventative strategies (youth education programmes, parenting classes, family therapy, stress management), provision of treatment services, and positive liaison with other drug service providers, community associations and leaders of the black community. The issues addressed by the IBCA are late entry into treatment, cultural pain and the economic effects of addiction in low-income areas. Other authors have argued the importance of culture in the assessment process as necessary in the planning of recovery services because the 'information obtained can identify patterns of belief and customs that can help or hinder recovery plans' (Carmell H. Woll). The Centre for Substance Abuse Treatment has funded a residential treatment program which utilises an Afrocentric perspective as its chief philosophical orientation, the key elements of which are: spirituality, respect for tradition, harmony with nature, the centrality of community, life as a series of passages, the importance of elders, and the creation of self-identity and dignity (M.S. Jackson et al.).

The only outcome study to date attempting to evaluate a culturally enhanced treatment programme (Weeks et al., 1997), is the preliminary analysis of PROJECT COPE 11 (the Community Outreach Prevention Effort), a community based AIDS prevention programme for drug users. COPE 11's efficacy study compares the standard intervention against two culturally targeted enhanced interventions, one for African-Americans and one for Hispanics. The three groups were compared at base line and six month follow up for changes in injection rates and proportionate user of new and pre-used needles. The results at follow-up showed an overall pattern of greater risk reduction in the enhanced intervention group with African-Americans, but not with Puerto Ricans. However, the high rates of attrition and low sample size limited the conclusions that could be drawn. The authors raise the question of the degree to which any improved outcome can be attributed to cultural content, location, the character of the intervention provider (staff were of the same ethnic group as participants), or simply providing an intervention of any kind over and above the standard protocol.

There is a need for further research to tease out the different components of culturally enhanced programmes that may be mediating a favourable effect It is important to bear in mind that black Americans comprise a heterogeneous group and represent diverse cultures, classes and backgrounds. Bell (1990) has categorised a number of major differences in African-Americans from acculturated blacks who have fully integrated into the majority culture at one end of the spectrum to traditional unacculturated blacks at the other end with various gradations in between. Each sub-group will have differing cultures, norms and values and it is therefore arguable what exactly a culturally sensitive programme should comprise given this heterogeneity. Concepts of the Afrocentric paradigm may have little relevance for a large section of the African-American population, and may be seen as patronising by some. While the black community has traditionally been mistrustful of treatment agencies, and attracting as well as retention in treatment is important, there is a danger that culturally targeted programmes will be seen as a panacea without adequate evaluation.

Great Britain

Britain has been enhanced by waves of immigration down through the centuries. The most recent significant wave of immigration was after the Second World War when black and other visible minorities were invited from the colonies due to acute labour shortages in Britain. Primary sources of immigration were the Caribbean colonies and the Indian subcontinent. Geographically, the majority of visible minorities live in urban areas, with nearly half residing in London. There is evidence from the Office of National Statistics of ongoing racial inequality in terms of employment, education, housing and health that concludes that despite the relative progress made by some of the black and other minority populations, the overall picture remains one of discrimination and disadvantage. (Social Focus on Ethnic Minorities, 1996).

Drug Services

The first drug dependency units were established in the 1960s under the auspices of the National Health Service with the voluntary sector setting up the first street drug agencies. Throughout the 1970s and 1980s these services proliferated. However, growth remained patchy and uneven with no one organisation invested with statutory obligation for the provision of drug treatment and care services. The late 1980s witnessed the advent of HIV and other drug-related infections with burgeoning public health concerns prompting the Government to set-up specialist Drug Dependency Units throughout the country. The Community Care Act (1990) lead to the introduction of the contract culture and internal market, with the cash-strapped local authority social services made responsible for the delivery of care in the community for drug treatment.

This ironically has led to more paperwork for providers with uncertainty about future funding and overall less choice for users of the services.

The Central Drugs Co-ordination Unit (CDCU) was set-up in 1994 to implement and monitor government drugs policy. The CDCU launched a strategic paper in 1995 called 'Tackling Drugs Together' which set out government policy for the succeeding five years and identified three strategic areas for intervention: crime, young people and public health. The 'Tackling Drugs Together' document is devoid of any mention of race or ethnic minority issues and fails to make specific recommendations for minimum standards of involvement from ethnic minorities in the local Drug Action Teams or Drug Reference Groups (inter-agency groups set up to tackle drug abuse at the local level). The government also funded a review of drug services called 'The Task Force Review of Drug Treatment Services'. The Task Force Review merely comments on the lack of information on requirements of black and other minority groups and the need for more. The situation currently facing drug purchasers and providers is one in which local authorities have not highlighted race as an important issue in drug services coupled with a National Health Service which has a poor track record in terms of race equality.

Prevalence

'This has been hard to gauge both because of the stereotypes that abound and because it is only lately that race has figured as a variable in any kind of prevalence studies', commented David Turner, former director of SCODA (Standing Conference on Drug Addiction) in 1989. Results from the 1992 British Crime Survey (a household survey) shows that among respondents aged 16–29 years around a third of white (29 per cent) and Afro-Caribbean respondents (30 per cent) reported ever taking any drug, compared with 10 per cent of Asians. A much smaller group had taken cocaine (3 per cent white and 2 per cent afro-Caribbean) or crack cocaine (1 per cent white and 2 per cent Afro-Caribbean). However these figures give no estimate of dependent drug use.

The 1991 Census is the only source of data on the population of London. At that time 20.2 per cent of resident Londoners self-reported as belonging to an ethnic minotiry group, representing 45 per cent of the ethnic minority population of Great Britain. The percentage reporting to drug treatment services are not substantially different to the population estimate. This concurs with the Office of Population Censuses and Surveys (OPCS) of Psychiatric Morbidity (referred to earlier in the chapter) which found no significant association between ethnicity and problem drug use. Ethnic minorities are not evenly distributed across London, with some groups concentrated in only a few boroughs. There may be an under-representation in statistics because culturally, some groups may be wary of seeking help. Also, some agencies may not be culturally sensitive to the needs of different ethnic groups.

Ethnic group	Number	%	** % population
White	7,546	78.8	79.8
Black (Caribbean)	460	4.8	4.4
Black (African)	76	0.8	2.4
Indian	225	2.3	5.2
Pakistani	49	0.5	1.3
Bangladeshi	54	0.6	0.8
Chinese	10	0.1	1.7
Other	723	7.5	3.5
Not known	2,349		
Valid total	9,576	100.0	

The Race and Drugs Project

The Race and Drugs Project (previously called the Four Cities Project) was a European funded initiative set up in 1995 to investigate drug service provision for black, migrant and other minority drug users who because of their different skin pigmentation or other visible distinguishing signs were likely to experience discrimination or racism. A literature search had revealed a dearth of information in the field, and hence the project was established with four core objectives:

- critical evaluation of selected European specialist drug services and their ability to meet the needs of their ethnic minority drug users;

- to establish a specialist network via links with existing networks in order to facilitate policy change and development in this whole area;
- to initiate support infrastructure for those agencies wishing to develop models of good practice;
- to contribute to the overall EC initiatives on drug abuse prevention, care and management.

The four countries selected – the United Kingdom, France, the Netherlands and Portugal – were chosen as they were historically the leading European colonising powers and therefore likely to have similar patterns of settlement of 'black and other visible minorities'.

Findings of the Project

United Kingdom

Due to time and resource constraints Greater London-based drug agencies only were interviewed, though this area alone represents 25 per cent of the drug treatment and care services in England. The results relate to interviews with staff, selected users and community groups (21 agencies). Two of the agencies were mainly staffed by black workers with a predominantly black client base. Though there was a high percentage of ethnic minority staff employed in the various drug agencies (more than 50 per cent), they by and large congregated at the lower end of the hierarchy providing front-line service provision with the management tiers predominantly comprised of those from the majority ethnic group. Overall a picture of unevenly resourced agencies in terms of staff, training and service output emerged from the interviews, together with low morale among staff particularly ethnic minority staff and patchy, piecemeal race equality initiatives. Another feature to emerge from the research was the extent to which agencies rely on client self-referral rather than engage in actively accessing local communities.

France

In France, individuals are divided into those who have French citizenship and those who do not (*étrangers*). The former category involves some black people from the former French colonies and the latter includes some whites and other 'foreigners'. As ethnic monitoring as it is practised in the UK is not permitted it is impossible to track second or third generation black people who are French nationals. Nevertheless the highest prevalence of black 'foreigners' emanate from Africa (Maghreb Africans comprise 39 per cent of 'foreigners'). There are no official statistics of drug use prevalence rates among the differing ethnic minority groups in France. However, the authors speculate that drug misuse is likely to be high in relation to the majority population due to the known association of drug use with urbanicity, unemployment, poverty, poorer educational performance and over-representation in the penal system, all of which are significantly higher in the ethnic minority population. There is a higher rate of conviction for drug use and/or trafficking offences among visible minorities compared with French nationals (9.2 per cent to 3.8 per cent), a 21 per cent consumption rate of stimulants by Maghrebien women compared with 14 per cent for French national women. These factors can lead to an expectation that levels of drug use amongst black and visible minority population will rise.

The Netherlands

Immigration has been a feature of Dutch society since the sixteenth century. There have been four main periods of immigration related to colonialism after the Second World War. Those from the former colonial Dutch Indies in the 1940s to 1950s, those from Surinam in the 1970s, from the Dutch Antilles and those from the Mediterranean countries in the 1960s. In 1990 the estimated proportion of the Dutch population who were 'non-native' was 14 per cent. The majority of these individuals were Surinamese.

Research conducted by the National Alcohol and Drugs Information System shows that Dutch agencies have proportionately more visible minority clients than white (Cruts, 1996). These figures relate to registered clients. It is likely that black drug users experiencing problems are less likely to be registered. More than 50 per cent of registered addicts are black. This means that one in 80 black people are addicts compared with one in 1,045 white Dutch (Lawalata, 1996). This growing problem relates to the disadvantaged socio-economic situation of black people not only in the Netherlands but also in the other three countries studies.

Portugal

Despite the absence of strongly differentiated groups in Portugal, there has been a small black population since the early 1900s. There is a large hidden population of illegal immigrants; hence official statistics pertaining to the number of black people is unreliable. Overall the number of foreigners resident in Portugal remains small (1 per cent). It is estimated that the visible minorities comprise 40 per cent of the non-national population. The largest group are from Africa (42,627 making up 44 per cent of the foreign population) (EC, 1992, Employment Department).

Up to 1994 there were no official studies of the prevalence of drug use in the adult population. Prevalence studies with Lisbon schoolchildren in 1988 showed that for the 12–18 age range 8.8 per cent had tried cannabis, 1.8 per cent heroin and 1.5 per cent cocaine, however, there are only limited figures on prevalence in general. There is little or no information about drug use in the black population. However, the socioeconomic conditions under which they live make it likely that drug misuse will be high relative to the indigenous population. Indications of this trend are emerging from agencies which are beginning to see more black clients from community groups who report increased use and dealing, especially amongst the young.

Conclusions

The project confirmed through examination of relevant literature, available statistics and interviews a pattern across the four countries of:

* discrimination in key areas such as employment, education and health among black and visible minorities.
* sparse research or information on prevalence rates of drug use/misuse among ethnic minorities.
* patchy implementation of equal opportunities policies with little ethnic minority representation at management level.
* little formal assessment of local ethnic minority needs in relation to drug services.
* services offered to black drug users seriously deficient (except for specialist minority or black agencies) in virtually all areas.

These findings combined with the other studies reviewed highlight the information gaps which must be targeted by research and future service development proposals.

References

Bell, P. (1990), *Chemical Dependency and the African American*, Hazeldon, Minneapolis.
Bell, P., Boissan, M., Moore, B. and Peterson, D. (1990), *Developing Chemical Dependency Services for Black People: a Manual*, Institute of Black Chemical Abuse, Minneapolis.
Bhopal, R. (1997), 'Is Research into Ethnicity and Health Racist, Unsound, or Important Science?', *British Medical Journal*, 314, p. 1751.
Braun, B.L., Murray, D., Hannan, P., Sidney, S. and Le, C. (1996), 'Cocaine Use and Characteristics of Young Adult Users from 1987 to 1992: the CARDIA Study', *American Journal of Public Health*, 86(12), pp. 1736–41.
Brown, B.S., Love, G.W. and Thompson, P. (1985), 'Minority Group Status and Treatment Retention', *International Journal of Addiction*, 20(2), pp. 319–35.
Coomber, R. (ed.) (1998), *The Control of Drugs and Drug Users: Reason or Reaction?*, Harwood Academic Publishers, Amsterdam.
Cruts, A. (1996), *Key Figures on Allochtonous Clients in the LADIS; the Dutch National Alcohol and Drugs Information System*, 1VV, Utrecht.
Department of Health (1996), *The Task Force to Review Services for Drug Misusers, HMSO, London. Home Office. Research and Planning Unit Paper 89, Self-reported Drug Misuse in England and Wales: Findings from the 1992 British Crime Survey, Specialist Drugs Services and Managing Change to Meet the Needs of Black, Other Minority and Migrant Drug Users*, The Four Cities Project, London, pp. 1–20.
Donald, J. and Rattansi, A. (1992), *Culture and Difference*, Sage, London.
Ensminger, M.E., Anthony, J.C. and McCord, J. (1997), 'The Inner City and Drug Use: Initial Findings from an Epidemiological Study', *Drug and Alcohol Dependence*, 48(3), pp. 175–84.
Harrison, E.R., Haaga, J. and Richards, T. (1993), 'Self-reported Drug Use Data: What do They Reveal?', *American Journal of Drug and Alcohol Abuse*, 19, pp. 423–41.
Home Office, Department of Health, Department of Education (1995), 'Tackling Drugs Together: a Strategy for England 1995–1998', HMSO, London.
Howard , D.L., LaVeist, T.A. and McCaughrin, W.C. (1996), 'Effect of Social Environment on Treatment Outcomes in Out-patient Substance Misuse Treatment Organisations: Does Race Matter?', *Substance Use and Misuse*, 31(5), pp. 617–38.
Jackson, M.S., Stephen, R.C. and Smith, R.L. (1997), 'Afrocentric Treatment in Residential Substance Abuse Care', *Journal of Substance Abuse Treatment*, 14(1), pp. 87–92.
Kandel, D., Chen, K., Warner, L.A. and Kessler, R.C. (1997), 'Grant B – Prevalence and Demographic Correlates of Symptoms of Last Year Dependence on Alcohol, Nicotine, Marijuanha and Cocaine in the US Population', *Drug and Alcohol Dependence*, 44(1), pp. 11–29
Lillie-Blanton, M., Anthony, J.C. and Schuster, C.R. (1993), 'Probing the Meaning of Racial/ Ethnic Group Comparisons in Crack Cocaine Smoking', *Journal of the American Medical Association*, 26(8).
Meltzer, H., Gill, B., Petticrew M. and Hinds, K. (1995), *OPCS Surveys of Psychiatric Morbidity in Great Britain, Report One: The Prevalence of Psychiatric Morbidity among adults living in Private Households*, HMSO, London.
Office for National Statistics (1996), *Social Focus on Ethnic Minorities*, HMSO, London.
Robins, L.N. and Regier, D.A. (1991), *Psychiatric Disorders in America: the Epidemiologic Catchment Area Study*, Free Press, New York.

Room, R., Janca, A., Bennett, L.A., Schmidt, L. and Sartorius, N. (1996) WHO Cross-cultural Applicability Research on Diagnosis and Assessment of Substance Use Disorders: an Overview of Methods and Selected Results', *Addiction*, 91(2), pp. 199–220.

Substance Abuse and Mental Health Service Administration (1995), *National Household Survey on Drug Abuse, Population Estimates 1994*, Office of Applied Studies, SAMHSA, Rockville, MD.

Warner, LA., Kessler, RC., Hughes, M., Anthony, J.C. and Nelson, C.B. (1995), 'Prevalence and Correlates of Drug Use and Dependence in the United States: Results from the National Co-morbidity Study', *Archives of General Psychiatry*, 52, pp. 219–29.

Weeks, M.R., Himmelgreen, D.A., Singer, M. , Woolley, S , Romero-Daza, N. and Grier, M. (1997), 'Community-based AIDS Prevention: Preliminary Outcomes of a Program for African American and Latino Injection Drug Users', *Drug Issues*, 26(3), pp. 561–90.

Woll, C.H. (1996), 'What Difference does Culture Make? Providing Treatment to Women Different from You', *Journal of Chemical Dependency Treatment*, 6(12) pp. 67–85.

Chapter 11

Alcohol Use in Black People of African Descent

Vincent Kirschner

Introduction

This chapter will concentrate on the epidemiological literature on patterns of drinking among black people originally of African descent in the UK and USA. Drinking patterns in women and adolescents is not specifically dealt with. Black people in the UK and USA are two populations identified purely by race, which does not give credit to the large variations within and between these populations. The black population in the USA has been well established for generations and their origins are largely from Africa during the time of slavery. Intra-ethnic differences among black people in the US are largely ignored and they are seen as a uniform group when political and social policies are decided, however, the point has to be recognised that there are inter-group interactions, socio-political contexts and intra-group pressures that contribute to the definition of an ethnic group (Herd and Grube, 1996). The black population in the UK mostly immigrated from the Caribbean after the Second World War for employment reasons. This population was also added to by immigrants from the ex-British colonies and refugees from various African countries. The UK black population thus still has large numbers of first and second generation immigrants whereas in the USA immigrants represent a much smaller proportion of the black population. Because African-Caribbeans are the largest single group of black people in the UK most research has been based on this group, again ignoring the other groups of people who are also of black African origin.

It makes sense that an individual's social context, which encompasses ethnicity, will affect attitudes in general, including those towards alcohol. Family organisation, social control, social roles, beliefs and norms are some of the ways in which ethnicity may influence patterns of alcohol use (Herd and Grube, 1996). This argument assumes that people tend to live in ethnically cohesive systems, which is a pattern that may not be true or may be in a state of constant change. It is important to develop appropriate models of drinking behaviour among different groups, including ethnic groups if ethnicity constitutes a true identifying characteristic in a particular group, to further understanding and so that more effective and appropriate interventions may be offered for alcohol related problems (Herd, 1991).

This chapter will discuss relevant research into alcohol use that has explored rates of alcohol use among black versus white people, associated social and demographic factors, ethnic identity and acculturation.

Search

A literature search was conducted using the databases Medline and Embase covering the years 1994 to 1999. Further information was obtained from Alcohol Concern, an organisation receiving government funding to improve the availability of alcohol advice and counselling services across England.

Aspects of Culture

The World Health Organisation (WHO) has attempted to address the issue that different cultures differ in their views on what constitutes psychiatric illness including substance use disorders. The Cross-Cultural Applicability Research (CAR) study compared the reliability and validity of two epidemiological instruments for the definition and detection of substance use disorders in nine different countries with diverse cultures and languages (Gureje et al., 1996). The following points were reported. The limits of what constitutes 'normal' drinking varies among cultures and within cultures especially cultures where regular consumption is common. Among Navajo Indians, alcohol consumption is widespread despite it being viewed as being an illicit substance so there is no concept of 'normal' drinking and any drinking is considered a problem. Where drinking is considered acceptable, an important indicator of normal drinking is the absence of socially disruptive behaviour. Heavy alcohol consumption without disruptive behaviour is even extolled in some cultures.

The use of other drugs is generally viewed as abnormal in different cultures except cannabis use, which ranged from being viewed as acceptable and normal to illegal. Alcohol has been used by humans for millennia and has been present in some cultures for a long time so its use is more likely to have been integrated into these cultures and have established criteria of normal use compared to other drugs and cultures that have not been exposed to alcohol. The CAR study found it is difficult to apply the same set of criteria for the definition of alcohol use disorders in different cultures (Cochrane and Howell, 1985).

Increased rates of alcohol-related problems have been found in small studies of black communities and the explanation for this finding has been that people who moved from rural societies in the Caribbean or Africa to urban settings in the USA or Britain may have experienced social disorganisation and discrimination making them vulnerable to alcohol abuse (Burke, 1984). In the USA the move from a rural setting into an urban one is more likely to be occurring among people living in the rural south migrating to economically more prosperous urban areas. This does not constitute moving into a new culture, but rather moving to a different environment within the same culture. This obviously does not negate the stress that such a move may induce. In the UK it is more likely that the move from a rural to urban setting has occurred by moving from one country to another. The assumption that such a move is necessarily associated with extreme stress has been challenged. Neff et al. (1992) used a language-based measure of acculturation in a community survey of 1,286 adult regular drinkers in San Antonio, Texas. The focus of this study was on Mexican Americans, although data on black Americans were analysed separately. Previous studies had consistently indicated that alcohol consumption was increased among more highly acculturated individuals in the USA. However, this study found the reverse. These authors found little evidence to support the theory that acculturation is inherently a stressful process. This investigation was of Mexican Americans as it is unlikely that black or white Americans would constitute a large group of immigrants. As an aside the black men included in this study had a lower mean alcohol consumption that white or Mexican Americans.

USA

In her editorial, Herd (1991) commented that drinking patterns in black Americans were generally neglected in research until the 1980s. It was presumed that black social patterns were similar to those of white Americans and thus cultural factors were largely ignored. Researchers tended to assume black communities were in a state of social disorganisation and that black drinking was deviant. Alcohol use was assumed, erroneously, to be common in areas of socioeconomic deprivation with adult drinking patterns being established in adolescence. These views were supported by studies based on small population segments and the fact was ignored that drinking patterns are highly variable depending on social, cultural, economic and fashion factors. This is illustrated in the change in attitude to alcohol that occurred during the early part of this century among black people. Prior to this abstinence was associated with the prevailing religious and antislavery movements, however, with the occurrence of prohibition alcohol became a symbol of freedom and leisure during a time of political conservatism and racism. Even now there are different patterns of alcohol use among people in different social contexts, for example, black people in the rural south are drinking more heavily than those in the urban north although traditionally the reverse has been the case (Herd, 1991).

Research done during the 1980s suggested that, if anything, black people's attitudes to alcohol are more conservative and alcohol plays a smaller role in the home. Alcohol consumption is also low among black youths at a time when there is concern at the high levels of drinking among young people in the general population (Herd, 1991).

The rates of alcohol use in the US were determined in the National Household Surveys on Drug Abuse (NHSDA) in 1991, 1992 and 1993. The sample size was 87,915 and was from the civilian, non-institutionalised population. Minority groups and youths were oversampled. White men and women had greater prevalence of last year of alcohol use than their black counterparts (white men 72.8 per cent (SE 0.8) vs black men 61.3 per cent (SE 1.1) and white women 65.2 per cent (SE 0.8) vs black women 50.5 per cent (SE 1.0)). The highest rates of drinking for black and white men were at ages 18–49 and women 18–34 and the drinking rates by age did not vary according to race (Kandel et al., 1997).

A subsample of 1,947 black men and women from the 1984 survey by the Alcohol Research Group was analysed by Herd and Grube (1996), looking specifically at the concept of ethnic identity and how it influences drinking patterns. This survey sampled the general population. A conclusion reached was that black ethnic identity is multidimensional and being black meant different things to different segments of the black population. The effects of black identity had complex interactions with drinking patterns, which were largely mediated through drinking norms and religiosity. Involvement in black social networks and greater black awareness was associated with lower levels of drinking because these factors were themselves associated with more conservative drinking norms and greater religiosity. One aspect of black ethnic identity that was associated with increased drinking was using black media, and this may have been due to the promotion of alcoholic drinks in the media. This was also evident as an age dependent effect in that black youths were greater users of black media. The effect of age on the form and nature of ethnic identity that an individual endorsed was seen in other ways, for example, older black people were more likely to have separatist beliefs (Herd and Grube, 1996).

Up until the mid-1980s it was generally believed that alcohol abuse had more severe consequences among black people than white even though rates of use were similar (Burke, 1984). This was because black drinkers were more likely to be labelled 'alcoholic' during hospital admissions and medical problems would thus be more frequently attributed to alcohol.

Rates of arrest for alcohol-related offences among black people have declined or grown more slowly to now equal those among white people. During the 1960s these arrest rates were much higher among black people, which does not necessarily reflect heavier alcohol use as it may be due to prevailing societal attitudes resulting in blacks being selectively arrested (Herd, 1991).

Jones-Webb et al. (1996) analysed data from the Coronary Artery Risk Development in Young Adults (CARDIA) study, which consisted of 1,214 black women, 905 black men, 1179 white women and 1,054 white men aged 21–41 years who completed the year 5 evaluation (1990–91). Black people were more likely to be younger, single, unemployed, less affluent, smokers and have higher body mass index. Black men had higher alcohol intake (19.2 ml/day) than white men (16.0 ml/day), but black women (5.9 ml/day) had the lowest intake (white women 6.3 ml/day). Depressive symptoms were positively correlated to alcohol intake in black people, but not whites and the same was found for anxiety symptoms except in white women there was no correlation. Alcohol intake was positively correlated with blood pressure in black people and effect was stronger in men than in women. The authors suggested that some of these variables like anxiety, depressive symptoms, blood pressure and alcohol, may all be measuring a similar construct and the racial differences found may be due to different responses to psychological distress for various reasons (Jones-Webb et al., 1996).

The Epidemiological Catchment Area (ECA) Study conducted in 1980 and 1985 included a one year observation period of people from various ethnic and racial backgrounds in five different metropolitan areas. DSM III criteria were used to determine alcohol abuse and dependence. The one year prevalence for black men was 11.51 per cent (SE 1.53) versus 11.69 per cent (SE 0.52) for white men and 2.11 per cent (SE 0.23) for white women versus 2.50 per cent (SE 0.68) for black women (Helzer et al., 1991). These figures show smaller differences along racial lines compared to epidemiological studies.

The 1992 National Longitudinal Alcohol Epidemiological Survey (NLAES) was a nationwide household survey sponsored by the National Institute on Alcohol Abuse and Alcoholism. Interviews were conducted with 42,862 respondents 18 years and older. Blacks and youths were over-sampled and DSM-IV criteria of alcohol use disorders were used. The prevalence of alcohol abuse and dependence in black men was 8.25 per cent (SE 0.72) and in men from the rest of the population it was 11.33 per cent (SE 0.34). In women these prevalence figures were 2.88 per cent (SE 0.32) and 4.25 per cent (SE 0.20) for black and other women respectively. Levels of alcohol use disorders among black people were thus significantly lower that the rest of the population. In the age group 18–29 years the prevalence of alcohol abuse and dependence was greater than the overall prevalence for all youths but racial differences were more pronounced. Black male youths had a prevalence of 12.3 per cent (SE 1.70) versus 23.48 per cent (SE 0.84) for other male youths. For female black youths the prevalence was 3.32 per cent (SE 0.60) versus 10.99 per cent (SE 0.64) for the rest of the population (Grant et al., 1994).

The 1992 National Alcohol Follow-up Survey (NAS), which included subjects from the 1984 NAS, examined the change in drinking patterns and problems among 1,151 black, 1,407 white and 1,149 Hispanic adult men. Black and Hispanic men were twice as likely to be in the lower socioeconomic classes and four times as likely to live in impoverished neighbourhoods. Black men were least likely to be married. Although black and Hispanic men reported more conservative drinking norms, they also reported greater alcohol consumption consequences and dependence symptoms than white men. Black men, but not Hispanic men, living in impoverished neighbourhoods reported more alcohol related problems than comparable white men, but these racial differences disappeared among affluent men. This suggests that the social experience of being black and living in an impoverished neighbourhood is different to that of whites and Hispanics. Poverty and race/ethnicity are thus important factors in alcohol related problems but the relationship is complex and probably best understood by examining the interaction of race/ethnicity with poverty (Jones-Webb et al., 1997).

The Woodlawn study is a developmental epidemiological study of black people from a relatively poor black community in Chicago. It was a one-age cohort of individuals from a single community. Data was collected over a 25 year period with subjects being evaluated in first grade, at age 16–17, via public school records, through age 25 and finally in their early 30s when 953 of the original 1,242 subjects were interviewed. The lifetime prevalence of alcohol use disorders was 13.5 per cent, which is similar to other surveys of inner city children. Men were twice as likely to have current lifetime diagnosis. Predictors of alcohol use disorders were under-achievement identified in first grade, few family rules about school, plans to limit education to high school during adolescence and failure to complete high school. Failure to complete college was not predictive. Cases were more likely to be single and unemployed. Some suggested reasons for alcohol use presented were individual tendency to deviance or using alcohol to cope with bad feelings and alienation. Explanations of findings were given in terms of individual experience rather than in terms of race. In the ECA study, education level and school drop out were found to be associated with the development of alcohol use disorders (Crum et al., 1998).

Ethnic differences for high quantity alcohol consumption were largely eliminated when education, escape drinking motives and solitary drinking were controlled for in an analysis of 481 adult male regular drinkers in San Antonio, Texas. Solitary drinking was more strongly related to heavy drinking among African-Americans than among white or Mexican-Americans. Social isolation was not a significant factor in solitary drinking in any of the race groups (Neff, 1997).

Herd (1997) analysed the data from 3,724 subjects from a national general population survey by the Alcohol Research Group and found there was a greater gender gap in drinking patterns among black people, although no race by sex interactions were significant. The greatest effect of heavier alcohol use resulting in drinking associated problems occurred in white women, a finding that has previously been explained by the difference in physiology among the sexes, however, this finding was not present among black women. These analyses showed that none of a range of indicators of social status, norms or social contexts had any effect on the interaction of gender, race and heavier drinking on alcohol dependence.

Darrow et al. (1992) undertook a household survey of stress, alcohol use and hypertension in an industrial area of New York and compared 654 African-American and 474 white women. Abstainers were more likely to attend church frequently, particularly fundamentalist religions, and have lower socioeconomic status. Abstention among white women was not associated with church attendance, but was associated with increased household density. In both groups older age was associated with abstention and a positive family history with heavier drinking.

Discussions of USA Studies

The national epidemiological studies undertaken in the USA indicate that compared to whites, black people drink less, have fewer alcohol use disorders and have a smaller problem of alcohol use among youths. Of all gender and ethnic groups, black women have the lowest rates of alcohol use and alcohol use disorders. When looking at specific drinking problems such as solitary drinking or escape drinking, race has little effect.

Among black people having conservative norms and values, religiosity, increasing age and lower socioeconomic status are associated with lower rates of alcohol use and alcohol use disorders. Higher rates of alcohol use and alcohol use disorders among black people are associated with the following demographic factors: being male, single, unemployed and having a family history of alcohol use disorders. Social factors include making use of black media, under-achievement in junior school, few family rules about school and plans to limit education to secondary school. Mental health factors include depressive and anxiety symptoms.

This body of research supports the view that black ethnic identity is a complex and variable construct, as is its effect on drinking patterns. Black ethnic identity seems to be influenced by factors like age, religiosity, current social and political influences and separatist versus acculturation beliefs. It is thus expected that black drinking patterns, like in other ethnic groups will be highly variable among individuals and communities. These patterns are difficult to predict and seem to depend on a particular community's norms and values. This is illustrated by the different lifestyles and pressures present in rural versus inner city communities, which suggests that the social environment affects norms and values probably independently to ethnicity.

UK

A review by McKeigue and Karmi (1993) examined alcohol consumption and alcohol related problems among African-Caribbean people living in the UK. Four studies, the General Household Survey (Balarajan and Yuen, 1986). The Birmingham Factory Study (Cruickshank et al., 1985), the Northwick Park Study (Meade et al., 1978) and the Craven Park Study (Haines et al., 1987) all showed lower rates of alcohol consumption among men and women who were African-Caribbean.

The General Household Survey was based on a nationally representative UK sample of people living in private households from 1978 until 1980. This sample included 300 African-Caribbean people. The rate of heavy alcohol use among African-Caribbean men was about half that of the average expected for age and socioeconomic status (Balarajan and Yuen, 1986). This finding was even more significant in the Craven Park Study of 1359 subjects registered in a general practice in northwest London between 1983 and 1986, which was comprised of 31 per cent African-Caribbeans (Haines et al., 1987).

The Northwick Park Study examined 553 men and women working in a food processing plant in North West London between 1972 and 1977. Of this sample, 25 per cent were African-Caribbean (Meade et al., 1978). The Birmingham Factory Study included 603 European and 274 African-Caribbean men and women (Cruickshank et al. 1985). The average rate of alcohol consumption for black men were 10–18 units per week and 15–22 units for white men. African-Caribbean women used 3–4 units per weeks and European women 3–7 units per week. Unlike in Europeans consumption was not higher in male African-Caribbean youths.

A study in 1984 by Taylor et al. (1986) found 6 per cent of African-Caribbeans admitted to a north London hospital were for alcohol-related problems compared to 10 per cent of admission of white Britons. Cochrane (1987, 1989) examined crude rates of admission to psychiatric hospitals in England and Wales. In 1971 alcohol-related problems accounted for 14 per 105 admissions to psychiatric hospitals for black men born in the Caribbean and 28 per 105 for black men born in the UK. These rates had increased by 75 per cent by 1981 but the racial differences were maintained. These differences were not apparent when comparing African-Caribbean born women and those born in England and Wales (Cochrane, 1977; Cochrane and Bal, 1989). McKeigue and Karmi (1993) conclude that there is a lot of evidence in support of alcohol consumption and related problems being less of a problem among African-Caribbeans living in England and Wales compared to white Britons.

Harrison et al. (1997) looked at the mortality rates in England and Wales for causes known to be associated with alcohol use among first generation immigrants from the Caribbean commonwealth for the period 1979–91. During the 1970s rates of death were lower than those for the national population, but since then rates have increase. This increase implies greater or heavier alcohol use and the authors felt it could be attributed to various factors including migration stress and acculturation (Harrison et al., 1997). It has been suggested that social stress continues to be a problem in second generation immigrants who continue to feel alienated having increased police contact, unemployment (Burke, 1984).

The effect of immigration on alcohol use disorders could be illustrated by comparing rates of admission to psychiatric hospitals for black people of Caribbean descent in the Caribbean and UK. Burke (1984) compared two such studies and the rates of admission were 3.5 times greater in the UK. Comparisons like this are not valid because medical services in the regions may be different with different thresholds and criteria for admission, diagnostic criteria may differ and the societies capacity to contain drinking related problems may also differ.

When comparing demographics and drinking habits between 170 white and 200 men of African-Caribbean origin in the West Midlands of England, Cochrane and Howell (1985) found that black men were significantly more likely to be single (48.0 per cent vs 25.3 per cent whites), unemployed (31.0 per cent vs 18.8 per cent whites) and belong to social classes IV and V (33.5 per cent vs 14.7 per cent whites). However, despite these social differences significantly fewer black men reported drinking more than twice a week (16.5 per cent vs 35.3 per cent whites) and 20.0 per cent described themselves as abstainers compared to 4.7 per cent of white men. Among regular drinkers black men consumed fewer units of alcohol per week (19 units vs 27 units in white men). This supports the previously described finding that heavy drinking is relatively rare among African-Caribbean men living in the UK. Interestingly, by far the majority of men in both groups believed their alcohol consumption was average or below average. The preferred beverage in both groups was beer and black men consumed slightly more spirits and did more of their drinking at home. Both groups did most of their drinking over the weekend (Cochrane and Howell, 1985).

Discussions of UK Studies

The UK epidemiological studies, like the US studies, show that black people of African-Caribbean descent have lower rates of alcohol use, including heavy use, with fewer admissions to hospital for alcohol related problems compared with white people. This is supported by findings that the rate of hospital admissions and mortality rates for alcohol related problems is significantly greater in black men born in the UK compared to those born in the Caribbean suggesting that African-Caribbean culture is associated with less alcohol abuse. With acculturation these rates are rising but remain lower than those for white Britons. This could be due to several reasons for example, increased drinking rates or increased acceptability of going to hospital with alcohol-related problems.

The theory of social, migration and acculturation stress being major factors in the pathogenesis of alcohol related disorders is not entirely supported by research findings, for example, Cochrane and Howell (1985) showed that despite several socioeconomic disadvantages African-Caribbean people drank less than white Britons. It is likely that societal norms and values have a strong effect.

Most studies show that drinking rates are lower among African-Caribbean people, but this does not negate the presence and extent of these problems which need to be addressed. It does show that drinking patterns are different in different communities depending on how these communities are defined and therefore may need different strategies of intervention.

Conclusion and Future Research

Population-based studies are useful in establishing the extent of alcohol use disorders and to determine resource allocations. These studies are also beneficial in picking up changes in drinking trends, which will need different strategies to reduce the impact of these changes on communities. What is unclear is how much of this kind of information can be generalised to local communities in a group of disorders that has such clear socioeconomic and cultural influences on its pathogenesis. The available information suggests that there are some trends. It is also not yet established whether information can be generalised between communities. Relevant research for local communities would look for specific risk factors and influences that affect drinking patterns applicable to that particular community. Research from other communities would help in directing research to what the likely influencing factors would be. There are individuals with specific drinking problems that probably have less to do with outside influences and more to do with their own inherent characteristics. These individuals would be less influenced by community-based interventions as they are often excluded and would benefit more from individual treatments. Future research needs to identify this group of individuals and explore whether they suffer from a specific disorder that makes them vulnerable to alcohol use disorders and what the prevalence is in different communities. It is probable that this group constitute a stable number in many communities.

Developmental studies are time consuming and expensive and often have high attrition rates, but the information they provide is probably the most valid and reliable because they give an idea of the effect of different socio-cultural influences occurring at different developmental stages. The large amount of epidemiological information available should be translated into models targeting specific problems that can be tested to see if interventions make a difference. Questions that require answering are whether public health drives reduce prevalence rates or is it more effective to target individuals with risk factors.

A criticism of the epidemiological studies is that they fail to define sufficiently the ethnic groups they are looking at ignoring the complexity of societies. It would be of interest to establish the criteria which people use to identify themselves with a particular group and then use these groups to determine the prevalence and aetological factors of alcohol use disorders. The study by Herb and Grube (1996) is one such study.

References

Balarajan, R. and Yuen, P. (1986), 'British Smoking and Drinking Habits: Variation by Country of Birth', *Community Medicine*, 8, pp. 237–9.

Burkes, A.W. (1984), 'Cultural Aspects of Drinking Behaviour among Migrant West Indians and Related Groups', in Krasner N., Madden J.S. and Walker R.J. (eds), *Alcohol-Related Problems: Room for Manoeuvre*, John Wiley, Chichester, pp. 197–205.

Cochrane, R. (1971), 'Mental Illness in Immigrants to England and Wales: an Analysis of Mental Hospital Admissions', *Social Psychiatry*, 12, pp. 25–35.

Cochrane, R. and Bal, S. (1989), 'Mental Hospital Admission Rates of Immigrants to England: a Comparison of 1971 and 1981', *Social Psychiatry and Psychiatric Epidemilogy*, 24, pp. 2–11.

Cochrane, R. and Howell, M. (1995), 'Drinking Patterns of Black and White Men in the West Midlands', *Social Psychiatry and Psychiatric Epidemiology*, 30, pp. 139–46.

Cruickshank, J.K., Jackson, S.H.D., Beevers, D.G., Bannan, L.T., Beevers, M. and Stewart, V.L. (1985), 'Similarity of Blood Pressure in Blacks, Whites and Asians in England: the Birmingham Factory Study', *Journal of Hypertension*, 3, pp. 365–71.

Crum, R.M., Ensminger, M.E. and Ro, M.J. (1998), 'The Association of Educational Achievement and School Dropout With risk of Alcoholism: a Twenty five-year Prospective Study of Inner City Children', *Journal of Studies on Alcohol*, 59, pp. 318–26.

Darrow, S.L., Russell, M., Cooper, M.L., Mudar, P. and Frone, M.R. (1992), 'Sociodemographic Correlates of Alcohol Consumption among African-American and White Women', *Women and Health*, 18(4), pp. 35–51.

Grant, B.F., Harford, T.C., Dawson, D.A., Chou, P., Dufour, M. and Pickering, R. (1994), 'Prevalence of DSM-IV Alcohol Abuse and Dependence', *NIAAA's Epidemiologic Bulletin*, 18(3), pp. 243–8.

Gureje, O., Vazquez-Barquero, J.L. and Janca, A. (1996), 'Comparisons of Alcohol and Other Drugs: Experience from the WHO Collaborative Cross-cultural Applicability Research (CAR) Study', *Addiction*, 91(10), pp. 1529–38.

Haines, A.P., Booroff, A., Goldenberg, E., Morgan, P., Singh, M. and Wallace, P. (1987), Blood Pressure, Smoking, Obesity and Alcohol Consumption in Black and White Patients in General Practice', *Journal of Hypertension*, 1, pp. 39–46.

Harrison, L., Sutton, M. and Gardiner, E. (1997), 'Ethnic Differences in Substance Use and Alcohol-use-related Mortality among First Generation Migrants to England and Wales', *Substance Use and Misuse*, 32(7 and 8), pp. 849–76.

Helzer, J.E., Burnam, A. and McEvoy, L.T. (1991), 'Alcohol Abuse and Dependence', in Robins, L.N. and Regier, D.A. (eds), *Psychiatric Disorders in America: the Epidemiologic Catchment Area Study*, Free Press, New York.

Herd, D. (1987), 'Rethinking Black Drinking', British Journal of Addiction, 82, pp. 219–23.

Herd, D. (1997), 'Sex Ratios of Drinking Patterns and Problems among Blacks and Whites: Results from a National Survey', *Journal of the Study of Alcohol*, 58, pp. 75–82.

Herd, D. and Grube, J. (1996), 'Black Identity and Drinking in the US: a National Study', *Addiction*, 91(6), pp. 845–57.

Jones-Webb, R., Jacobs, D.R., Flack, J.M. and Liu, K. (1996), 'Relationships between Depressive Symptoms, Anxiety, Alcohol Consumption, and Blood Pressure: Results from the CARDIA Study', *Alcoholism Clinical and Experimental Research*, 20(3), pp. 420–27.

Jones-Webb, R., Snowden, L., Herd, D., Short, B. and Hannan, P. (1997), 'Alcohol-related Problems among Black, Hispanic and White Men: the Contribution of Neighbourhood Poverty', *Journal of Studies on Alcohol*, 58, pp. 539–45.

Kandel, D., Chen, K., Warner, L.A., Kessler, R.C. and Grant, B. (1997), 'Prevalence and Demographic Correlates of Symptoms of Last Year Dependence on Alcohol, Nicotine, Marijuana and Cocaine in the US Population', *Drug and Alcohol Dependence*, 44, pp. 11–29.

McKeigue, P.M. and Karmi, G. (1993), 'Alcohol Consumption and Alcohol-related Problems in Afro-Caribbeans and South Asians in the United Kingdom', *Alcohol and Alcoholism*, 28(1), pp. 1–10.

Meade, T.W., Brozovic, M., Chakrabarti, R., Haines, A.P., North, W.R.S. and Stirling, Y. (1978), 'Ethnic Group Comparisons of Variables associated with Ischaemic Heart Disease', *British Heart Journal*, 40, pp. 789-795.

Neff, J.A. (1997), 'Solitary Drinking, Social Isolation, and Escape Drinking Motives as Predictors of High Quantity Drinking, among Anglo, African American and Mexican American Males', *Alcohol and Alcoholism*, 32(1), pp. 33–41.

Neff, J.A. and Hoppe, S.K. (1992), 'Acculturation and Drinking Patterns among US Anglos, Black and Mexican Americans', *Alcohol and Alcoholism*, 27(3), pp. 293–308.

Taylor, C.L., Kilbane, P., Passmore, N. and Davies, R. (1986), 'Prospective Study of Alcohol-related Admissions in an Inner-city Related Hospital', *The Lancet*, 2, pp. 265–8.

Index